Skin Cancer Treatment

Editor

JEFFREY S. MOYER

FACIAL PLASTIC SURGERY CLINICS OF NORTH AMERICA

www.facialplastic.theclinics.com

Consulting Editor
J. REGAN THOMAS

February 2019 • Volume 27 • Number 1

ELSEVIER

1600 John F. Kennedy Boulevard • Suite 1800 • Philadelphia, Pennsylvania, 19103-2899

http://www.theclinics.com

FACIAL PLASTIC SURGERY CLINICS OF NORTH AMERICA Volume 27, Number 1
February 2019 ISSN 1064-7406, ISBN-13: 978-0-323-65455-5

Editor: Jessica McCool
Developmental Editor: Sara Watkins

Facial Plastic Surgery Clinics of North America (ISSN 1064-7406) is published quarterly by Elsevier Inc., 360 Park Avenue South, New York, NY 10010-1710. Months of issue are February, May, August, and November. Business and Editorial Offices: 1600 John F. Kennedy Blvd., Suite 1800, Philadelphia, PA 19103-2899. Periodicals postage paid at New York, NY, and additional mailing offices. Subscription prices are $408.00 per year (US individuals), $659.00 per year (US institutions), $454.00 per year (Canadian individuals), $820.00 per year (Canadian institutions), $535.00 per year (foreign individuals), $820.00 per year (foreign institutions), $100.00 per year (US students), and $255.00 per year (foreign students). Foreign air speed delivery is included in all *Clinics* subscription prices. All prices are subject to change without notice. POSTMASTER: Send address changes to *Facial Plastic Surgery Clinics*, Elsevier Health Sciences Division, Subscription Customer Service, 3251 Riverport Lane, Maryland Heights, MO 63043. **Customer service: 1-800-654-2452 (US and Canada); 1-314-447-8871 (outside US and Canada); Fax: 314-447-8029; E-mail: journalscustomerservice-usa@elsevier.com (for print support); journalsonline support-usa@elsevier.com (for online support).**

Reprints. For copies of 100 or more of articles in this publication, please contact the Commercial Reprints Department, Elsevier Inc., 360 Park Avenue South, New York, NY 10010-1710. Tel.: 212-633-3874; Fax: 212-633-3820; E-mail: reprints@elsevier.com.

Facial Plastic Surgery Clinics of North America is covered in *MEDLINE/PubMed* (*Index Medicus*).

Contributors

CONSULTING EDITOR

J. REGAN THOMAS, MD
Professor, Facial Plastic and Reconstructive
Surgery, Department of Otolaryngology–Head
and Neck Surgery, Northwestern University
Feinberg School of Medicine, Chicago, Illinois,
USA

EDITOR

JEFFREY S. MOYER, MD, MS, FACS
Professor and Division Chief, Division of Facial
Plastic and Reconstructive Surgery,
Department of Otolaryngology–Head and Neck
Surgery, University of Michigan, Ann Arbor,
Michigan, USA

AUTHORS

FAISAL I. AHMAD, MD
Fellow, Department of Head and Neck Surgery,
The University of Texas MD Anderson Cancer
Center, Houston, Texas, USA

EILEEN AXIBAL, MD
Department of Dermatology, University of
Colorado Hospital and School of Medicine,
Aurora, Colorado, USA

SHAN R. BAKER, MD
Professor, Department of Otolaryngology–
Head and Neck Surgery, University of Michigan
Medical School, Ann Arbor, Michigan, USA

CHRISTOPHER K. BICHAKJIAN, MD
Professor, Department of Dermatology,
University of Michigan Medical School,
University of Michigan, Ann Arbor, Michigan,
USA

BENJAMIN D. BRADFORD, MD
Clinical Instructor, Department of
Otolaryngology–Head and Neck Surgery,
Division of Facial Plastic and Reconstructive
Surgery, NYU School of Medicine, New York,
New York, USA

MICHAEL G. BRANDT, MD, FRCSC
Assistant Professor, Division of Facial Plastic
and Reconstructive Surgery, Department of
Otolaryngology–Head and Neck Surgery,
Faculty of Medicine, University of Toronto,
Toronto, Ontario, Canada

MARIAH BROWN, MD
Department of Dermatology, University of
Colorado Hospital and School of Medicine,
Aurora, Colorado, USA

PATRICK J. BYRNE, MBA, MD
Director, Division of Facial Plastic
and Reconstructive Surgery,
Professor, Department of
Otolaryngology–Head and Neck Surgery,
Johns Hopkins School of Medicine, Baltimore,
Maryland, USA

NATHAN D. CASS, MD
Resident Physician, Department of
Otolaryngology, University of Colorado
School of Medicine, Aurora, Colorado,
USA

JOSEPH MADISON CLARK, MD, FACS
Associate Professor, Division of Facial Plastic and Reconstructive Surgery, Department of Otolaryngology–Head and Neck Surgery, University of North Carolina at Chapel Hill, Chapel Hill, North Carolina, USA

GREGORY A. DANIELS, MD, PhD
Division of Hematology-Oncology, University of California, San Diego, Moores Cancer Center, La Jolla, California, USA

KATIE GEELAN-HANSEN, MD
Facial Plastic and Reconstructive Surgery Fellow, Division of Facial Plastic and Reconstructive Surgery, Department of Otolaryngology–Head and Neck Surgery, University of North Carolina at Chapel Hill, Chapel Hill, North Carolina, USA

NEIL D. GROSS, MD, FACS
Professor, Department of Head and Neck Surgery, The University of Texas MD Anderson Cancer Center, Houston, Texas, USA

SCOTT J. HOLLISTER, PhD
Wallace H. Coulter Department of Biomedical Engineering, Professor and Patsy and Alan Dorris Chair in Pediatric Technology, Georgia Institute of Technology, Atlanta, Georgia, USA

ANDREW W. JOSEPH, MD, MPH
Assistant Professor, Department of Otolaryngology–Head and Neck Surgery, University of Michigan Medical School, Ann Arbor, Michigan, USA

JUDY W. LEE, MD
Assistant Professor, Department of Otolaryngology–Head and Neck Surgery, Division of Facial Plastic and Reconstructive Surgery, NYU School of Medicine, New York, New York, USA

MICHELLE L. MIERZWA, MD
Assistant Professor, Department of Radiation Oncology, University of Michigan, Ann Arbor, Michigan, USA

COREY C. MOORE, MD, MSc, FRCSC, FACS
Associate Professor, Division of Facial Plastic and Reconstructive Surgery, Department of Otolaryngology–Head and Neck Surgery, Schulich School of Medicine, Western University, St Joseph's Hospital, London, Ontario, Canada

CHRISTINE C. NELSON, MD, FACS
Bartley R. Frueh, MD and Frueh Family Professorship in Eye Plastics and Orbital Surgery, Kellogg Eye Center, Michigan Medicine, Ann Arbor, Michigan, USA

CRISTEN E. OLDS, MD
Resident, Department of Otolaryngology–Head and Neck Surgery, Stanford University, Palo Alto, California, USA

JON-PAUL PEPPER, MD
Assistant Professor, Department of Otolaryngology–Head and Neck Surgery, Stanford University, Palo Alto, California, USA

MARIA J. QUINTANILLA-DIECK, MD
Clinical Lecturer, Department of Dermatology, University of Michigan Medical School, University of Michigan, Ann Arbor, Michigan, USA

ASSUNTINA G. SACCO, MD
Division of Hematology-Oncology, University of California, San Diego, Moores Cancer Center, La Jolla, California, USA

KIRA L. SEGAL, MD
Clinical Lecturer, Kellogg Eye Center, Michigan Medicine, Ann Arbor, Michigan, USA

WILLIAM W. SHOCKLEY, MD, FACS
W. Paul Biggers Distinguished Professor, Chief, Division of Facial Plastic and Reconstructive Surgery, Department of Otolaryngology–Head and Neck Surgery, University of North Carolina at Chapel Hill, Chapel Hill, North Carolina, USA

RYAN M. SMITH, MD
Clinical Fellow, Division of Facial Plastic and Reconstructive Surgery, Department of Otolaryngology–Head and Neck Surgery, Johns Hopkins School of Medicine, Baltimore, Maryland, USA

SHIRLEY Y. SU, MBBS, FRACS
Assistant Professor, Department of Head and Neck Surgery, The University of Texas MD Anderson Cancer Center, Houston, Texas, USA

ADAM M. TERELLA, MD
Assistant Professor, Departments of Otolaryngology and Dermatology, University of Colorado School of Medicine, Aurora, Colorado, USA

CARL TRUESDALE, MD
Resident, Department of Otolaryngology–Head
and Neck Surgery, University of
Michigan Medical School, Ann Arbor,
Michigan, USA

KYLE K. VANKOEVERING, MD
Assistant Professor, Department of
Otolaryngology–Head and Neck Surgery,
University of Michigan Medical Center, Ann
Arbor, Michigan, USA

EMILY WONG, MD
Department of Dermatology, University of
Colorado Hospital and School of Medicine,
Aurora, Colorado, USA

DAVID A. ZOPF, MD
Assistant Professor, Department of
Otolaryngology–Head and Neck Surgery,
Division of Pediatric Otolaryngology, University
of Michigan Medical Center, Ann Arbor,
Michigan, USA

Contributors

CARL TRUESDALE, MD
Resident, Department of Otolaryngology–Head and Neck Surgery, University of Michigan Medical School, Ann Arbor, Michigan, USA

KYLE K. VANKOEVERING, MD
Assistant Professor, Department of Otolaryngology–Head and Neck Surgery, University of Michigan Medical Center, Ann Arbor, Michigan, USA

EMILY WONG, MD
Department of Dermatology, University of Colorado Hospital and School of Medicine, Aurora, Colorado, USA

DAVID A. ZOPF, MD
Assistant Professor, Department of Otolaryngology–Head and Neck Surgery, Division of Pediatric Otolaryngology, University of Michigan Medical Center, Ann Arbor, USA

Contents

This article reviews the most common nonmelanoma skin cancers affecting the head and neck region. Although the most common of these malignancies rarely result in mortality, local morbidity caused by the tumors and their extirpation cannot be underestimated. Complete tumor extirpation with pathologically confirmed negative margins is the gold standard. Regional and distant metastases are rare, but must be treated appropriately should they occur. Although reconstructive surgery can be life changing for the patients and rewarding for the clinicians, it behooves the treating surgeons to remain true to oncologic principles above all else.

Mohs micrographic surgery (MMS) is the gold standard for treating various cutaneous tumors. MMS has evolved into a single-day, outpatient procedure. The tumor is excised, mapped, and processed with frozen, horizontal sections for immediate histologic evaluation. The process is repeated as necessary until the tumor is completely removed, with maximal conservation of normal tissue. Evaluation of 100% of the surgical margin allows for exceptional cure rates. The Mohs surgeon is trained in tumor excision, histopathology interpretation, and surgical reconstruction. The use of MMS is often part of a multidisciplinary approach to treating cutaneous tumors.

Melanoma is a potentially aggressive skin cancer with a steadily rising incidence. Most melanomas are diagnosed at an early stage and associated with an excellent prognosis when treated appropriately. Primary treatment for melanoma is surgical. Wider surgical margins and a variety of techniques for comprehensive histologic margin assessment may be considered for lentigo maligna type melanoma on the head and neck, due to characteristic broad subclinical extension. For invasive melanoma, sentinel lymph node biopsy may be indicated for staging, and to guide further management and follow-up. Appropriate treatment guidelines for early-stage melanoma are reviewed and discussed.

Nasal reconstructive techniques have advanced significantly over the past 50 years. Modern techniques in nasal reconstruction are based on the nasal aesthetic subunits. In order to achieve ideal outcomes, reconstructive surgeons must consider differences in tissue qualities across the nasal aesthetic subunits and formulate reconstructive plans based on these differences. Local flaps, skin grafts, and several types of interpolated flaps comprise the most commonly used techniques for nasal reconstruction. Defects that involve structural or internal lining defects require reconstruction of significantly higher complexity.

outcomes are achieved by assessing regional contours, skin type, and facial aesthetic units. Like tissue should replace like tissue; for example, skin with skin, tarsus with tarsus (or equivalent material, eg, hard palate, ear cartilage, or autologous substitute), and conjunctiva with mucous membrane or like substitute (buccal mucous membrane, amniotic membrane). Patient characteristics including wound care needs, transportation needs, smoking status, and history of radiation can influence the reconstruction plan. Techniques most commonly used in our practice are reviewed.

Sentinel lymph node biopsy uses the concept of selective lymphatic drainage and the lymphatic microvasculature to identify first-echelon nodes draining a given malignancy. Although initially considered difficult and unreliable in the head and neck, experience with the technique has improved and evolved significantly over the last 3 decades. It is now recognized to be accurate and reliable for regional nodal staging and detection of occult nodal metastasis in the head and neck. Although initially described for nodal staging of melanoma, the usefulness of sentinel lymph node biopsy continues to expand and is now extended to other cutaneous malignancies as well as mucosal malignancies of the oral cavity and oropharynx.

Radiotherapy plays a role in the definitive or adjuvant management of early and late stage skin cancers including nonmelanoma basal cell carcinoma and cutaneous squamous cell carcinoma, melanoma, and Merkel cell carcinoma. The role of radiotherapy in skin cancers of the head and neck is reviewed including early and advanced-stage nonmelanoma skin cancers, melanoma, and Merkel cell carcinoma. In particular, the indications, oncologic outcomes, and technical aspects of radiotherapy for these diseases are discussed.

Skin cancer represents a broad classification of malignancies, which can be further refined by histology, including basal cell carcinoma, squamous cell carcinoma and melanoma. As these three cancers are distinct entities, we review each one separately, with a focus on their epidemiology, etiology including relevant genomic data, and the current evidence-based recommendations for adjuvant and neoadjuvant therapy. We also discuss future directions and opportunities for continued therapeutic advances.

Three-dimensional (3D) printing has transformed craniofacial reconstruction over the last 2 decades. For cutaneous oncologic surgeons, several 3D printed technologies are available to assist with craniofacial bony reconstruction and preliminary soft tissue reconstructive efforts. With improved accessibility and simplified design software, 3D printing has opened the door for new techniques in anaplastology. Tissue engineering has more recently emerged as a promising concept for complex auricular and nasal reconstruction. Combined with 3D printing, several groups have demonstrated promising preclinical results with cartilage growth. This article highlights the applications and current state of 3D printing and tissue engineering in craniofacial reconstruction.

As cutaneous cancers are the most common malignancies affecting US citizens, they represent a significant public health problem and health care cost burden. There are a variety of treatment options available to manage cutaneous malignancies, but limited data are available regarding outcomes, including quality of life, recurrence, and mortality. Here, we examine outcomes of skin cancer surgery as they relate to sociodemographic data and treatment factors.

FACIAL PLASTIC SURGERY CLINICS OF NORTH AMERICA

THE CLINICS ARE AVAILABLE ONLINE!
Access your subscription at:
www.theclinics.com

FACIAL PLASTIC SURGERY CLINICS
OF NORTH AMERICA

Preface
State-of-the-Art in Skin Cancer Surgery

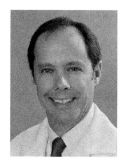

Jeffrey S. Moyer, MD, MS, FACS
Editor

Skin cancer remains the most common cancer in the United States, affecting approximately 20% of Americans during their lifetime. Despite major advances in care delivery, including targeted drug therapies and immunotherapy, the primary treatment for early nonmelanoma skin cancer (NMSC) and melanoma continues to be careful surgical extirpation with clear margins, along with meticulous reconstruction that optimally addresses functional and aesthetic deficits.

The care of patients with skin cancers of the face is uniquely challenging, and this issue of *Facial Plastic Surgery Clinics of North America* addresses the contemporary management of facial NMSC and melanoma as well as up-to-date reconstruction of the resultant defects. In cases of advanced skin cancer, adjuvant treatment is often required, and this issue reviews the tremendous advances in this area over the last 10 years. Looking to the future, the state of tissue engineering and 3D modeling is examined, along with the increasing role these technologies have in facial reconstructive surgery—they are becoming more refined and readily available as methods and techniques. Measuring our reconstructive outcomes is also critically important, and this issue illustrates numerous opportunities where future research might be impactful.

The management of skin cancer continues to evolve, and it is important that surgeons remain current with the latest advances. It is our hope that this issue succeeds in keeping the reader current with state-of-the-art methodologies and technologies in the field, along with the direction the discipline is currently moving.

Jeffrey S. Moyer, MD, MS, FACS
Division of Facial Plastic and
Reconstructive Surgery
Department of Otolaryngology—
Head and Neck Surgery
University of Michigan
1500 East Medical Center Drive, TC 1904
Ann Arbor, MI 48109, USA

E-mail address:
jmoyer@med.umich.edu

Facial Plast Surg Clin N Am 27 (2019) xiii
https://doi.org/10.1016/j.fsc.2018.08.015
1064-7406/19/© 2018 Published by Elsevier Inc.

Nonmelanoma Skin Cancer

Michael G. Brandt, MD, FRCSC[a],*, Corey C. Moore, MD, MSc, FRCSC[b]

KEYWORDS

- Nonmelanoma • Skin cancer • Keratinocyte carcinoma • Basal cell • Squamous cell • Merkel cell
- Adnexal carcinomas of the skin • Sarcomas of the skin

KEY POINTS

- Nonmelanoma skin cancers include a broad group of cutaneous malignancies.
- Keratinocyte carcinomas, including both basal cell and squamous cell carcinomas, are the most common malignancies worldwide.
- Less common nonmelanoma skin cancers include Merkel cell carcinoma, adnexal carcinomas of the skin, and sarcomas of the skin.
- The National Comprehensive Cancer Network (NCCN) provides up-to-date and evidence-based clinical practice guidelines for the evaluation and management of nonmelanoma cancers.

Nonmelanoma skin cancer represents a broad group of cutaneous malignancies. Included in this category are common keratinocyte carcinomas (KCs) and rare neoplasms such as Merkel cell carcinoma (MCC), adnexal carcinomas, and cutaneous sarcomas. Although divergent in cell lineage and presentation, these malignancies occur in the head and neck region and result in some degree of facial morbidity. It has been well established that a defect or lesion of the face negatively affects quality of life and affect display.[1,2] Facial plastic surgeons have the unique opportunity to both cure these patients of potentially life-threatening malignancies and also improve their quality of life through well-executed postablative reconstruction. This article provides a contemporary overview of cutaneous neoplasms that present in the head and neck region.

KERATINOCYTE CARCINOMAS

Basal cell carcinoma (BCC) and squamous cell carcinoma (SCC) represent the 2 most common skin malignancies and are frequently grouped together under the umbrella term nonmelanoma skin cancer. These two cutaneous malignancies share a cellular lineage with keratinocytes and are thus more accurately termed KC.[3] KCs are the most common malignancies worldwide, with an annual incidence that exceeds all other malignancies combined.[4] The incidence of KC continues to increase with more than 3 million treatments for KC in the United States each year.[4] Although KCs are typically well managed and only rarely metastasize, they can result in substantial morbidity.

CAUSE

Although the risk of developing KC depends on genotypic, phenotypic, and environmental factors, it is well established that ultraviolet (UV) solar radiation is the greatest single risk factor for the development of KC.[5] UVB (290–320 nm) is considered more carcinogenic than UVA (320–400 nm) because it is completely absorbed in the skin

Disclosure: Dr M.G. Brandt and Dr C.C. Moore have no conflicts of interest.
[a] Division of Facial Plastic and Reconstructive Surgery, Department of Otolaryngology–Head and Neck Surgery, Faculty of Medicine, University of Toronto, 190 Elizabeth Street, Room 3S-438, TGH RFE Building, Toronto, Ontario M5G 2C4, Canada; [b] Division of Facial Plastic and Reconstructive Surgery, Department of Otolaryngology–Head and Neck Surgery, Schulich School of Medicine, Western University, St Joseph's Hospital, 268 Grosvenor Street 2nd Floor, London, Ontario N6A 4V2, Canada
* Corresponding author.
E-mail address: drmbrandt@gmail.com

Facial Plast Surg Clin N Am 27 (2019) 1–13
https://doi.org/10.1016/j.fsc.2018.08.001

and results in the mutation of tumor suppressor genes.[6] UVA, which penetrates deeper than UVB, also plays a role because it activates the signal transduction molecule protein C kinase, and also impairs the activity of tumor suppressor T cells, leading to tumor expansion and a failed immune response.[7,8] Cumulative sun exposure may be more causally related to the development of SCC in that it results in UV-induced DNA damage and subsequent p53 gene mutations.[5,9] Mutations of the p53 gene can also be found in up to 50% of BCCs.[10] In contrast with SCC, intense intermittent recreational sun exposure (ie, resulting in sun burns) and exposure during childhood may be more central to the development of BCCs.[5,9] BCCs frequently show mutations of chromosome 9q resulting in Patched (PTCH) gene mutations and subsequently induced hedgehog (Hh) signaling.[9] It is this Hh signaling pathway that is targeted by the systemic Hh inhibitors vismodegib and sonidegib, which are US Food and Drug Administration approved for the treatment of advanced BCC.[11,12] Other risks factors for the development of KC are listed in **Box 1**.

CLINICAL FEATURES AND WORK-UP

Common clinical features of KCs are listed in **Box 2**. Because of the relationship between KCs and UV light exposure, these lesions occur most frequently in the head and neck region. Of the KCs, approximately 75% are BCCs and 25% are SCCs. BCCs are clinically categorized as nodular, superficial, and infiltrative or sclerosing subtypes (**Figs. 1–7**). Nodular BCCs are most common and present as waxy, raised papules or nodules with telangiectasias (see **Figs. 1–3**).[9] Superficial BCCs increase horizontally and present as thin, erythematous plaques with variable scale and telangiectasias (see **Figs. 4** and **5**).[9] Sclerosing BCCs are ill-defined, indurated red or white plaques that can be slightly elevated or depressed and atrophic (see **Figs. 6** and **7**).[9]

Invasive SCC of the skin frequently presents as an erythematous, keratotic papule, plaque, or nodule occurring in a background of actinic damage (**Figs. 8–12**).[9] These lesions can show ulceration and patients often describe a history of an intermittently bleeding and nonhealing sore. Actinic keratosis and Bowen disease (SCC in situ) are considered precursor lesions to invasive SCC and frequently present as a well-demarcated erythematous, scaly plaque.[3]

Any clinically suspicious lesion should be biopsied. Although multiple biopsy techniques have been advocated, a 3-mm full-thickness punch biopsy provides the greatest histologically

Box 1
Risk factors for the development of keratinocyte carcinomas

Risk factor

UV radiation (sun exposure, tanning beds)

Ionizing radiation

Immunosuppression

Human papillomavirus

Smoking

Chronic scarring/inflammation

Exposure to polycyclic hydrocarbons

Phototherapy with psoralens (PUVA [psoralen and UVA] therapy)

Photosensitizing drugs (ie, fluoroquinolones)

Arsenic ingestion

Syndromes

Xeroderma pigmentosum

Oculocutaneous albinism

Nevoid BCC syndrome/Gorlin syndrome/basal cell nevus syndrome

Epidermodysplasia verruciformis

Dystrophic epidermolysis bullosa

Muir-Torre syndrome

KID (keratosis, ichthyosis, deafness)

Fanconi anemia

Rothmund-Thompson syndrome

Werner syndrome

Data from Madan V, Lear JT, Szeimies R-M. Nonmelanoma skin cancer. Lancet 2010;375(9715):673–85; and Lee DA, Miller SJ. Nonmelanoma skin cancer. Facial Plast Surg Clin North Am 2009;17(3):309–24.

diagnostic information and is thus recommended by the authors for any suspicious lesion. Diagnostic imaging is reserved for clinically aggressive lesions to determine the extent of invasion or to help evaluate for distant metastasis from clinical suspicion or clinically palpable adenopathy. It is important to recognize that SCC of the lip is considered an oral cancer and accordingly requires prudent clinical examination and may necessitate radiographic evaluation of regional lymphatics.

MANAGEMENT
Resection of the Primary Malignancy

The primary goal in the treatment of BCC and SCC is to cure the patient of the malignancy while

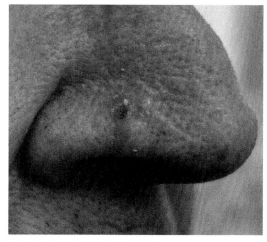

Fig. 2. Nodular BCC of the right alar margin.

limiting both tumor and iatrogenic morbidity. Further to these goals, the National Comprehensive Cancer Network (NCCN) provides clinical practice guidelines for the evaluation and management of nonmelanoma skin cancers. These guidelines are up to date and established by group consensus based on currently available evidence. Guidelines are available at www.NCCN.org.[13,14]

Because most facial plastic and reconstructive surgeons manage cutaneous malignancies isolated to the head and neck region, this article focuses on cutaneous malignancies arising in this area. The treatment of BCC and SCC is guided principally by the risk of local recurrence and/or disease progression. The NCCN indicates that, within the head and neck, nonmelanoma skin cancers that are most likely to recur present in the central face, are more than 1 cm in diameter, are

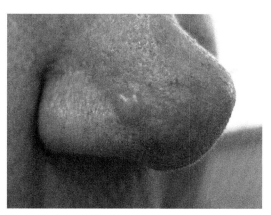

Fig. 1. Nodular BCC of the right ala.

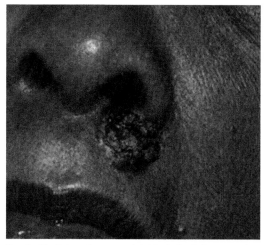

Fig. 3. Nodular pigmented BCC of the left upper lip.

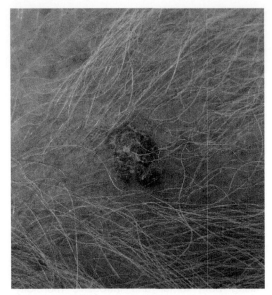

Fig. 4. Superficial pigmented BCC of the scalp.

Fig. 6. Sclerosing BCC of the forehead.

clinically poorly defined, are recurrent lesions, occur in areas of previous radiation, or occur among patients who are immunosuppressed. In the case of SCC, tumors larger than 6 mm in the central face, rapidly growing tumors, or those that show neurologic symptoms (ie, anesthesia, motor dysfunction) are also considered high risk.[13,14]

For high-risk BCCs and SCCs (with no evidence of metastasis) the NCCN recommends management via Mohs micrographic surgery, resection with complete circumferential margin assessment (ie, intraoperative frozen section analysis), standard excision with wide margins (4–6 mm), and postoperative margin assessment, or radiation

therapy for nonsurgical candidates.[13,14] For standard surgical excision, Wolf[15] and Bordland and Zitelli[16] showed that, for well-defined BCCs less than 2 cm in diameter, excision with 4-mm clinical margins resulted in complete removal in more than 95% of cases. Wider surgical margins are recommended for SCCs whereby high-risk SCCs measuring less than 1 cm, 1 to 1.9 cm, or more than 2 cm in diameter require clinical margins of 4, 6, and 9 mm respectively when treated via standard surgical excision with postoperative margin assessment.[16]

As per the NCCN guidelines, low-risk BCCs and SCCs can be managed via electrodessication and curettage (excluding terminal hair-bearing areas) or via standard excision with 4-mm to 6-mm margins and postoperative margin assessment.[13,14] For nonsurgical candidates, radiation therapy is recommended.

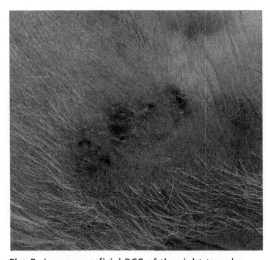

Fig. 5. Large superficial BCC of the right temple.

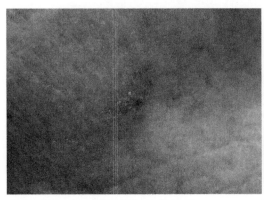

Fig. 7. Sclerosing BCC of the right neck.

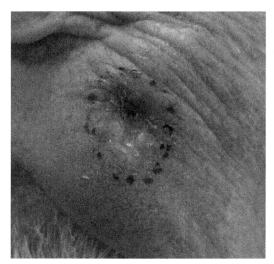

Fig. 8. SCC of the left cheek.

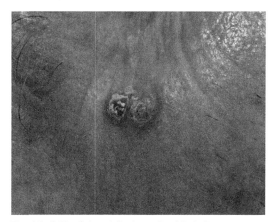

Fig. 10. SCC of the right lateral orbital rim.

INCOMPLETE EXCISIONS AND AGGRESSIVE FEATURES ON PATHOLOGY

Reexcision via Mohs micrographic surgery or resection with complete circumferential margin assessment (ie, intraoperative frozen section analysis) is recommended for any BCC or SCC that has been incompletely excised in the head and neck region.[13,14] For those patients who are nonsurgical candidates or among those lesions for which further surgery is not possible, radiation therapy is recommended.[13,14] Adjuvant radiation therapy is also recommended for BCCs or SCCs showing perineural or lymphovascular involvement.[13,14]

ADVANCED DISEASE

Patients presenting with advanced BCCs or SCCs, including those with regional lymphatic involvement, benefit from evaluation and management by a multidisciplinary tumor board. The authors recommend reviewing the latest NCCN guidelines at www.NCCN.org to direct management of advanced KCs.

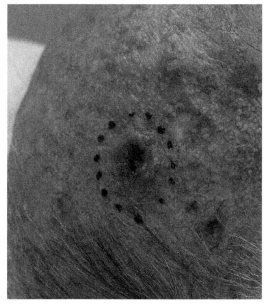

Fig. 9. SCC of the scalp in a background of actinic damage.

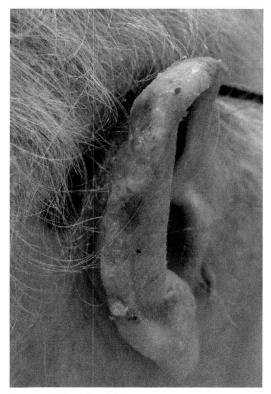

Fig. 11. SCC of the right ear.

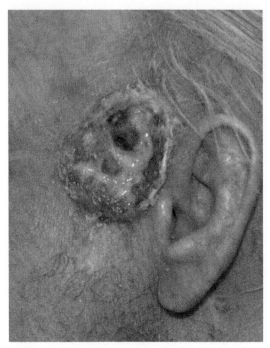

Fig. 12. SCC of the left temple/cheek.

The incidence of metastatic BCC ranges from 0.0028% to 0.55%.[10] Systemic therapy in the form of Hh pathway inhibitors (ie, vismodegib, sonidegib) can be considered for any patient presenting with nodal or distant metastatic BCC.[13] This treatment is also an option for patients with recurrent BCC following resection and adjuvant radiation, or for patients who are not candidates for either surgery or radiation.[13]

Metastatic SCC of the skin occurs with an incidence of approximately 2% to 6%.[17] The lip and ear represent the sites at highest risk for metastasis in primary SCC, with an incidence of 10% to 14%.[17] Note that recurrent SCC has a 30% incidence of metastasis, emphasizing the need for adequate primary control. Neck dissection and adjuvant radiation therapy are recommended for SCCs with regional lymph node involvement, and the extent of dissection depends on lymph node size, lymph node number, and node location (ie, parotid, ipsilateral neck, contralateral neck).[14] Concurrent systemic chemotherapy is recommended for any patient showing extracapsular extension of tumor on lymphadenectomy.[14]

LESS COMMON NONMELANOMA SKIN CANCERS
Merkel Cell Carcinoma

MCC is an uncommon cutaneous neuroendocrine carcinoma. Although it remains uncommon, the annual incidence has risen 5-fold over the past

30 years.[18] In 2011, the incidence in the United States was 7.9 cases per 1 million persons.[18] MCC primarily affects white men at sites of chronic sun exposure in their seventh to ninth decade of life.[18] Immunosuppression is also considered a major risk factor for the development of MCC.[18] MCC is an aggressive malignancy with a 5-year survival rate of 50.6% for those with primary disease, 35.4% for those with regional lymph node involvement, and 13.5% for those with distant metastases.[19]

The cell of origin of MCC is unknown and potentially includes epidermal stem cells, B cells, and fibroblasts. A novel human polyomavirus named Merkel cell polyomavirus (MCPyV) can be detected in 60% to 80% of Merkel cell tumors.[20] MCPyV works through a variety of mechanisms, resulting in inhibited tumor suppressor function and carcinomatous cellular proliferation.[18]

Clinical features and work-up

MCC presents as an asymptomatic, rapidly growing, firm, red, pink, purple, or skin-colored nodule (**Figs. 13–15**).[21] Heath and colleagues[21] proposed the AEIOU acronym to represent lesions that are asymptomatic and expanding rapidly among immunosuppressed fair-skinned individuals older than 50 years at UV-exposed sites. In spite of awareness of MCC and clinical vigilance, its varied appearance results in most MCCs being diagnosed histopathologically on biopsy when differentiated from other small blue cell tumors on positive cytokeratin 20 (CK20) and negative thyroid transcription factor 1 (TTF-1) immunohistochemistry, differentiating it from small cell lung cancer. At time of presentation, 65% of patients present with local disease, 26% of patients

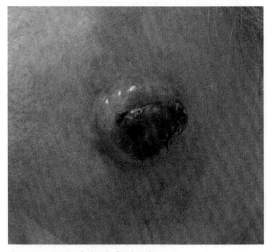

Fig. 13. MCC of the left cheek.

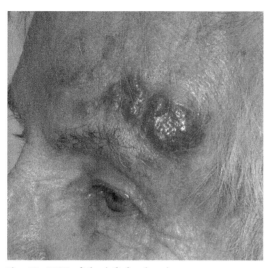

Fig. 14. MCC of the left forehead.

present with regional lymph node metastases, and 8% present with distant metastases.[18]

Work-up and management are guided by the most up-to-date NCCN guidelines available from www.NCCN.org. The authors recommend diagnostic imaging to evaluate for regional lymph node involvement and distant metastasis for any patient diagnosed with MCC. For patients presenting with clinically palpable lymph nodes, these should be biopsied via fine-needle aspiration biopsy (FNAB) or core biopsy. Evaluation by a multidisciplinary tumor board should be strongly considered.

Management

The latest NCCN guidelines recommend sentinel lymph node biopsy (SLNB) before definitive surgical excision.[22] One-third of patients presenting with clinically negative lymph nodes are found to have micrometastases on SLNB.[23] Recurrence occurred in 56% of SLNB-positive and 39% of

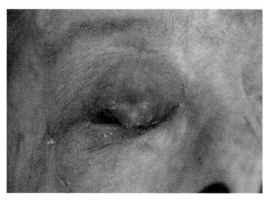

Fig. 15. MCC of the right upper eyelid.

SLNB-negative patients.[23] Note that SLNB is less consistent in the head and neck region because of variability in nodal drainage, which can result in a false-negative SLNB.[24] However, SLNB does remain useful in guiding the dose and region of adjuvant radiation that is recommended for all patients with MCC, except perhaps for those presenting in immunocompetent patients with lesions less than 1 cm that have been widely excised with no lymphovascular or perineural invasion.

Once SLNB has been performed, the primary tumor requires resection with 1-cm to 2-cm margins to the investing fascia (when possible).[22] In the head and neck region, this is typically best performed via Mohs surgery, modified Mohs surgery, or complete circumferential peripheral and deep-margin assessment.[25] Neck dissection should be considered for any patient presenting with regional lymph node involvement diagnosed on FNAB, core biopsy, or SLNB; these patients require evaluation by a multidisciplinary tumor board.[22] Radiation to the primary site and involved nodal basin is recommended for any patient with nodal involvement.[22]

Radiation therapy is recommended for most patients presenting with MCC in an adjuvant fashion to the primary tumor site.[22] For patients with head and neck region MCC, radiation to the nodal basin should be considered even among those with negative SLNB because of the aforementioned risk of a false-negative result. These recommendations are based on the NCCN guidelines, which indicate that adjuvant radiation therapy decreases local recurrence and significantly improves overall survival.[22]

Adnexal Carcinomas of the Skin

Adnexal carcinomas are rare, with an annual incidence of approximately 1 per 20 million persons in the United States.[26,27] Although rare, the incidence of these tumors has tripled over the past 30 years.[26] Similar to MCC, adnexal carcinomas occur most frequently among elderly white men. This category of tumor includes carcinomas of the eccrine and apocrine glands, carcinomas of the hair follicle, and carcinomas of the sebaceous glands. This review of these lesions focuses on those most frequently affecting the head and neck region and are summarized in **Tables 1–3**.

Sarcomas of the Skin

Sarcomas of the skin are a broad group of rare, nonepithelial, primary skin neoplasms. These cutaneous neoplasms are classified according to the mature cell type they resemble. This article

Table 1
Eccrine and apocrine gland carcinomas stratified by area of involvement, gender, age at incidence, clinical features, notable features, and management

	Common Site	Gender	Decade	Clinical Features	Keep in Mind	Management
Mucinous carcinoma	Face/eyelid	F>M	Third to eighth	Asymptomatic, slow-growing, flesh colored soft/spongy nodule	Rule out metastatic mucinous carcinoma from breast or GI tract	Standard surgical excision or MMS
Microcystic adnexal carcinoma	Face/upper lip	F>M	Sixth	Slow-growing neoplasm. Indurated firm plaque or discrete nodule Yellowish to flesh colored Epidermal surface is smooth or crusted	Perineural invasion is common	Standard surgical excision or MMS for the primary tumor RT ± chemotherapy with perineural invasion
Adenoid cystic carcinoma	Scalp	F>M	Fifth	Asymptomatic crusted verrucous plaque or deep-seated nodule	Perineural invasion is common	MMS or resection with complete circumferential margin assessment for the primary tumor RT for perineural invasion
Acrospirocarcinoma	Face	F>M	>Fifth	Large, ulcerated mass or nodule or an infiltrative plaque	Frequently metastasize to regional lymph nodes + distant sites	Standard surgical excision + sentinel node biopsy or neck dissection
Cylindrocarcinoma	Scalp	F>M	>Fifth	Typically arise from a preexisting cylindroma with associated rapid growth, tenderness, ulceration, discoloration, and/or bleeding	Aggressive tumors	Standard surgical excision or MMS for the primary tumor. RT for metastatic disease or inoperable tumors
Syringocystadenocarcinoma papilliferum	Scalp	M = F	Sixth	Exophytic verrucous plaque or nodule	Metastasis is rare	Standard surgical excision or MMS for the primary tumor

Abbreviations: F, female; GI, gastrointestinal; M, male; MMS, Mohs micrographic surgery; RT, radiation therapy.
Data from Walsh SN, Santa Cruz DJ. Adnexal carcinomas of the skin. In: Rigel DS, Robinson JK, Ross M, et al, editors. Cancer of the skin. 2nd edition. Saunders; 2011. p. 140–9.

Table 2
Carcinomas of the hair follicle stratified by area of involvement, gender, age at incidence, clinical features, notable features, and management

	Common Site	Gender	Decade	Clinical Features	Keep in Mind	Management
Trichilemmal carcinoma	Head and neck	M>F	70th	Slow-growing papule or nodule	Metastasis is rare	Conservative standard surgical excision or MMS
Proliferating/malignant trichilemmal cystic carcinomas	Scalp	F>M	Sixth	Long-standing subcutaneous mass that has grown rapidly. Firm, painless nodule with overlying alopecia or ulceration	Aggressive tumors with a high rate of metastasis	Standard surgical excision with wide margins or MMS for the primary tumor. Neck dissection, RT, and chemotherapy have variable to limited success for disseminated tumors
Matrical carcinoma/malignant pilomatricoma	Head and neck	M>F	Fourth	Slow-growing, firm, nontender nodule. Clinically mistaken as a benign pilomatricoma or inclusion cyst	Metastasis is common	Standard surgical excision with 0.5–1 cm margins or MMS. RT for metastatic disease or inoperable tumors

Data from Walsh SN, Santa Cruz DJ. Adnexal carcinomas of the skin. In: Rigel DS, Robinson JK, Ross M, et al, editors. Cancer of the skin. 2nd edition. Saunders; 2011. p. 140–9.

Table 3
Carcinomas of the sebaceous glands stratified by area of involvement, gender, age at incidence, clinical features, notable features, and management

	Common Site	Gender	Decade	Clinical Features	Keep in Mind	Management
Sebaceous carcinoma	Head and neck, eyelid	M>F	70th	Slow-growing firm subcutaneous nodule with occasional ulceration. Yellow hue is common at extraocular sites	Classified as ocular or extraocular Associated with Muir-Torre syndrome (especially if diagnosed in younger patients). Can metastasize	Standard surgical excision with wide margins or MMS for the primary tumor. Sentinel node biopsy may be useful for poorly differentiated and ocular lesions

Data from Walsh SN, Santa Cruz DJ. Adnexal carcinomas of the skin. In: Rigel DS, Robinson JK, Ross M, et al, editors. Cancer of the skin. 2nd edition. Saunders; 2011. p. 140–9.

focuses on 3 of these neoplasms: the most common sarcoma of the skin, dermatofibrosarcoma protuberans (DFSP); the most common cutaneous sarcoma of the head and neck, atypical fibroxanthoma (AFX); and the most common vascular sarcoma of the head and neck, cutaneous angiosarcoma of the face and scalp.

Dermatofibrosarcoma Protuberans

DFSP is the most common sarcoma of the skin. Its annual incidence has been estimated at 4.5 cases per 1 million persons in the United States, making DFSP nearly half as common as MCC.[28,29] Unlike other rare skin malignancies, this tumor most frequently occurs in the second to fifth decade of life and affects individuals of African American heritage twice as frequently as white people.[28,29]

DFSP is a low-grade sarcoma of fibroblast origin. DFSP is characterized by a translocation between chromosomes 17 and 22, resulting in the overexpression of platelet-derived growth factor receptor β.[30] It is differentiated from a common dermatofibroma on immunohistochemistry, being positive for CD34 and negative for factor XIIIa. Given the characteristically slow growth of these lesions, they typically present as large tumors. Microscopically, many deep, fingerlike projections are present, resulting in indistinct borders and recurrence rate as high as 60%.[31,32] Metastatic disease is uncommon.

Clinical features and work-up
DFSP typically presents as a slow-growing, flesh-colored or pink, nodular lesion of the trunk or extremities. Presentation in the head and neck is rare. Over time, the tumor develops a more protuberant appearance. The latest NCCN guidelines

recommend a deep subcutaneous punch or incisional biopsy because superficial biopsies may mistakenly suggest the lesion is a benign dermatofibroma.[33] Given the low rate of metastasis, imaging is not routinely performed. The NCCN suggests MRI if extensive extracutaneous extension is suspected.[33]

Management
Management is directed by the most recent NCCN guidelines available from www.NCCN.org.[33] Mohs micrographic surgery or surgical excision down to the level of investing fascia with 2-cm to 4-cm peripheral margins is recommended with subsequent complete circumferential margin assessment (ie, intraoperative frozen section analysis).[33] Reresection is recommended should final pathology show positive margins.[33] Given the characteristic microscopic extension of DFSP, undermining and/or flap reconstruction should only be considered once all margins have been histologically cleared.[33] Radiation therapy and consultation with a multidisciplinary tumor board should be considered among patients with recurrent disease or if complete surgical excision is not possible.[33] Chemotherapy can be considered in the rare event of metastatic disease, and multidisciplinary tumor board consultation is recommended in this circumstance.[33]

Atypical Fibroxanthoma

AFX is a very rare, low-grade sarcoma of fibroblastic origin. It typically presents in the head and neck region among white men in their seventh decade of life.[31,34] Similar to other cutaneous malignancies, AFX presents with increased frequency among immunosuppressed patients.

Because AFX typically occurs in areas of chronic UV exposure, a history of previous KC is common, and frequently the AFX is misdiagnosed clinically as a keratinocyte carcinoma. Because of the rarity of the tumor, there are no incidence data.[31]

Similar to KC, AFX is thought to arise from UV-induced mutations of the p53 tumor suppressor gene.[35] AFX is histologically similar to other spindle cell neoplasms, such as cutaneous malignant fibrous histiocytoma (MFH). The distinction between AFX and MFH has been controversial and, in 2002, the World Health Organization recommended the term MFH be replaced by undifferentiated pleomorphic sarcoma (UPS); AFX is considered a distinct pathologic diagnosis to UPS.[36] In contrast with AFX, UPS is considered a diagnosis of exclusion and typically presents as an aggressive subfascial mass of the extremities among older adults. UPS is discussed herein because previous reports of aggressive AFX lesions may have been incorrectly categorized and would now be considered UPS.

Clinical features and work-up

AFX typically presents as a slow-growing ulcerated nodule and, as previously mentioned, clinically resembles keratinocyte carcinoma. On histopathology, the lesion is typically confined to the dermis and thus has limited metastatic potential.[36] More aggressive features on histopathology raise suspicion that the lesion may be an alternative sarcoma such as UPS. AFX is a diagnosis of exclusion on immunohistochemical analysis and is negative for S100 protein, cytokeratins, and desmin, differentiating it from melanoma, SCC, and leiomyosarcoma.[36]

Management

Mohs micrographic surgery or surgical excision down to the level of investing fascia with 1-cm to 2-cm peripheral margins is recommended with subsequent complete circumferential margin assessment (ie, intraoperative frozen section analysis). The recurrence rate is approximately 10% for wide local excision and may be lower with Mohs micrographic surgery.[31] To reiterate, nodal or distant metastases do not occur with AFX and these findings suggest a more aggressive soft tissue sarcoma.

Angiosarcomas

Angiosarcomas are very rare vascular sarcomas that include cutaneous angiosarcoma of the face and scalp. This lesion is considered a high-grade angiosarcoma and most frequently presents at the scalp or forehead among white men in their seventh decade of life.[37] These lesions are highly aggressive and often multicentric with a high metastasis rate, recurrence rate, and mortality.[37] Prognosis is poor, with perhaps 12% of patients surviving 5 years or more.[37]

Vascular endothelial growth factor (VEGF) is involved in the regulation of endothelial cell proliferation, and VEGF-D levels are significantly increased among patients with cutaneous angiosarcoma of the face and scalp.[38]

Clinical features and work-up

Cutaneous angiosarcoma of the face and scalp presents as an ill-defined bruiselike lesion (similar to a hematoma) or as broad facial edema, especially of the eyelids with minimal erythema.[39] Induration and ulceration may occur in more advanced lesions, with some lesions presenting multifocally.[39]

Tissue sampling can show immunohistochemical positivity for the endothelial markers CD34 and CD31, as well as positive VEGF receptor-3, podoplanin, and the proliferation marker K-67.[40] Tissue biopsies of the periphery of the lesion with testing for the aforementioned immunohistochemical markers can help determine the extent of the tumor.[39] Given the vascular origin of the tumor and the high propensity for metastasis, imaging of regional lymph nodes and screening for distant metastases is prudent.

Management

Ideal treatment involves wide excision of the lesion with subsequent complete circumferential margin assessment (ie, intraoperative frozen section analysis) and adjuvant radiotherapy.[39] This is frequently not possible because of wide extension at the time of diagnosis. Thus, primary radiation and potentially adjuvant systemic chemotherapy may be the only options. Nevertheless, referral to a multidisciplinary tumor board is recommended.

SUMMARY

Nonmelanoma skin cancers are an extensive group of malignancies. The most common malignancy is BCC; however, it is one of the least aggressive and best managed of the group. Clinical vigilance is paramount and a biopsy is always the right investigation when confronted with an unusual facial lesion. Although the aesthetic outcome of a facial reconstruction is important, the first priority is ensuring pathologic clearance of the malignancy.

REFERENCES

1. Godoy A, Ishii M, Dey J, et al. Facial lesions negatively impact affect display. Otolaryngol Head Neck Surg 2013;149(3):377–83.

2. Godoy A, Ishii M, Byrne PJ, et al. How facial lesions impact attractiveness and perception: differential effects of size and location. Laryngoscope 2011; 121(12):2542–7.

3. Albert MR, Weinstock MA. Keratinocyte carcinoma. CA Cancer J Clin 2003;53(5):292–302.

4. Rogers HW, Weinstock MA, Feldman SR, et al. Incidence estimate of nonmelanoma skin cancer (keratinocyte carcinomas) in the US population, 2012. JAMA Dermatol 2015;151(10):1081.

5. Madan V, Lear JT, Szeimies R-M. Non-melanoma skin cancer. Lancet 2010;375(9715):673–85.

6. Gailani MR, Leffell DJ, Ziegler A, et al. Relationship between sunlight exposure and a key genetic alteration in basal cell carcinoma. J Natl Cancer Inst 1996;88(6):349–54.

7. Matsui MS, DeLeo VA. Longwave ultraviolet radiation and promotion of skin cancer. Cancer Cells 1991;3(1):8–12.

8. Nghiem DX, Kazimi N, Mitchell DL, et al. Mechanisms underlying the suppression of established immune responses by ultraviolet radiation. J Invest Dermatol 2002;119(3):600–8.

9. Lee DA, Miller SJ. Nonmelanoma skin cancer. Facial Plast Surg Clin North Am 2009;17(3):309–24.

10. Rubin AI, Chen EH, Ratner D. Basal-cell carcinoma. N Engl J Med 2005;353(21):2262–9.

11. Sekulic A, Migden MR, Oro AE, et al. Efficacy and safety of vismodegib in advanced basal-cell carcinoma. N Engl J Med 2012;366(23):2171–9.

12. Chen L, Silapunt S, Migden MR. Sonidegib for the treatment of advanced basal cell carcinoma: a comprehensive review of sonidegib and the BOLT trial with 12-month update. Future Oncol 2016; 12(18):2095–105.

13. Cited (?with permission) from the NCCN clinical practice guidelines in oncology (NCCN Guidelines) for basal cell carcinoma V1.2018. 2018 national comprehensive cancer network, Inc. All rights reserved. The NCCN guidelines and illustrations herein may not be reproduced in any form for any purpose without the express written permission of the NCCN. To view the most recent and complete version of the NCCN Guidelines, go online to www.NCCN.org. National Comprehensive Cancer Network, NCCN, NCCN Guidelines, and all other NCCN Content are trademarks owned by the National Comprehensive Cancer Network, Inc.

14. Cited (?with permission) from the NCCN Clinical Practice Guidelines in Oncology (NCCN Guidelines) for Squamous Cell Skin Cancer V2.2018. 2018 National Comprehensive Cancer Network, Inc. All rights reserved. The NCCN Guidelines and illustrations herein may not be reproduced in any form for any purpose without the express written permission of the NCCN. To view the most recent and complete version of the NCCN Guidelines, go online to www.NCCN.org. National Comprehensive Cancer Network, NCCN, NCCN Guidelines, and all other NCCN Content are trademarks owned by the National Comprehensive Cancer Network, Inc.

15. Wolf DJ. Surgical margins for basal cell carcinoma. Arch Dermatol 1987;123(3):340–4.

16. Bordland DG, Zitelli JA. Surgical margins for excision of primary cutaneous squamous cell carcinoma. J Am Acad Dermatol 1992;27:241–8.

17. Rudolph R, Zelac DE. Squamous cell carcinoma of the skin. Plast Reconstr Surg 2004;114(6):82e–94e.

18. Tetzlaff MT, Nagarajan P. Update on Merkel cell carcinoma. Head Neck Pathol 2018;12(1):31–43.

19. Harms KL, Healy MA, Nghiem P, et al. Analysis of prognostic factors from 9387 Merkel cell carcinoma cases forms the basis for the new 8th edition AJCC staging system. Ann Surg Oncol 2016;23(11): 3564–71.

20. Feng H, Shuda M, Chang Y, et al. Clonal integration of a polyomavirus in human Merkel cell carcinoma. Science 2008;319(5866):1096–100.

21. Heath M, Jaimes N, Lemos B, et al. Clinical characteristics of Merkel cell carcinoma at diagnosis in 195 patients: the AEIOU features. J Am Acad Dermatol 2008;58(3):375–81.

22. Cited (?with permission) from the NCCN Clinical Practice Guidelines in Oncology (NCCN Guidelines) for Merkel Cell Carcinoma V2.2018. 2018 National Comprehensive Cancer Network, Inc. All rights reserved. The NCCN Guidelines and illustrations herein may not be reproduced in any form for any purpose without the express written permission of the NCCN. To view the most recent and complete version of the NCCN Guidelines, go online to www.NCCN.org. National Comprehensive Cancer Network, NCCN, NCCN Guidelines, and all other NCCN Content are trademarks owned by the National Comprehensive Cancer Network, Inc.

23. Santamaria-Barria JA, Boland GM, Yeap BY, et al. Merkel cell carcinoma: 30-year experience from a single institution. Ann Surg Oncol 2012;20(4): 1365–73.

24. Willis AI, Ridge JA. Discordant lymphatic drainage patterns revealed by serial lymphoscintigraphy in cutaneous head and neck malignancies. Head Neck 2007;29(11):979–85.

25. O'Connor WJ, Roenigk RK, Brodland DG. Merkel cell carcinoma. Comparison of Mohs micrographic surgery and wide excision in eighty-six patients. Dermatol Surg 1997;23:929–33.

26. Blake PW, Bradford PT, Devesa SS, et al. Cutaneous appendageal carcinoma incidence and survival patterns in the United States. Arch Dermatol 2010; 146(6).

27. Walsh SN, Santa Cruz DJ. Adnexal carcinomas of the skin. In: Cancer of the skin. Elsevier; 2011. p. 140–9.

28. Rouhani P, Fletcher CDM, Devesa SS, et al. Cutaneous soft tissue sarcoma incidence patterns in the U.S. Cancer 2008;113(3):616–27.

29. Criscione VD, Weinstock MA. Descriptive epidemiology of dermatofibrosarcoma protuberans in the United States, 1973 to 2002. J Am Acad Dermatol 2007;56(6):968–73.

30. McArthur G. Molecularly targeted treatment for dermatofibrosarcoma protuberans. Semin Oncol 2004; 31:30–6.

31. Reinstadler DR, Sinha UK. Uncommon cutaneous neoplasms of the head and neck. Facial Plast Surg Clin North Am 2012;20(4):483–91.

32. Stojadinovic A, Karpoff HM, Antonescu CR, et al. Dermatofibrosarcoma protuberans of the head and neck. Ann Surg Oncol 2000;7(9):696–704.

33. Cited (?with permission) from the NCCN Clinical Practice Guidelines in Oncology (NCCN Guidelines) for Dermatofibrosarcoma Protuberans V1.2018. 2018 National Comprehensive Cancer Network, Inc. All rights reserved. The NCCN Guidelines and illustrations herein may not be reproduced in any form for any purpose without the express written permission of the NCCN. To view the most recent and complete version of the NCCN Guidelines, go online to www.NCCN.org. National Comprehensive Cancer Network, NCCN, NCCN Guidelines, and all other NCCN Content are trademarks owned by the National Comprehensive Cancer Network, Inc.

34. Ang GC, Roenigk RK, Otley CC, et al. More than 2 decades of treating atypical fibroxanthoma at Mayo Clinic. Dermatol Surg 2009;35(5):765–72.

35. Dei Tos AP, Maestro R, Doglioni C, et al. Ultraviolet-induced p53 mutations in atypical fibroxanthoma. Am J Pathol 1994;145(1):11–7.

36. Bowles TL, Ross MI, Lazar AJ. Sarcomas of the skin. In: Rigel DS, editor. Cancer of the skin. 2nd edition. Elsevier; 2011. p. 157–67.

37. Holden CA, Spittle MF, Jones EW. Angiosarcoma of the face and scalp, prognosis and treatment. Cancer 1987;59(5):1046–57.

38. Mendenhall WM, Mendenhall CM, Werning JW, et al. Cutaneous angiosarcoma. Am J Clin Oncol 2006;29: 524–8.

39. Sangueza OP, Requena LC. Malignant neoplasms: vascular differentiation. In: Rigel DS, editor. Cancer of the skin. 2nd edition. Elsevier; 2011. p. 186–95.

40. Orchard GE, Zelger B, Jones EW, et al. An immunohistochemical assessment of 19 cases of cutaneous angiosarcoma. Histopathology 1996;28:235–40.

Mohs Micrographic Surgery

Emily Wong, MD, Eileen Axibal, MD, Mariah Brown, MD*

KEYWORDS

- Mohs micrographic surgery • Margin control • Surgical excision • Tissue sparing • Mohs technique
- Basal cell carcinoma • Squamous cell carcinoma • Melanoma

KEY POINTS

- Mohs micrographic surgery (MMS) has evolved since the 1930s to become the standard of care for the treatment of many types of cutaneous tumors, both primary and recurrent.
- MMS is a methodical technique that examines 100% of the tumor margin. Precise mapping and staged removal result in the highest cure rates for skin cancers, while sparing normal, uninvolved tissue.
- The surgical technique is a low-risk and cost-effective single-day procedure that is performed in the outpatient setting.
- The Mohs surgeon serves 2 roles: surgeon (excising the tumor) and pathologist (interpreting the horizontally oriented frozen sections).
- MMS is used to treat basal cell carcinomas, squamous cell carcinomas, dermatofibrosarcoma protuberans, atypical fibroxanthoma, and numerous rare cutaneous tumors.

INTRODUCTION

Mohs micrographic surgery (MMS) is the gold standard for treating a variety of cutaneous tumors. Dr Frederic Mohs developed the technique in the 1930s with the guiding principle of complete microscopically controlled excisions. MMS has evolved over the years into a single-day, outpatient procedure for treating primary and recurrent cutaneous tumors. The tumor is excised, precisely mapped, and processed with frozen, horizontal sections for immediate histologic evaluation. The Mohs surgeon serves as both surgeon and pathologist for the procedure. The process is repeated with tissue excised only at the positive margin, allowing for complete tumor removal while sparing normal tissue. Evaluation of 100% of the margin leads to the highest cure rates for skin cancer. The Mohs surgeon is trained in reconstruction of the surgical defects or collaborates with other

surgical specialties. The use of MMS is often part of a multidisciplinary approach to treating cutaneous tumors.

HISTORY OF MOHS SURGERY
Origins

MMS is named after its founder, Dr Frederic E. Mohs (1910–2002). In medical school, Dr Mohs first conceived of the idea of complete microscopic control of excisions while working with animal tumor models.[1–3] Standard tissue processing for skin pathology uses vertical, or breadloaf, sections, which do not completely evaluate the peripheral or deep surgical margins in most cases.[4] Dr Mohs proposed using a tissue fixative and then removing the tissue in horizontal layers so that the entire deep and peripheral margins could be examined microscopically until a tumor-free plane had been achieved.[2,5] Zinc chloride

Disclosures: No relevant financial disclosures for any authors.
Department of Dermatology, University of Colorado Hospital and School of Medicine, Mail Stop F703, 1665 North Aurora Court, Aurora, CO 80045, USA
* Corresponding author.
E-mail address: Mariah.brown@ucdenver.edu

Facial Plast Surg Clin N Am 27 (2019) 15–34
https://doi.org/10.1016/j.fsc.2018.08.002

possesses unique properties that made it the most useful fixative for such purposes: it provided excellent in situ histologic preservation, penetrated tissue in a controlled manner, was nontoxic and odorless, and left a healthy bed of granulation tissue after necrotic tissue sloughed.[1,6] The zinc chloride was compounded into a paste consisting of granular stibnite and *Sanguinaria canadensis* (bloodroot powder).[2] This combination allowed the zinc chloride to be released in a predictable manner, where the depth of penetration was precisely controlled, from 1 mm to 1 cm or more, based on the thickness of the applied paste.[1]

Chemosurgery

Dr Mohs termed his new technique "chemosurgery," which denoted the chemical fixation and surgical excision of tissue.[1,6] However, the name omitted the most important concept: complete microscopic control of surgical margins. Dr Mohs believed "...the essential feature of the chemosurgical method lies in the microscopically controlled technic (sic) by which cancer tissue is removed."[7]

Dr Mohs started treating patients with chemosurgery in 1936 at Wisconsin General Hospital[2] (**Box 1**). He published his first article on chemosurgery in 1941 in the *Archives of Surgery*.[5,7] The article described the chemosurgery process and reported on 440 skin cancers treated with the technique. Follow-up ranged from 1.0 to 4.5 years with a 93% cure rate.[7] With limited interest from general surgeons, Dr Mohs presented his techniques to dermatologists at the American Academy of Dermatology meeting in 1946 and was well-received.[2,8] Although Dr Mohs trained physicians in general surgery, vascular surgery, and plastic surgery in his technique, ultimately Mohs surgery became a subspecialty of dermatology, integrating with the specialty's existing focus on both skin malignancies and pathology.[2,5]

Fresh-Tissue Technique

As the chemosurgical technique gained popularity, certain aspects were problematic. Each stage of chemosurgery lasted 1 day, as zinc chloride took 18 hours to fix tissue.[7] Patients requiring multiple stages of excision were treated over numerous consecutive days. The paste was painful, causing significant swelling and at times requiring hospitalization for pain control.[9] Surgical defects could not be repaired the same day, as it took up to 7 to 10 days for the fixed tissue to slough off the wound bed.[9–11] Over time, a new method, known as the fresh-tissue technique, was developed and ushered in the method of micrographic surgery as it is performed today.

In 1953, Dr Mohs filmed surgery for a basal cell carcinoma (BCC) on the eyelid. To hasten the filming of multiple stages, Dr Mohs injected the area with local anesthetic and completed the second stage excision immediately, without using a chemical fixative. The procedure was such a success that Dr Mohs continued using this new fresh-tissue technique for all surgeries on the eyelid.[3,5] At the 1971 American College of Chemosurgery (ACC) meeting, Dr Theodore Tromovitch and Dr Samuel Stegman promoted the fresh-tissue technique,[9] and later published a series of 102 head and neck BCCs treated with the fresh-tissue technique, reporting equivalent cure rates to the chemosurgical technique.[12] The fresh-tissue technique, also known as microscopically controlled excision, offered important advantages over the fixed tissue, chemosurgery method.[13] Using a local anesthetic eliminated the need for and the discomfort of the zinc chloride fixative. The tumor was immediately excised and processed, resulting in significant time-savings for both patient and physician. Numerous tissue stages could be done in 1 day and the wound could be reconstructed immediately.[13] The most promising aspect was that more patients could be treated earlier in their disease state with the efficiency and comfort of the modified procedure.[12]

In 1974, Dr Daniel Jones, trained by Dr Mohs, introduced the term "micrographic surgery" to highlight the microscopic evaluation and tumor mapping of the technique.[14] The procedure was officially named "Mohs micrographic surgery" in 1985.[14] The ACC changed its name to the American College of Mohs Micrographic Surgery and Cutaneous Oncology in 1986 and established standards for an accredited, 1-year fellowship training program for MMS.[2,3,14] There are currently more than 70 Micrographic Surgery and Dermatologic Oncology Fellowship Programs approved by the Accreditation Council for Graduate Medical Education.[15] Fellowship training is not required to perform MMS. However, the College's efforts over the years have established standardized, high-quality fellowship training requirements in MMS and reconstruction, resulting in distinct expertise for fellowship-trained Mohs surgeons.[14]

The current MMS technique has several important advantages:

1. High cure rates resulting from complete evaluation of the deep and peripheral surgical margins using horizontal frozen sections. Traditional vertical, or breadloaf, sectioning of tissue evaluates less than 1% of the true surgical margin, leaving significant room for residual tumor and sampling error.[16]

Box 1
Dr Mohs' original chemosurgery process

1. Application of a keratolytic (dichloroacetic acid) to the tumor, causing the skin to turn white and allowing penetration of zinc chloride.
2. Application of zinc chloride paste to the desired thickness.
3. Placement of a moisture-tight dressing using cotton and petrolatum.
4. The next day, surgical excision of fixed tissue, inking the tissue to orient and precisely map the tumor, examination under the microscope.
5. If tumor was seen, more fixative as applied to the site.
6. Excision of the second tissue layer the following day and the process repeated until the cancer was completely removed.
7. Most defects healed by second intention, the exceptions were those needing immediate repair for functional purposes.

Data from Mohs FE. Chemosurgery in cancer, gangrene and infections. Cancer 1957;10(3):644; and Mohs FE. Chemosurgical treatment of cancer of the face: a microscopically controlled method of excision. Arch Derm Syphilol 1947;56(2):143–56.

2. MMS conserves normal, uninvolved tissue and often results in the smallest and shallowest surgical defect.[6,17]
3. The physician functions as both the surgeon and pathologist for the Mohs procedure, ensuring integrated, precise removal of the tumor without the potential errors introduced by tissue handoffs.
4. Reconstruction is performed only after tumor-free surgical margins are confirmed with 100% margin evaluation.[17] This minimizes the risk of having positive surgical margins after tumor excision with immediate tissue transfer.

Limitations of MMS include potentially prolonged surgical days for patients, inability to perform the procedure on patients who cannot tolerate surgery under local anesthesia, and difficulty in clearing margins for aggressive tumor involving deep structures, such as bone or parotid gland.

MOHS SURGERY TECHNIQUE
Preoperative Evaluation

Preoperatively, the patient should undergo either a separate-day or same-day surgical consultation.[18]

The consultation includes a thorough medical record review and provides the patient with an explanation of the tumor etiology and prognosis, treatment options and risk factors, reconstructive possibilities, postoperative wound care instructions (including activity limitation, pain control, and medication management), and a general overview of the day of surgery.[19] Written informed consent should be obtained on the day of the procedure.

The medical history review should focus on identifying comorbidities that may complicate surgery, including diabetes, hypertension, liver failure, renal failure, immunosuppression, inherited bleeding disorders, inflammatory skin conditions, and prior radiation therapy.[20,21] Patients also should be screened for antibiotic prophylaxis indications, but most Mohs patients do not require preoperative or postoperative antibiotics. Based on a 2008 advisory statement updating the indications for antibiotic prophylaxis in dermatologic surgery, patients with specific cardiac or joint conditions undergoing a dermatologic procedure involving the oral mucosa or infected skin (class II wounds) should receive prophylactic antibiotics to prevent infective endocarditis and hematogenous total joint infection, respectively.[21] Antibacterial prophylaxis may also be warranted in high-risk patients undergoing dermatologic surgery on sites with increased rates of infection (below the knee, in the groin, flaps on the ear and nose, wedge excisions or grafts); however, no specific antibiotic guidelines exist.[22] Given the risks associated with occupational exposure to communicable diseases, such as hepatitis B virus, hepatitis C virus, and human immunodeficiency virus, it is prudent to inquire about these infections. Patients also should be screened for smoking and alcohol consumption, as both can increase the risk of complications and even minor decreases in consumption can improve postoperative results.[23,24] Identifying patients with implantable electrical cardiac devices or other implantable electric devices is important to ensure the safe use of electrosurgery.[25] Allergies, particularly medication reactions and prior reactions to latex or other medical materials, should be noted.

A thorough list of the patient's medications and supplements should be reviewed, with a focus on identifying drugs that may increase the risk of bleeding complications; commonly implicated therapies include warfarin, aspirin (ASA), clopidogrel, factor Xa inhibitors, and nonsteroidal anti-inflammatory drugs (NSAIDs). Herbal supplements that may potentiate bleeding include ginkgo biloba, garlic, ginger, ginseng, feverfew, dong quai, vitamin E, and others.[26,27] For patients with increased bleeding risk, pertinent preoperative laboratory data, such as prothrombin time/International Normalized Ratio (INR) and platelet count should be reviewed. A platelet count less than 50,000 is widely considered a relative contraindication to an invasive procedure, and studies suggest that it is safe to proceed with dermatologic surgery if the INR is less than 3.5 within 1 week of the operation.[28] The current consensus is that patients should not stop any medically necessary anticoagulants or antiplatelet medications before dermatologic surgery, as the risk of catastrophic thrombotic complications exceeds the risk of bleeding.[29] If not medically indicated, it is recommended to discontinue ASA or NSAIDs 7 to 10 days before surgery.[30] There may be instances in which reduction or cessation of anticoagulation is warranted; in such cases, the decision is best made in conjunction with the prescribing provider.[31]

A preoperative focused physical examination is then performed. Most patients will have a skin biopsy performed before Mohs surgery to confirm the diagnosis of skin cancer. In some cases, where the suspicion of cutaneous malignancy is high, a biopsy with frozen section analysis can be performed the same day as Mohs surgery. In either case, the tumor site should be confirmed with the patient, measured and photographed for reference.[32] The pathology report from the biopsy should be reviewed and, if there is any uncertainty about the diagnosis or histologic features, the original biopsy site slides should be obtained for examination by the Mohs surgeon before the procedure.[33] Regional lymph nodes and other surrounding anatomic structures should be examined and palpated. Large, aggressive, or high-risk tumors may warrant preoperative radiologic imaging with ultrasound, lymphoscintigraphy, computed tomography, MRI, or PET.[34] Complex cases requiring a multidisciplinary approach should be evaluated preoperatively by other subspecialties, as indicated.[35]

On the day of surgery, vital signs should be obtained as part of the physical examination. One comprehensive review suggests that for patients with a systolic pressure ≤180 mm Hg, diastolic pressure ≤100 mm Hg, and no other medical contraindications, cutaneous surgery may proceed.[36] Higher blood pressures often warrant surgical deferment. Surgery should be avoided on actively inflamed or infected skin. Some patients may require a preoperative oral anxiolytic medication such as diazepam, alprazolam, or midazolam. During MMS, midazolam has been shown to cause amnesia and reduced alertness, with no clinically significant adverse effects.[37] Informed consent should always be obtained before administration of the anxiolytic.

Surgical Technique

Mohs surgery is typically performed under local anesthesia in a nonsterile procedure room in the outpatient setting. Most physicians operate under clean rather than sterile technique when performing Mohs surgery. Multiple studies, including a 2016 meta-analysis of more than 12,000 patients undergoing outpatient dermatologic, dental, and emergency room surgery, suggest that clean, nonsterile technique for resection and reconstruction is adequate for achieving an exceedingly low rate of skin and soft tissue infection.[38] In 2006, Rhinehart and colleagues[39] first demonstrated no statistical difference in infection rates with sterile versus nonsterile gloves during the tumor extirpation phase of MMS. Since that time, studies by Mehta and colleagues[40] and Xia and colleagues[41] support the safety and cost-effectiveness of nonsterile gloves during both MMS and surgical reconstruction, although many Mohs surgeons continue to perform all surgical reconstruction with sterile technique.

The first step of the Mohs procedure is identifying the biopsy site, which can be a challenge, as many sampled tumors are small, may be partially or fully healed scars due to a lag time between biopsy and MMS, and occur within a background of actinic damage with prior procedural scars.[32] One study revealed that 16.6% of patients and 5.9% of physicians incorrectly identify biopsy sites on examination alone, but that the ability to review preoperative photographs almost completely mitigates this risk.[42] The general consensus among Mohs surgeons is that photographs, augmented with anatomic landmarks and diagrams if available, are the best way to confirm a biopsy site.[43] Several additional strategies may be used to aid in correct site identification: patient biopsy site "selfies," dermatology smart phone applications, ultraviolet-fluorescent tattoos, procedural techniques (gauze dermabrasion, alcohol wipes, injection-induced blisters, tangential lighting, Wood light, dermoscopy), re-biopsy, and finally contacting or returning the patient to the referring physician.[44]

After biopsy site confirmation, the patient should be placed in a recumbent position and draped. The clinically apparent tumor or biopsy site margin should be outlined with a surgical marking pen, measured and photographed. It is important to mark the tumor before injection of local anesthesia, as the fluid tumescence will distort the tissue and obscure the visible margin. Marking nearby cosmetic subunit boundaries, anatomic landmarks, and rhytids before anesthesia is also helpful for optimizing reconstruction.[45] The site should then be cleansed. Although there are a variety of antiseptic techniques available, a 2015 survey revealed that most Mohs surgeons use 4.0% chlorhexidine gluconate when taking a Mohs layer and during defect reconstruction for all locations except the periocular area, where povidone-iodine of 7.5% to 10.0% was the most commonly reported antiseptic.[46] Local or regional anesthesia with 1% or 2% lidocaine with epinephrine 1:100,000 or 1:200,000 is most commonly used. Lidocaine has a maximum weight-based dose of 4.5 mg/kg without epinephrine and 7.0 mg/kg with epinephrine and has been found to be safe for all anatomic locations in most cases.[47] Lidocaine toxicity is rare in dermatologic surgery. Alam and colleagues[48] demonstrated that the perioperative peak lidocaine levels during MMS do not result in serum levels approaching toxic limits, even when relatively high total lidocaine doses (up to 50 mL) are used.

Once anesthetized, the surgeon may or may not use curettage to delineate tumor involvement from normal surrounding skin (**Fig. 1**). BCCs and squamous cell carcinomas (SCCs) are often more friable than normal surrounding skin, allowing curettage to detect tumor extensions that are not clinically visible. Although curettage may increase the size of the initial surgical defect, several studies have reported the need for fewer Mohs stages with this technique.[49–51] The surgeon may also debulk the visible tumor with a surgical blade and submit for vertical histopathologic sections in the Mohs laboratory, as this can help characterize tumor growth patterns or high-risk features.[52]

A 1-mm to 5-mm surgical margin, depending on tumor type, should be drawn around the clinically apparent tumor with a marking pen. An incision is then made with a scalpel (most typically a #15 blade) along the outlined margin, beveled at a 30° to 45° angle, and the tissue is then sharply excised to an appropriate depth along a flat horizontal plane[53,54] (**Fig. 2**). The beveled edges result in a saucer-shaped specimen that can be flattened, thus allowing for the deep and peripheral margins to be sectioned in the same histologic plane. Scalpel tissue nicks, suture, staples, gentian violet, and methylene blue have all been used to orient the specimen and adjacent tissue before its removal.[55] Once removed, the orientation of the specimen should be vigilantly maintained in preparation for mapping. Hemostasis is then most commonly achieved with electrosurgery, electrocautery, chemical cautery, or direct pressure. Finally, the patient is temporarily bandaged and instructed to wait for 0.5 to 2.0 hours in a comfortable area during the mapping, slide preparation, and histopathology interpretation.

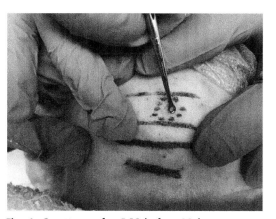

Fig. 1. Curettage of a BCC before Mohs surgery to define the clinical borders. Note the linear purple marking pen delineating the relaxed skin tension lines of the forehead.

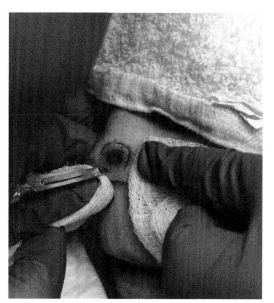

Fig. 2. First-stage Mohs procedure for BCC on the nose; tissue is removed with 45° blade angle.

Mohs Mapping

The Mohs map allows for correlation of the surgical site, specimen, and histopathology. Detail and accuracy of the map are paramount, as they serve to guide future stages of tumor extirpation if any surgical margins are involved[56] (**Fig. 3**). Tissue from the first stage of Mohs should be transferred from the patient to a separate clinical area for grossing of the specimen, maintaining tissue orientation at all times. In the case of large tumors, the excised tissue should be divided into pieces small enough fit on a microscope slide. Due to the increased risk of false-positive and false-negative margins with each additional subdivision, the Mohs tissue should be cut into as few tissue blocks as possible.[57] The sequence of numbering the tissue specimens should be made clear on the map and should be consistent from patient to patient. The tissue should then be inked and mapped with a drawn or digital image to document the exact tumor location and orientation[58,59] (**Fig. 4**). A variety of effective inking patterns have been

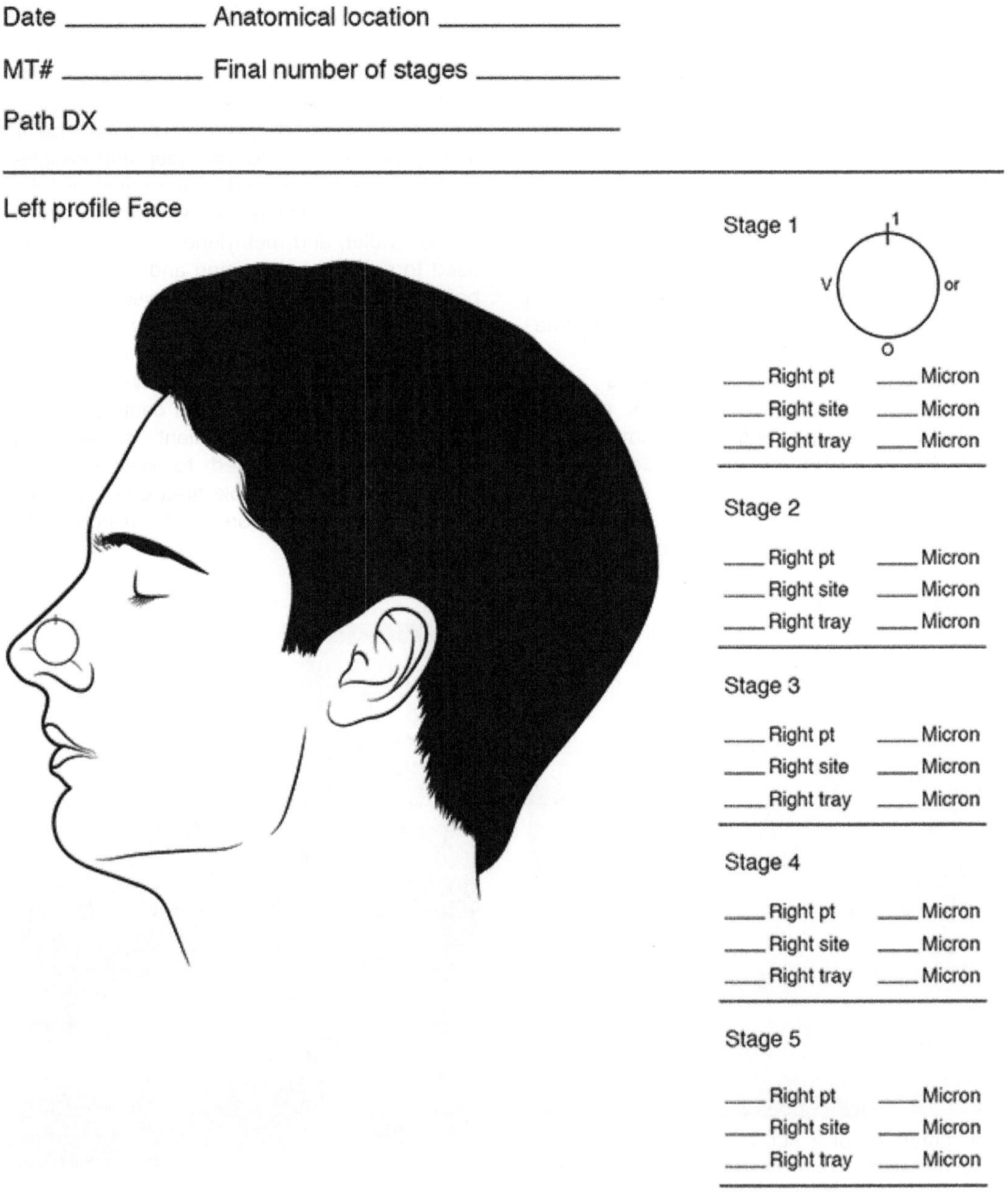

Fig. 3. Mohs map indicating the location of the tumor and inking pattern for stage 1.

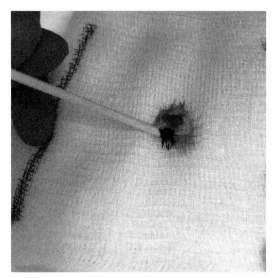

Fig. 4. Inking the specimen for precise mapping. Note the horizontal black line that denotes the 12 o'clock position and helps maintain tissue orientation.

described, including inking 2 adjacent nonepidermal edges with different colors and color-coding the 12, 3, 6, and 9 o'clock positions.[55,60,61] Regardless of technique, consistency is imperative. Any atypical features of the specimen, such as presence of cartilage, bone, or subcutaneous tissue lacking an epidermal edge, should be indicated on the map. In order for the epidermis to lie evenly in the same plane as the deep margin, the specimen should be flattened with shallow relaxing cuts made parallel and distant to the epidermal edge, as needed. The specimen can then be transferred via nonstick pad, filter paper in a Petri dish, glass slide, or gauze pad to the Mohs technician for sectioning and staining.[55]

Tissue Processing

The fresh frozen technique with horizontal sections, allowing complete margin visualization, is what distinguishes MMS from wide local excision. Classic histopathology uses a breadloaf technique in which tissue is sectioned in a vertical orientation at several intervals along the specimen. The amount of tissue visualized depends on the number of sections evaluated, but is typically limited to less than 0.01% to 1.0% of the true surgical margin.[16] If the sections fail to capture tumor extensions, false-negative margins and tumor recurrences occur. MMS does not rely on the intervals of sampled margins, but instead allows for 100% microscopic margin control (**Fig. 5**). In select high-risk skin cancers, vertical paraffin sections may be used in conjunction with frozen sections,

to aid in determining tumor diagnosis, tumor staging, and evaluation of high-risk features.[62]

Once in the laboratory, the flattened specimen, which may require additional manipulation by the technician to ensure the epidermal margin lies in the same plane as the deep margin, is preserved in an embedding medium and attached to the specimen-holder button or chuck used to hold the specimen during sectioning in the cryostat[63] (**Fig. 6**). Although numerous embedding media exist, all are generally composed of some combination of polyvinyl alcohol and polyethylene glycol and work optimally between $-15°C$ and $-30°C$.[64] Because slow freezing can result in ice crystal formation in the tissue (freeze artifact), the tissue should be frozen as rapidly as possible.[65] After the specimen is embedded and frozen in the medium, it is placed bottom-side up toward the microtome stage in the cryostat, so that horizontal sections are taken from the deep surface (**Fig. 7**). "Facing the block" is defined as trimming tissue on a microtome from the peripheral or deep surgical margins before sectioning; this is associated with a 39% increased false-positive margin rate and should not be performed.[66] The first section obtained is the "true margin." The number of sections cut per piece of tissue and the average thickness of each section vary depending on surgeon preference; a 2004 survey found that most Mohs surgeons prefer between 3 and 6 sections for review (range 1–9), and an average section thickness of 5 μm to 6 μm (range 4 μm–9 μm).[67] The first cut is placed either closest to or farthest from the frosted edge of the glass slide, depending on surgeon and technician preference, and additional sections are placed sequentially on the slides (**Fig. 8**). The preferred placement of sections differs between practices, but should be predetermined and consistent within each laboratory. The process is repeated for each tissue specimen.

Once all tissue has been processed, the slides are stained, either manually or with an automatic slide stainer. The same survey found that most laboratories used hematoxylin-eosin (H&E) as the routine staining method for MMS, but 6% of the respondents used toluidine blue to evaluate BCCs.[67] Most tumors are stained with H&E during MMS. However, with advancements in immunohistochemical (IHC) stains, many Mohs laboratories now perform IHC stains for melanoma in situ (MIS), rare tumors, and aggressive tumors.[68] Melanoma antigen recognized by T cells, (MART-1), and other melanoma markers are commonly used to aid in diagnosis of melanoma on frozen sections during MMS. Pancytokeratin, an IHC stain that incorporates both low and high

| Mohs Micrographic Surgery Technique | Routine Breadloafing Sectioning Technique |

Cutaneous tumors frequently extend beyond the clinically evident borders. The tumor (red) is first excised (black) with a margin of visibly unaffected skin.

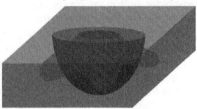
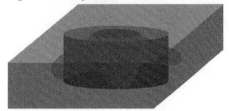

a. The Mohs excision is removed with a beveled angle, therefore allowing the deep and peripheral margin to be processed in the same plane.

a. The breadloafed section is excised with the edges at 90 degrees. The tissue is then sliced vertically in intervals along the specimen and these sections are examined.

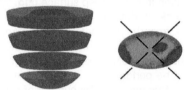
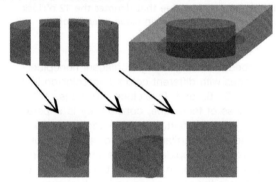

b. The Mohs section is processed horizontally, allowing for identification of 100% of the surgical margin. The positive margins are readily identified in the Mohs sections as shown above.

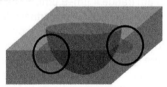

True positive   True positive   False negative

b. Examples of sampling errors from breadloafing tissue.

c. For Mohs tissue, additional layers are then taken from the mapped areas to ensure complete removal of the tumor, allowing for high cure rates. This technique allows for optimal tissue sparing of normal, uninvolved skin for smaller scars and more reconstructive options.

c. The breadloading technique sections the tissue in a vertical orientation. Typically, less than 1% of the specimen margin is evaluated. This may result in a higher rate of sampling error.

Fig. 5. Comparison of Mohs micrographic pathology technique compared with traditional vertical pathology sectioning. (*Courtesy of* Julia Kreger, MD, Aurora, CO.)

molecular weight keratins, is helpful for distinguishing SCC. Carcinoembryonic antigen has been used to detect extramammary Paget disease during MMS. After staining with H&E and/or IHC stains, the slides are rinsed and mounted with coverslips and transferred to the Mohs surgeon for interpretation. For most cases, the tissue blocks from MMS are discarded after the procedure. The Mohs slides are preserved for a minimum of 10 years, as guided by the Clinical Laboratory Improvement Amendments standard retention requirement.[69]

Histopathology Interpretation

The slides are examined methodically by the Mohs surgeon, who also functions as the pathologist, in the outpatient surgical suite. Two studies

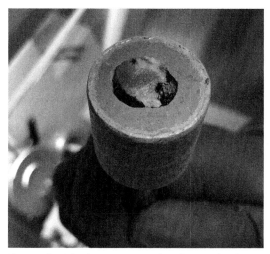

Fig. 6. The inked specimen is placed onto the frozen chuck to hold the specimen during sectioning. Great care is taken to ensure all of the epidermal edges are touching the chuck.

demonstrated a greater than 99% concordance between Mohs surgeons and dermatopathologists in reading MMS histology slides.[70,71] The Mohs surgeon should first review the slides macroscopically. Tissue shrinkage reliably occurs during frozen section processing, approximately 16.3% on the trunk and extremities and 10.2% on the head and neck, but any larger size discrepancy raises a concern for technical error.[72] If applicable, the debulk specimen should then be examined to gather information about the tumor's unique histopathologic characteristics. Each mounted Mohs section should be subsequently examined in sequential order corresponding to the map. The sections should contain full epidermis, dermis,

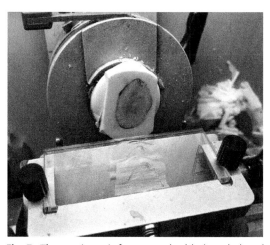

Fig. 7. The specimen is frozen, embedded, and placed on the microtome for sectioning.

and subcutaneous fat (if applicable), with no overlap of successive layers of skin and subcutis in the 2-dimensional plane on the slide.[63] In the 360° representation of Mohs tissue, the superficial epidermis and dermis are visualized at the periphery and the deeper subcutis is visualized centrally (**Fig. 9**). Any positive margin should be noted on the Mohs map. Areas of calcification, perineural or lymphovascular invasion, scar, and other incidental skin neoplasms should be noted. Sections need to be carefully examined because rete ridges, hair follicles, transposed epidermis, adnexal structures, and deposition artifact can mimic tumor.[73] Inflammation in histologic frozen sections may be predictive of adjacent tumor, and taking an additional layer may be warranted; in one study, the most common attributable cause of recurrence after MMS was failure to excise additional tissue when dense inflammation was present.[74–76] Floaters, or dislodged pieces of tumor tissue embedded in unaffected tissue, can also complicate margin assessment.[77]

When the first or most-peripheral section, the "true margin," reveals tumor or when all sections are tumor-free, margin status is immediately determined. In some cases, though, no tumor is present in the initial section but cancer becomes apparent in "deeper" tissue cuts.[78] To ensure tumor clearance, it is important that the excision has a margin of normal skin beyond the observed neoplasm. Varying opinions exist on how much normal tissue represents a clear margin, and the threshold may differ based on clinical and histologic factors, such as tumor type, primary versus recurrent status, thickness of section, level of inflammation, and quality of slides. A 2013 survey found that most respondents would not take an additional Mohs layer with 4 clear sections.[78]

If the surgical margins are clear, the excision is complete. If tumor is identified at the margins or there is poor visualization of the specimen despite cutting additional sections off the tissue block, a second Mohs stage is required. The precise tumor location and subtype should be indicated on the Mohs map for reference during the next stage of the procedure (**Fig. 10**).

Subsequent Stages

The patient is returned to the procedure room. The Mohs map is examined to determine the areas of tumor positivity and where this corresponds to on the patient's surgical defect. The second Mohs layer is performed in a similar fashion to the first, but often does not require complete reexcision of all surgical margins. Tumor identified in the epidermis or dermis requires focal extension

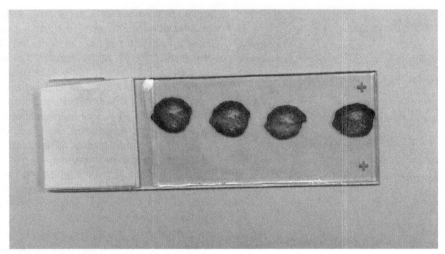

Fig. 8. A Mohs micrographic slide with 4 cuts of tissue for review. The piece closest to the frosted, yellow edge is the first cut, and the true margin at this particular laboratory.

of the periphery of the surgical defect, whereas residual tumor isolated to the subcutaneous tissue requires a deeper excision. When laterally extending the defect, the layer should be obtained in a crescentic, rather than rectangular, shape that extends beyond the edge of the tumor margin; this prevents false-negative margins due to incomplete visualization of the vertical edges of a rectangular specimen[79] (**Fig. 11**). The specimen containing the area of residual tumor and a small amount (1–2 mm) of surrounding tissue is removed, oriented, mapped, and processed. This cycle is repeated until no residual tumor is identified: each cycle of tissue removal is called a "Mohs stage." Alam and colleagues[80] demonstrated that BCCs and SCCs required an average

number of 1.92 and 1.66 stages for clearance, respectively, and that tumors on the nose and ear required a higher number of stages relative to other anatomic sites. After confirmation of clear margins, the defect is measured, photographed, and the patient most commonly undergoes surgical reconstruction the same day. **Fig. 12** shows examples of frozen section Mohs histology. **Fig. 13** shows preoperative photos and the final defect after MMS.

Complications

A large, multicenter, prospective study of more than 20,000 MMS patients demonstrated a 0.72% complication rate, with 0.02% serious

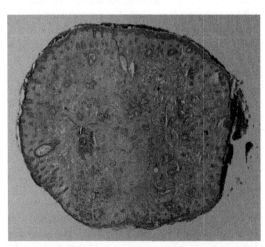

Fig. 9. A Mohs micrographic tissue piece showing 360° of epidermis and dermis at the periphery and the deeper subcutis centrally. (hematoxylin-eosin, original magnification ×2).

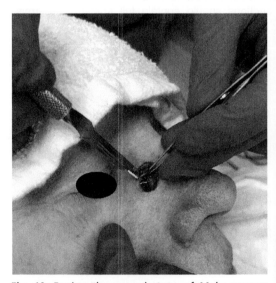

Fig. 10. During the second stage of Mohs surgery, only the area of positivity is excised.

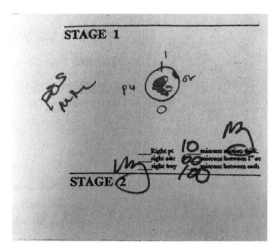

Fig. 11. Mohs map indicating the area of positivity in the deep and lateral margin from stage 1 with a red marker.

events and no deaths.[81] Postoperative complications, when they occur, most often result from surgical reconstruction rather than MMS itself. Documented complications include infection, bleeding, hematoma formation, wound dehiscence, tissue necrosis, scar contracture/hypertrophy, and suboptimal cosmetic outcome. These risks can be minimized with meticulous surgical technique and wound care.

USE OF MOHS SURGERY

MMS is indicated for numerous cutaneous tumors, depending on their clinical appearance, size, location, histologic findings, prior treatment, and patient immune status and/or genetic syndromes.[82] Most tumors treated with Mohs surgery are BCCs and SCCs. In 2012, the American Academy of Dermatology, in collaboration with the American College of Mohs Surgery, the American Society for Dermatologic Surgery Association, and the American Society for Mohs Surgery, established appropriate use criteria (AUC) for MMS to minimize overuse of the procedure.[83] The document presents 270 clinical scenarios and rates each scenario as inappropriate, uncertain, or appropriate for MMS. The tumors evaluated are listed in **Box 2**. Invasive melanoma was not included in the AUC due to the complexities of treatment with MMS. The location on the body, patient characteristics, and tumor characteristics should be taken into consideration when determining if MMS is appropriate[83] (**Table 1**). MMS allows for the complete removal of tumors with poorly defined borders, extensive subclinical spread, or aggressive pathology. MMS also should be considered for any tumor with a high risk of

recurrence or whose treatment may result in cosmetic or functional impairment.[82]

MMS is particularly useful on certain special sites, such as the eyelids, lips, genitalia, and nail units, where the anatomy is unique and functional considerations are paramount. Skin cancers on the eyelids (5%–10%), lips (3%–4%), penis (0.5% of all cancer), vulva (1% of all cancers in women), and the nail unit (0.3%) are all considered high-risk tumors.[83,84] BCC (90%), sebaceous carcinoma (5%), and SCC (4%) are the most common eyelid tumors.[84] BCC and SCC are the most common tumors on the lips. SCC of the lip is of particular risk, with a reported 3% to 20% metastasis rate.[85] MMS has been shown to have higher cure rates than surgical excision in treating tumors of the eyelid and lip.[84] Genital cancers are most commonly SCC (>95%) and the recurrence rate in these sites can be high with any treatment modality[84]; however, MMS is often used due to the tissue conservation, particularly to avoid partial penectomy in men.[86] Cancer in the nail unit is quite rare, but when found, it is most commonly SCC, followed by melanoma and BCC. Most data for MMS of the nail unit is for SCC, with cure rates ranging from 92% to 96%.[87,88] For all of these cancer sites, a multidisciplinary approach may be needed for large and aggressive tumors.

Although the Mohs AUC establishes the appropriateness of MMS, it does not compare the efficacy between various treatment modalities, nor does it determine which treatment is preferred.[83] The choice of treatment ultimately depends on the physician's clinical judgment and the patient's individual situation and preferences. The Mohs AUC does not explicitly integrate cost into the appropriateness ratings; however, cost was considered secondary to the degree of potential clinical improvement.[83]

MMS is cost-effective in the treatment of nonmelanoma skin cancer (NMSC).[89–93] With the Mohs surgeon serving as both surgeon and pathologist, the MMS billing codes include all of the following: entire surgical procedure, anesthesia, pathology processing and evaluation, and cost of supplies.[17] Cook and Zitelli[89] evaluated the cost of treating 400 consecutive tumors with MMS. They found MMS comparable to excision with permanent section analysis and significantly less than office-based and ambulatory surgical facility excision with frozen section analysis.[89] Bialy and colleagues[90] found similar results comparing 98 patients with primary nonmelanoma skin cancer on the face and ears treated with MMS versus traditional surgical excision. Although office-based traditional surgical excision with permanent sections is the least expensive, the study found

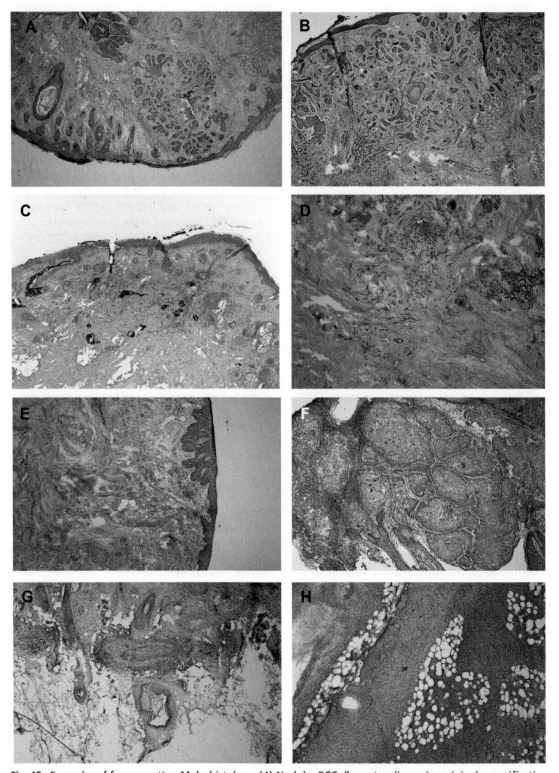

Fig. 12. Examples of frozen section Mohs histology. (*A*) Nodular BCC. (hematoxylin-eosin, original magnification ×4). (*B*) Desmoplastic BCC. (hematoxylin-eosin, original magnification ×4). (*C*) Desmoplastic trichoepithelioma. (hematoxylin-eosin, original magnification ×4). (*D*) Microcystic adnexal carcinoma. (hematoxylin-eosin, original magnification ×10). (*E*) SCC in situ. (hematoxylin-eosin, original magnification ×4). (*F*) SCC, well-differentiated. (hematoxylin-eosin, original magnification ×4). (*G*) SCC with perineural invasion. (hematoxylin-eosin, original magnification ×4). (*H*) Dermatofibrosarcoma protuberans. (hematoxylin-eosin, original magnification ×10).

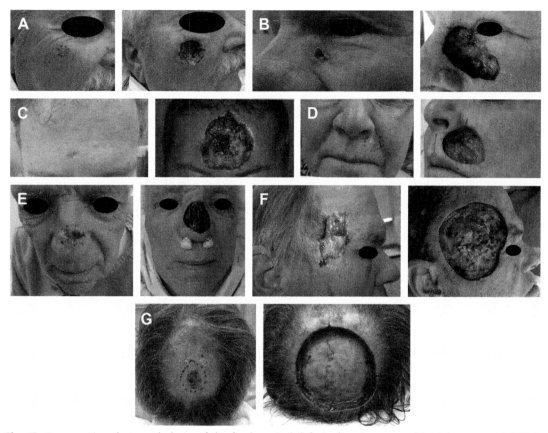

Fig. 13. Preoperative photo and photo of the final surgical defect after clearance with Mohs surgery. (*A*) Right cheek squamous cell carcinoma with perineural invasion. (*B*) Left lower eyelid BCC. (*C*) Forehead dermatofibrosarcoma protuberans. (*D*) Left upper cutaneous lip microcystic adnexal carcinoma. (*E*) Nasal dorsum SCC in a transplant patient. (*F*) Right temple desmoplastic BCC. (*G*) Vertex scalp.

that 32% of cases had surgical margins positive for tumor and needed further treatment, thus resulting in increased costs. Including the cost of retreating the positive surgical margin, MMS is cost comparable. Rogers and Coldiron[91] also found the cost of MMS comparable to office-based surgical excision with permanent sections, noting that procedures in the operating room or radiation treatment were significantly more expensive. Most recently, Ravitskiy and colleagues[92] analyzed 406 tumors and estimated the cost of MMS to be $805 per tumor. This was less expensive than surgical excision with permanent sections or frozen sections and surgical excision in an ambulatory surgical center. MMS is the preferred treatment for many cutaneous tumors, especially certain BCCs[94] and SCCs.[95]

Mohs Surgery for Nonmelanoma Skin Cancer

NMSCs, also known as keratinocyte carcinomas, are the most common malignancies in humans.

The incidence of NMSC in 2012 was more than 5.4 million, with 3.3 million people in the United States receiving treatment.[96] From 2006 to 2012, the incidence of NMSC rose 35% in the Medicare population in the United States.[96] The cost of treating NMSC is estimated at $426 million per year.[97] Surgical treatment, particularly MMS, is the mainstay of treatment for many NMSCs.

BCC comprises most NMSCs. These tumors typically have a slow, indolent clinical course with low risk of metastasis. However BCCs can be locally invasive, causing extensive tissue destruction.[98] MMS results in very high cure rates for primary BCC: 98% to 99% compared with 91% to 95% for non-Mohs modalities.[10,99–101] Recurrent BCC treated with MMS has a 94% to 98% cure rate compared with 80% to 88% for non-Mohs modalities.[99,100,102] MMS is the treatment of choice for high-risk BCC and tumors in locations where tissue conservation is of utmost importance.[94,98] It is particularly clear that MMS has distinct treatment advantages when treating recurrent BCC.[99]

Cutaneous SCC (cSCC) is the second-most common skin cancer in the United States, with an estimated incidence of 186,157 to 419,843.[103] Most cSCCs are low-risk tumors, but high-risk cSCCs have the potential for significant destruction of local tissues, perineural invasion, nodal metastasis, and death.[104] It is estimated that 3932 to 8791 deaths occurred due to cSCC in the United States in 2012, with death rates nearing those of melanoma in the southern and central United States.[103] MMS has superior cure rates for cSCC to non-Mohs treatments, including electrodesiccation and curettage, surgical excision, and radiation therapy, regardless of location, size, histologic findings, prior treatment, and neurotropism.[105] MMS is recommended as the gold standard treatment for high-risk cSCC.[95,104] As more data emerge, there also may be a role for sentinel lymph node biopsy in certain high-risk cSCCs.[106]

A study by Schell and colleagues[107] determined the margins necessary to completely extirpate 95% of NMSCs based on MMS findings. For low-risk BCC and SCC, surgical margins were found to be 4.75 mm and 5.0 mm, respectively. For high-risk BCC and SCC, recommended surgical margins were 8.0 mm and 13.25 mm, respectively. Given that skin biopsies may incompletely sample tumors and that MMS often reveals high-risk features that are not seen on initial biopsy, MMS can help avoid taking unnecessarily large or inadequate surgical margins for NMSC.[107–109]

Mohs Surgery for Melanoma In Situ

The incidence of MIS has continued to rise over the past several decades.[110] Lentigo maligna is a subtype of MIS found on sun-damaged skin, typically on the head and neck of elderly patients, and can have extensive subclinical spread.[111] Although MIS has no significant mortality, patients with MIS are at higher risk to develop a secondary tumor, most commonly invasive melanoma.[110] Lentigo maligna has been found to have a 5% risk of progression to invasive lentigo maligna melanoma.[111] Therefore, adequate treatment of MIS is warranted. Surgical treatment is recommended for MIS when possible and the standard margin for a wide local excision is at least 0.5 cm.[112] Kunishige and colleagues[113] evaluated 1072 patients with 1120 MISs treated with MMS and found a minimum surgical margin of 9 mm was required to remove 98.9% of tumors. Melanoma tumor cells are difficult to visualize on H&E frozen sections. As result, MMS has been used to treat MIS with great success using IHC stains and allows for 100% margin evaluation.[111,113–116] Most Mohs surgeons use the MART-1 IHC stain for MMS for MIS, but other IHC stains used for MMS for MIS include microphthalmia transcription factor (MITF),[117] human melanoma black-45 (HMB-45), and MEL-5.[68,118] Although many of these IHC stains are negative for desmoplastic melanoma, S-100 staining is preferred in such cases.[68] Recurrence rates using MMS for MIS have been reported as ranging from 0% to 10%.[112] Multiple studies document high cure rates of thin melanomas with MMS using IHC staining,[114,116] but the use of MMS for invasive melanoma remains less common.[115] It should be noted that using and interpreting IHC stains requires surgical and histopathologic expertise, as well as meticulous laboratory processing.[112]

Mohs Surgery for Other Head and Neck Cutaneous Tumors

MMS can also be used to treat rare cutaneous tumors. Atypical fibroxanthoma (AFX) is a spindle cell tumor typically arising in sun-damaged skin

Table 1
Mohs micrographic surgery appropriate use criteria

Body areas	Area H	Central face, eyelids, eyebrows, nose, lips, chin, ears, periauricular
		Genitalia (perineal, perianal)
		Nipples/areola, hands, feet, ankles, nail units
	Area M	Cheeks, forehead, scalp, neck, jawline
		Pretibial surface
	Area L	Trunk and extremities (excluding pretibial surface, hands, feet, ankles, nail units)
Patient characteristics	Immunocompromised	Human immunodeficiency virus, organ transplant, hematologic malignancy, pharmacologic immunosuppression
	Genetic syndromes	Basal cell nevus syndrome, xeroderma pigmentosum, other syndromes at high risk for skin cancer
	Healthy	No immunosuppression, prior radiation therapy, chronic infections, or genetic syndromes
	Prior radiated skin	Skin has been treated with therapeutic radiation
	History of high-risk tumors	Patient is known to have a history of aggressive tumors
Tumor characteristics	Positive margin on excision	Tumor involvement at lateral and/or deep margins after excision
	Aggressive features	Basal cell carcinoma (BCC): morpheaform, fibrosing, sclerosing, infiltrating, perineural, metatypical, keratotic, micronodular
		Squamous cell carcinoma: sclerosing, basosquamous (excluding keratotic BCC), small cell, poorly or undifferentiated, perineural, perivascular, spinkle cell, Pagetoid, infiltrating, keratoacanthoma type: central facial, single cell, clear cell, lymphoepithelial, sarcomatoid, Breslow depth 2 mm or greater, Clark level IV or greater

Data from Connolly SM, Baker DR, Coldiron BM, et al. AAD/ACMS/ASDSA/ASMS 2012 appropriate use criteria for Mohs micrographic surgery: a report of the American Academy of Dermatology, American College of Mohs Surgery, American Society for Dermatologic Surgery Association, and the American Society for Mohs Surgery. Dermatol Surg 2012;38(10):1582–603.

on elderly white patients. MMS is the preferred treatment for AFX, with cure rates approaching 100%.[119–121] Pleomorphic dermal sarcoma (PDS) is similar clinically and histologically to AFX, but with deeper extension and more aggressive behavior.[122] PDS has also been termed undifferentiated pleomorphic sarcoma.[122] MMS can also be used for PDS, but due to its deeper invasion and higher risk of metastasis, sentinel lymph node biopsy and multidisciplinary care may be considered as well.[122]

Dermatofibrosarcoma protuberans (DFSP) is an indolent tumor that can have extensive subclinical spread in the skin and soft tissues and potentially high-grade, aggressive fibrosarcomatous change.[123] MMS is reported to have significantly lower recurrence rates for DFSP when compared with wide local excision.[124,125] In a meta-analysis, MMS was found to have a 1% recurrence rate for DFSP and was particularly recommended for tumors of the head and neck,

where recurrence rates are the highest.[121] CD34 immunostaining can be helpful for frozen or permanent section evaluation of DFSP.[68] Merkel cell carcinoma (MCC) is a neuroendocrine tumor, primarily associated with Merkel cell polyoma virus and secondarily by ultraviolet radiation, with significant risk of metastasis and recurrence.[126] Recent retrospective data indicate that MMS may be at least as effective as wide local excision in reducing the risk of local persistence and regional metastasis of disease for MCC, but additional studies are needed to assess the potential role of MMS in treating this high-risk malignancy.[127,128]

MMS is also used for the surgical treatment of adnexal carcinomas.[129] Microcystic adnexal carcinoma is frequently treated with MMS due to considerable local subclinical spread and perineural invasion.[130] Recurrence rates after MMS range from 4.3% to 5.7%,[129–131] whereas wide local excision recurrence rates range from 17% to

60%.[129] Sebaceous carcinoma, both periocular and extraocular, has been successfully treated with MMS.[129] A recent study of 45 sebaceous carcinomas treated with MMS had no recurrence or metastasis after an average follow-up of 3.6 years.[132] The investigators recommend a complete workup to evaluate the risk of Muir-Torre syndrome, including a comprehensive history, up-to-date cancer screening, and immunostaining with MLH1, MSH2, and MSH6.[132] Other adnexal carcinomas treated with MMS include primary cutaneous mucinous carcinoma, trichilemmal carcinoma, hidradenocarcinoma, eccrine porocarcinoma, squamoid eccrine duct tumor, pilomatrix carcinoma, and spiradenocarcinoma.[129]

SUMMARY

MMS is a precise, methodical procedure to treat skin cancer that examines the complete surgical margin and conserves the maximum amount of healthy tissue. Contiguous cutaneous tumors can be accurately tracked with the technique, resulting in the highest cure rates. MMS is the treatment of choice for many tumors, such as BCC, SCC, MIS, and other less common tumors. The Mohs surgeon can be a valuable addition to a multidisciplinary approach to treating cutaneous tumors.

REFERENCES

1. Mohs F. Chemosurgery in cancer, gangrene, and infections. Springfield (IL): Charles C. Thomas; 1956.
2. Mohs FE. Frederic E. Mohs, M.D. J Am Acad Dermatol 1983;9(5):806–14.
3. Mohs FE. Mohs micrographic surgery. A historical perspective. Dermatol Clin 1989;7(4):609–11.
4. Rapini RP. Comparison of methods for checking surgical margins. J Am Acad Dermatol 1990;23(2 Pt 1):288–94.
5. Mohs F. Origin and progress of Mohs micrographic surgery. In: Snow S, Mikhail G, editors. Mohs micrographic surgery. 2nd edition. Madison (WI): University of Wisconsin Press; 2004. p. 3–13.
6. Mohs FE. Chemosurgery in cutaneous malignancy. Calif Med 1949;71(3):173–7.
7. Mohs FE. Chemosurgery: a microscopically controlled method of cancer excision. Arch Surg 1941;42(2):279–95.
8. Mohs FE. Chemosurgical treatment of the face: a microscopically controlled method of excision. Arch Derm Syphilol 1947;56(2):143–56.
9. Stegman SJ, Tromovitch TA. Fresh tissue chemosurgery for tumors of the nose. Eye Ear Nose Throat Mon 1976;55(2):26–30, 32.
10. Robins P. Chemosurgery: my 15 years of experience. J Dermatol Surg Oncol 1981;7(10):779–89.
11. Mohs FE. Chemosurgery for skin cancer: fixed tissue and fresh tissue techniques. Arch Dermatol 1976;112(2):211–5.
12. Tromovitch TA, Stegeman SJ. Microscopically controlled excision of skin tumors. Arch Dermatol 1974;110(2):231–2.
13. Stegman SJ, Tromovitch TA. Modern chemosurgery—microscopically controlled excision. West J Med 1980;132(1):7–12.
14. Brodland DG, Amonette R, Hanke CW, et al. The history and evolution of Mohs micrographic surgery. Dermatol Surg 2000;26(4):303–7.
15. Micrographic surgery and dermatologic oncology. Accreditation Council for Graduate Medical Education 2017-2018. Available at: https://apps.acgme.org/ads/Public/Reports/ReportRun?ReportId=1&CurrentYear=2017&SpecialtyCode=081&IncludePreAccreditation=false. Accessed March 28, 2018.
16. Abide JM, Nahai F, Bennett RG. The meaning of surgical margins. Plast Reconstr Surg 1984;73(3):492–7.
17. Tolkachjov SN, Brodland DG, Coldiron BM, et al. Understanding Mohs micrographic surgery: a review and practical guide for the nondermatologist. Mayo Clin Proc 2017;92(8):1261–71.
18. Sharon VR, Armstrong AW, Jim On SC, et al. Separate- versus same-day preoperative consultation in dermatologic surgery: a patient-centered investigation in an academic practice. Dermatol Surg 2013;39(2):240–7.
19. Knackstedt TJ, Samie FH. Shared medical appointments for the preoperative consultation visit of Mohs micrographic surgery. J Am Acad Dermatol 2015;72(2):340–4.
20. Delaney A, Diamantis S, Marks VJ. Complications of tissue ischemia in dermatologic surgery. Dermatol Ther 2011;24(6):551–7.
21. Wright TI, Baddour LM, Berbari EF, et al. Antibiotic prophylaxis in dermatologic surgery: advisory statement 2008. J Am Acad Dermatol 2008;59(3):464–73.
22. Rosengren H, Dixon A. Antibacterial prophylaxis in dermatologic surgery: an evidence-based review. Am J Clin Dermatol 2010;11(1):35–44.
23. Tønnesen H, Nielsen PR, Lauritzen JB, et al. Smoking and alcohol intervention before surgery: evidence for best practice. Br J Anaesth 2009;102(3):297–306.
24. Goldminz D, Bennett RG. Cigarette smoking and flap and full-thickness graft necrosis. Arch Dermatol 1991;127(7):1012–5.
25. Voutsalath MA, Bichakjian CK, Pelosi F, et al. Electrosurgery and implantable electronic devices: review and implications for office-based procedures. Dermatol Surg 2011;37(7):889–99.
26. Chang LK, Whitaker DC. The impact of herbal medicines on dermatologic surgery. Dermatol Surg 2001;27(8):759–63.

27. Dinehart SM, Henry L. Dietary supplements: altered coagulation and effects on bruising. Dermatol Surg 2005;31(7 Pt 2):819–26 [discussion: 826].

28. Ah-Weng A, Natarajan S, Velangi S, et al. Preoperative monitoring of warfarin in cutaneous surgery. Br J Dermatol 2003;149(2):386–9.

29. Callahan S, Goldsberry A, Kim G, et al. The management of antithrombotic medication in skin surgery. Dermatol Surg 2012;38(9):1417–26.

30. Henley J, Brewer JD. Newer hemostatic agents used in the practice of dermatologic surgery. Dermatol Res Pract 2013;2013:279289.

31. O'Neill JL, Taheri A, Solomon JA, et al. Postoperative hemorrhage risk after outpatient dermatologic surgery procedures. Dermatol Surg 2014;40(1):74–6.

32. Nemeth SA, Lawrence N. Site identification challenges in dermatologic surgery: a physician survey. J Am Acad Dermatol 2012;67(2):262–8.

33. Butler ST, Youker SR, Mandrell J, et al. The importance of reviewing pathology specimens before Mohs surgery. Dermatol Surg 2009;35(3):407–12.

34. Humphreys TR, Shah K, Wysong A, et al. The role of imaging in the management of patients with nonmelanoma skin cancer: when is imaging necessary? J Am Acad Dermatol 2017;76(4):591–607.

35. Wee E, Goh MS, Estall V, et al. Retrospective audit of patients referred for further treatment following Mohs surgery for non-melanoma skin cancer. Australas J Dermatol 2018. [Epub ahead of print].

36. Bunick CG, Aasi SZ. Hemorrhagic complications in dermatologic surgery. Dermatol Ther 2011;24(6):537–50.

37. Ravitskiy L, Phillips PK, Roenigk RK, et al. The use of oral midazolam for perioperative anxiolysis of healthy patients undergoing Mohs surgery: conclusions from randomized controlled and prospective studies. J Am Acad Dermatol 2011;64(2):310–22.

38. Brewer JD, Gonzalez AB, Baum CL, et al. Comparison of sterile vs nonsterile gloves in cutaneous surgery and common outpatient dental procedures: a systematic review and meta-analysis. JAMA Dermatol 2016;152(9):1008–14.

39. Rhinehart MB, Murphy MM, Farley MF, et al. Sterile versus nonsterile gloves during Mohs micrographic surgery: infection rate is not affected. Dermatol Surg 2006;32(2):170–6.

40. Mehta D, Chambers N, Adams B, et al. Comparison of the prevalence of surgical site infection with use of sterile versus nonsterile gloves for resection and reconstruction during Mohs surgery. Dermatol Surg 2014;40(3):234–9.

41. Xia Y, Cho S, Greenway HT, et al. Infection rates of wound repairs during Mohs micrographic surgery using sterile versus nonsterile gloves: a prospective randomized pilot study. Dermatol Surg 2011;37(5):651–6.

42. McGinness JL, Goldstein G. The value of preoperative biopsy-site photography for identifying cutaneous lesions. Dermatol Surg 2010;36(2):194–7.

43. Alam M, Lee A, Ibrahimi OA, et al. A multistep approach to improving biopsy site identification in dermatology: physician, staff, and patient roles based on a Delphi consensus. JAMA Dermatol 2014;150(5):550–8.

44. St John J, Walker J, Goldberg D, et al. Avoiding medical errors in cutaneous site identification: a best practices review. Dermatol Surg 2016;42(4):477–84.

45. Tajirian A, Tsui M. Central forehead reconstruction with a simple primary vertical linear closure. J Clin Aesthet Dermatol 2016;9(8):47–9.

46. Collins LK, Knackstedt TJ, Samie FH. Antiseptic use in Mohs and reconstructive surgery: an American College of Mohs Surgery member survey. Dermatol Surg 2015;41(1):164–6.

47. Kouba DJ, LoPiccolo MC, Alam M, et al. Guidelines for the use of local anesthesia in office-based dermatologic surgery. J Am Acad Dermatol 2016;74(6):1201–19.

48. Alam M, Ricci D, Havey J, et al. Safety of peak serum lidocaine concentration after Mohs micrographic surgery: a prospective cohort study. J Am Acad Dermatol 2010;63(1):87–92.

49. Huang CC, Boyce S, Northington M, et al. Randomized, controlled surgical trial of preoperative tumor curettage of basal cell carcinoma in Mohs micrographic surgery. J Am Acad Dermatol 2004;51(4):585–91.

50. Chung VQ, Bernardo L, Jiang SB. Presurgical curettage appropriately reduces the number of Mohs stages by better delineating the subclinical extensions of tumor margins. Dermatol Surg 2005;31(9 Pt 1):1094–9 [discussion: 1100].

51. Ratner D, Bagiella E. The efficacy of curettage in delineating margins of basal cell carcinoma before Mohs micrographic surgery. Dermatol Surg 2003;29(9):899–903.

52. Singh B, Dorelles A, Konnikov N, et al. Detection of high-risk histologic features and tumor upstaging of nonmelanoma skin cancers on debulk analysis: a quantitative systematic review. Dermatol Surg 2017;43(8):1003–11.

53. Tromovitch TA, Stegman SJ. Microscopic-controlled excision of cutaneous tumors: chemosurgery, fresh tissue technique. Cancer 1978;41(2):653–8.

54. Bouzari N, Olbricht S. Histologic pitfalls in the Mohs technique. Dermatol Clin 2011;29(2):261–72, ix.

55. Li JY, Silapunt S, Migden MR, et al. Mohs mapping fidelity: optimizing orientation, accuracy, and tissue identification in Mohs surgery. Dermatol Surg 2018;44(1):1–9.

56. Mansouri B, Bicknell LM, Hill D, et al. Mohs micrographic surgery for the management of cutaneous malignancies. Facial Plast Surg Clin North Am 2017;25(3):291–301.

57. Ellis JI, Khrom T, Wong A, et al. Mohs math—where the error hides. BMC Dermatol 2006;6:10.

58. Lin BB, Taylor RS. Digital photography for mapping Mohs micrographic surgery sections. Dermatol Surg 2001;27(4):411–4.

59. Alcalay J. Mohs mapping in the cloud: an innovative method for mapping tissue in Mohs surgery. J Drugs Dermatol 2015;14(10):1127–30.

60. Cottel WI, Proper S. Mohs' surgery, fresh-tissue technique. Our technique with a review. J Dermatol Surg Oncol 1982;8(7):576–87.

61. Randle HW, Zitelli J, Brodland DG, et al. Histologic preparation for Mohs micrographic surgery. The single section method. J Dermatol Surg Oncol 1993;19(6):522–4.

62. Ebede TL, Lee EH, Dusza SW, et al. Clinical value of paraffin sections in association with Mohs micrographic surgery for nonmelanoma skin cancers. Dermatol Surg 2012;38(10):1631–8.

63. Benedetto PX, Poblete-Lopez C. Mohs micrographic surgery technique. Dermatol Clin 2011; 29(2):141–51, vii.

64. Cocco C, Melis GV, Ferri GL. Embedding media for cryomicrotomy: an applicative reappraisal. Appl Immunohistochem Mol Morphol 2003;11(3): 274–80.

65. Erickson QL, Clark T, Larson K, et al. Flash freezing of Mohs micrographic surgery tissue can minimize freeze artifact and speed slide preparation. Dermatol Surg 2011;37(4):503–9.

66. Taylor BR, Groover JA, Cook J. Facing the block and false positives in Mohs surgery: a retrospective study of 2,198 cases. Dermatol Surg 2013; 39(11):1662–70.

67. Silapunt S, Peterson SR, Alcalay J, et al. Mohs tissue mapping and processing: a survey study. Dermatol Surg 2004;30:961. United States.

68. El Tal AK, Abrou AE, Stiff MA, et al. Immunostaining in Mohs micrographic surgery: a review. Dermatol Surg 2010;36(3):275–90.

69. Thornton SL, Beck B. Setting up the Mohs surgery laboratory. Dermatol Clin 2011;29(2):331–40, xi.

70. Semkova K, Mallipeddi R, Robson A, et al. Mohs micrographic surgery concordance between Mohs surgeons and dermatopathologists. Dermatol Surg 2013;39(11):1648–52.

71. Mariwalla K, Aasi SZ, Glusac EJ, et al. Mohs micrographic surgery histopathology concordance. J Am Acad Dermatol 2009;60(1):94–8.

72. Gardner ES, Sumner WT, Cook JL. Predictable tissue shrinkage during frozen section histopathologic processing for Mohs micrographic surgery. Dermatol Surg 2001;27(9):813–8.

73. Desciak EB, Maloney ME. Artifacts in frozen section preparation. Dermatol Surg 2000;26(5): 500–4.

74. Alam M, Khan M, Veledar E, et al. Correlation of inflammation in frozen sections with site of nonmelanoma skin cancer. JAMA Dermatol 2016;152(2): 173–6.

75. Macdonald J, Sneath JR, Cowan B, et al. Tumor detection after inflammation or fibrosis on Mohs levels. Dermatol Surg 2013;39(1 Pt 1):64–6.

76. Zabielinski M, Leithauser L, Godsey T, et al. Laboratory errors leading to nonmelanoma skin cancer recurrence after Mohs micrographic surgery. Dermatol Surg 2015;41(8):913–6.

77. Alam M, Shah AD, Ali S, et al. Floaters in Mohs micrographic surgery. Dermatol Surg 2013;39(9): 1317–22.

78. Cartee TV, Monheit GD. How many sections are required to clear a tumor? Results from a web-based survey of margin thresholds in Mohs micrographic surgery. Dermatol Surg 2013;39(2): 179–86.

79. Yu Y, Finn DT. Crescent versus rectangle: is it a true negative margin in second and subsequent stages of Mohs surgery? Dermatol Surg 2010; 36(2):171–6.

80. Alam M, Berg D, Bhatia A, et al. Association between number of stages in Mohs micrographic surgery and surgeon-, patient-, and tumor-specific features: a cross-sectional study of practice patterns of 20 early- and mid-career Mohs surgeons. Dermatol Surg 2010;36(12):1915–20.

81. Alam M, Ibrahim O, Nodzenski M, et al. Adverse events associated with Mohs micrographic surgery: multicenter prospective cohort study of 20,821 cases at 23 centers. JAMA Dermatol 2013;149(12):1378–85.

82. Asgari MM, Olson JM, Alam M. Needs assessment for Mohs micrographic surgery. Dermatol Clin 2012;30(1):167–75, x.

83. Connolly SM, Baker DR, Coldiron BM, et al. AAD/ACMS/ASDSA/ASMS 2012 appropriate use criteria for Mohs micrographic surgery: a report of the American Academy of Dermatology, American College of Mohs Surgery, American Society for Dermatologic Surgery Association, and the American Society for Mohs Surgery. Dermatol Surg 2012;38(10):1582–603.

84. Horner KL, Gasbarre CC. Special considerations for Mohs micrographic surgery on the eyelids, lips, genitalia, and nail unit. Dermatol Clin 2011; 29(2):311–7, x.

85. Holmkvist KA, Roenigk RK. Squamous cell carcinoma of the lip treated with Mohs micrographic surgery: outcome at 5 years. J Am Acad Dermatol 1998;38(6 Pt 1):960–6.

86. Shindel AW, Mann MW, Lev RY, et al. Mohs micrographic surgery for penile cancer: management

and long-term followup. J Urol 2007;178(5): 1980–5.

87. Dika E, Fanti PA, Patrizi A, et al. Mohs surgery for squamous cell carcinoma of the nail unit: 10 years of experience. Dermatol Surg 2015;41(9): 1015–9.

88. Goldminz D, Bennett RG. Mohs micrographic surgery of the nail unit. J Dermatol Surg Oncol 1992; 18(8):721–6.

89. Cook J, Zitelli JA. Mohs micrographic surgery: a cost analysis. J Am Acad Dermatol 1998;39(5 Pt 1):698–703.

90. Bialy TL, Whalen J, Veledar E, et al. Mohs micrographic surgery vs traditional surgical excision: a cost comparison analysis. Arch Dermatol 2004; 140(6):736–42.

91. Rogers HW, Coldiron BM. A relative value unit-based cost comparison of treatment modalities for nonmelanoma skin cancer: effect of the loss of the Mohs multiple surgery reduction exemption. J Am Acad Dermatol 2009;61(1):96–103.

92. Ravitskiy L, Brodland DG, Zitelli JA. Cost analysis: Mohs micrographic surgery. Dermatol Surg 2012; 38(4):585–94.

93. Sebaratnam DF, Choy B, Lee M, et al. Direct cost-analysis of Mohs micrographic surgery and traditional excision for basal cell carcinoma at initial margin clearance. Dermatol Surg 2016;42(5): 633–8.

94. Kim JYS, Kozlow JH, Mittal B, et al. Guidelines of care for the management of basal cell carcinoma. J Am Acad Dermatol 2018;78(3):540–59.

95. Kim JYS, Kozlow JH, Mittal B, et al. Guidelines of care for the management of cutaneous squamous cell carcinoma. J Am Acad Dermatol 2018;78(3): 560–78.

96. Rogers HW, Weinstock MA, Feldman SR, et al. Incidence estimate of nonmelanoma skin cancer (Keratinocyte Carcinomas) in the U.S. population, 2012. JAMA Dermatol 2015;151(10): 1081–6.

97. Chen JG, Fleischer AB Jr, Smith ED, et al. Cost of nonmelanoma skin cancer treatment in the United States. Dermatol Surg 2001;27(12):1035–8.

98. Kauvar AN, Cronin T Jr, Roenigk R, et al. Consensus for nonmelanoma skin cancer treatment: basal cell carcinoma, including a cost analysis of treatment methods. Dermatol Surg 2015; 41(5):550–71.

99. Mosterd K, Krekels GA, Nieman FH, et al. Surgical excision versus Mohs' micrographic surgery for primary and recurrent basal-cell carcinoma of the face: a prospective randomised controlled trial with 5-years' follow-up. Lancet Oncol 2008;9(12): 1149–56.

100. Leibovitch I, Huilgol SC, Selva D, et al. Basal cell carcinoma treated with Mohs surgery in Australia

II. Outcome at 5-year follow-up. J Am Acad Dermatol 2005;53(3):452–7.

101. Rowe DE, Carroll RJ, Day CL Jr. Long-term recurrence rates in previously untreated (primary) basal cell carcinoma: implications for patient follow-up. J Dermatol Surg Oncol 1989;15(3): 315–28.

102. Rowe DE, Carroll RJ, Day CL Jr. Mohs surgery is the treatment of choice for recurrent (previously treated) basal cell carcinoma. J Dermatol Surg Oncol 1989;15(4):424–31.

103. Karia PS, Han J, Schmults CD. Cutaneous squamous cell carcinoma: estimated incidence of disease, nodal metastasis, and deaths from disease in the United States, 2012. J Am Acad Dermatol 2013;68(6):957–66.

104. Kauvar AN, Arpey CJ, Hruza G, et al. Consensus for nonmelanoma skin cancer treatment, part II: squamous cell carcinoma, including a cost analysis of treatment methods. Dermatol Surg 2015; 41(11):1214–40.

105. Rowe DE, Carroll RJ, Day CL. Prognostic factors for local recurrence, metastasis, and survival rates in squamous cell carcinoma of the skin, ear, and lip. Implications for treatment modality selection. J Am Acad Dermatol 1992;26(6): 976–90.

106. Navarrete-Dechent C, Veness MJ, Droppelmann N, et al. High-risk cutaneous squamous cell carcinoma and the emerging role of sentinel lymph node biopsy: a literature review. J Am Acad Dermatol 2015;73(1):127–37.

107. Schell AE, Russell MA, Park SS. Suggested excisional margins for cutaneous malignant lesions based on Mohs micrographic surgery. JAMA Facial Plast Surg 2013;15(5):337–43.

108. Genders RE, Kuizinga MC, Teune TM, et al. Does biopsy accurately assess basal cell carcinoma (BCC) subtype? J Am Acad Dermatol 2016;74(4): 758–60.

109. Izikson L, Seyler M, Zeitouni NC. Prevalence of underdiagnosed aggressive non-melanoma skin cancers treated with Mohs micrographic surgery: analysis of 513 cases. Dermatol Surg 2010; 36(11):1769–72.

110. Higgins HW 2nd, Lee KC, Galan A, et al. Melanoma in situ: part I. Epidemiology, screening, and clinical features. J Am Acad Dermatol 2015;73(2):181–90 [quiz: 191–2].

111. McKenna JK, Florell SR, Goldman GD, et al. Lentigo maligna/lentigo maligna melanoma: current state of diagnosis and treatment. Dermatol Surg 2006;32(4):493–504.

112. Higgins HW 2nd, Lee KC, Galan A, et al. Melanoma in situ: part II. Histopathology, treatment, and clinical management. J Am Acad Dermatol 2015; 73(2):193–203 [quiz: 203–4].

113. Kunishige JH, Brodland DG, Zitelli JA. Surgical margins for melanoma in situ. J Am Acad Dermatol 2012;66(3):438–44.

114. Etzkorn JR, Sobanko JF, Elenitsas R, et al. Low recurrence rates for in situ and invasive melanomas using Mohs micrographic surgery with melanoma antigen recognized by T cells 1 (MART-1) immunostaining: tissue processing methodology to optimize pathologic staging and margin assessment. J Am Acad Dermatol 2015;72(5):840–50.

115. Hui AM, Jacobson M, Markowitz O, et al. Mohs micrographic surgery for the treatment of melanoma. Dermatol Clin 2012;30(3):503–15.

116. Valentin-Nogueras SM, Brodland DG, Zitelli JA, et al. Mohs micrographic surgery using MART-1 immunostain in the treatment of invasive melanoma and melanoma in situ. Dermatol Surg 2016;42(6): 733–44.

117. Christensen KN, Hochwalt PC, Hocker TL, et al. Comparison of MITF and Melan-A immunohistochemistry during Mohs surgery for lentigo maligna-type melanoma in situ and lentigo maligna melanoma. Dermatol Surg 2016;42(2): 167–75.

118. Thosani MK, Marghoob A, Chen CS. Current progress of immunostains in Mohs micrographic surgery: a review. Dermatol Surg 2008;34(12): 1621–36.

119. Seavolt M, McCall M. Atypical fibroxanthoma: review of the literature and summary of 13 patients treated with Mohs micrographic surgery. Dermatol Surg 2006;32(3):435–41 [discussion: 439–41].

120. Ang GC, Roenigk RK, Otley CC, et al. More than 2 decades of treating atypical fibroxanthoma at mayo clinic: what have we learned from 91 patients? Dermatol Surg 2009;35(5):765–72.

121. Love WE, Schmitt AR, Bordeaux JS. Management of unusual cutaneous malignancies: atypical fibroxanthoma, malignant fibrous histiocytoma, sebaceous carcinoma, extramammary Paget disease. Dermatol Clin 2011;29(2): 201–16, viii.

122. Soleymani T, Tyler Hollmig S. Conception and management of a poorly understood spectrum of dermatologic neoplasms: atypical fibroxanthoma, pleomorphic dermal sarcoma, and undifferentiated pleomorphic sarcoma. Curr Treat Options Oncol 2017;18(8):50.

123. Hoesly PM, Lowe GC, Lohse CM, et al. Prognostic impact of fibrosarcomatous transformation in dermatofibrosarcoma protuberans: a cohort study. J Am Acad Dermatol 2015;72(3): 419–25.

124. Buck DW 2nd, Kim JY, Alam M, et al. Multidisciplinary approach to the management of dermatofibrosarcoma protuberans. J Am Acad Dermatol 2012;67(5):861–6.

125. Nelson RA, Arlette JP. Mohs micrographic surgery and dermatofibrosarcoma protuberans: a multidisciplinary approach in 44 patients. Ann Plast Surg 2008;60(6):667–72.

126. Tello TL, Coggshall K, Yom SS, et al. Merkel cell carcinoma: an update and review: current and future therapy. J Am Acad Dermatol 2018;78(3): 445–54.

127. Kline L, Coldiron B. Mohs micrographic surgery for the treatment of Merkel cell carcinoma. Dermatol Surg 2016;42(8):945–51.

128. Singh B, Qureshi MM, Truong MT, et al. Demographics and outcomes of stage I and II Merkel cell carcinoma treated with Mohs micrographic surgery compared with wide local excision in the national cancer database. J Am Acad Dermatol 2018;79(1):126–34.e3.

129. Tolkachjov SN. Adnexal carcinomas treated with Mohs micrographic surgery: a comprehensive review. Dermatol Surg 2017;43(10): 1199–207.

130. Leibovitch I, Huilgol SC, Selva D, et al. Microcystic adnexal carcinoma: treatment with Mohs micrographic surgery. J Am Acad Dermatol 2005;52(2): 295–300.

131. King BJ, Tolkachjov SN, Winchester DS, et al. Demographics and outcomes of microcystic adnexal carcinoma. J Am Acad Dermatol 2018;79(4): 756–8.

132. Brady KL, Hurst EA. Sebaceous carcinoma treated with Mohs micrographic surgery. Dermatol Surg 2017;43(2):281–6.

Management of Early-Stage Melanoma

Maria J. Quintanilla-Dieck, MD[a], Christopher K. Bichakjian, MD[b],*

KEYWORDS

- Melanoma • Melanoma in situ • Lentigo maligna • Sentinel lymph node biopsy

KEY POINTS

- Melanoma incidence continues to rise, particularly among young individuals with early-stage disease.
- Early-stage melanoma has excellent prognosis when appropriately treated.
- The primary treatment for melanoma is surgery.
- Surgical techniques for comprehensive histologic margin control may be considered for lentigo maligna–type melanoma on the head and neck, where subclinical extension can be prominent.
- For invasive melanoma, sentinel lymph node biopsy may be indicated for staging, based on histologic parameters.

INTRODUCTION

Melanoma is one of the most aggressive forms of skin cancer, originating from melanocytes in the basal layer of the epidermis. The incidence of melanoma has doubled in the United States from 1982 to 2011, constituting an important public health concern.[1] In the past decade, the incidence of melanoma has increased by 2.6% annually, more rapidly than any other malignancy. This is largely attributed to a drastic rise in the rate of melanoma in situ, which has increased annually in the United States by 9.5%, particularly among younger individuals (20–49 years of age).[2] According to the American Cancer Society, 178,560 new melanomas will be diagnosed in the United States in 2018, of which 91,270 will be invasive and 87,290 will be noninvasive (in situ). An estimated 9320 people will die of metastatic melanoma in 2018.[3]

Risk factors for melanoma include lighter skin type, male sex, the presence of multiple melanocytic nevi, dysplastic nevi, immunosuppression, a personal or family history of melanoma, and exposure to ultraviolet radiation (UVR). The latter has come to light as the primary risk factor associated with the development of melanoma and is thought to be primarily responsible for the rising incidence. The nature and timing of UVR exposure is thought to influence the development of melanoma.[4,5] Melanomas that develop in areas exposed to intermittent UVR (trunk and limbs) are associated with sunburns acquired during childhood or young adulthood. Melanomas that develop on the head and neck are usually associated with lifelong chronic UVR exposure, and are generally of the lentigo maligna (LM) histologic subtype. Whereas UVR appears to play a significant role in the development of most melanomas, some subtypes, including acral lentiginous and mucosal melanoma, occur independently of UVR exposure.

Although sunlight is the main source of UVR, indoor tanning devices have also been conclusively

Disclosure Statement: No financial interests to disclose.

a Department of Dermatology, University of Michigan Medical School, University of Michigan, 1500 East Medical Center Drive, UH South Room F7679, Ann Arbor, MI 48109-5218, USA; b Department of Dermatology, University of Michigan Medical School, University of Michigan, 1500 East Medical Center Drive, UH South Room F7680, Ann Arbor, MI 48109-5218, USA
* Corresponding author.
E-mail address: chriskb@med.umich.edu

facialplastic.theclinics.com

linked to an increased, dose-dependent risk of melanoma, particularly in women younger than 35.[6,7] Women who have ever used an indoor tanning device are 6 times more likely to be diagnosed with melanoma in their 20s, than those who have never tanned indoors. Ultraviolet tanning devices were reclassified by the Food and Drug Administration from Class I (low risk), to Class II (moderate to high risk) devices in September 2014. In the United States, 15 states plus the District of Columbia now prohibit people younger than 18 from using indoor tanning devices.[8]

STAGING

Accurate staging is crucial to direct treatment recommendations, provide a framework for clinical decision-making, and stratify patients into prognostic categories. The eighth edition American Joint Committee on Cancer melanoma staging system was recently implemented.[9] In this system, stage 0 refers to melanoma in situ (MIS) confined to the epidermis, stages I and II represent invasive, but localized disease, and stages III and IV refer to melanoma with regional nodal or distant metastases, respectively. Early-stage melanoma T classification includes T0 (MIS), T1a (<0.8 mm Breslow depth *without* ulceration), T1b (<0.8 mm *with* ulceration, or 0.8–1.0 mm with or without ulceration), and T2a (>1.0–2.0 mm depth without ulceration).[9]

With appropriate treatment, early-stage melanoma is associated with a very favorable prognosis. Although stage 0 disease generally has no direct associated mortality, occult microinvasion has been identified in as many as one-third of in situ melanomas, which may explain rare metastatic events.[10] Patients with stage I melanoma still have an excellent prognosis, with 5-year and 10-year melanoma-specific survival rates of 98% and 95%, respectively. Stages II and III melanoma are associated with 5-year and 10-year melanoma-specific survival rates of 90% and 84%, and 77% and 69%, respectively.[9] For the purpose of this review, early-stage melanoma is defined as stage 0 and I.

In recent years, major progress has been made in the treatment of patients with metastatic melanoma, specifically the development of targeted immunotherapy, which has significantly improved prognosis for these patients. However, the vast majority of patients are diagnosed with early-stage melanoma. It is projected that nearly half of all new melanoma cases diagnosed in 2018 will be in situ (stage 0) disease. It is therefore crucial to ensure that this large number of patients is treated appropriately, to reduce the risk of local recurrence and potential metastasis, and prevent the need for systemic therapy, ensuring a favorable long-term prognosis.

TREATMENT AND MANAGEMENT

The primary treatment for early-stage melanoma is surgery, which is considered standard of care and provides excellent long-term prognosis. The goal of wider and deeper excision around the primary tumor site is to prevent local recurrence from persistent disease, by complete removal of the tumor with histologically negative margins. For MIS, nonsurgical treatment modalities may be considered for patients who are not surgical candidates or when resection is not reasonable based on patient and/or tumor characteristics.[11]

Melanoma In Situ

The most common subtype of MIS encountered on the head and neck is the LM subtype, which usually occurs on chronically sun-exposed skin of elderly fair-skinned individuals (**Fig. 1**). It is characterized histologically by the presence of atypical melanocytes in the basal layer of the epidermis with a background of solar elastosis. This slow-growing subtype of MIS is estimated to progress to invasive melanoma (ie, LM melanoma [LMM]) in 5% of cases.[12] Although other subtypes of melanoma can develop on the head and neck (eg, superficial spreading, nodular), LM/LMM comprise most melanomas in this anatomic region. LM differs from most other histologic subtypes of melanoma, based on the tendency of the tumor cells to exhibit lentiginous spread, that is, solitary tumor cells (rather than nests) within the epidermis, as well as extension within the epithelium of adnexal

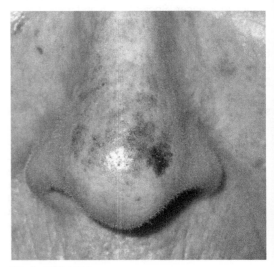

Fig. 1. MIS, LM type.

structures, particularly hair follicles. MIS-LM type is characterized by poorly defined clinical margins, unpredictable subclinical peripheral tumor extension, and adjacent multifocal subclinical disease, which is often asymmetric.[13] Further complicating this issue, the lesion is frequently surrounded by sun-damaged melanocytes (actinic melanocytic hyperplasia), which may be difficult to differentiate histopathologically from MIS-LM.[14]

Surgical treatment
Surgery is the primary treatment modality for MIS, which provides several distinct advantages: (1) permits histopathologic margin assessment to ensure complete removal; (2) allows detection of an unsuspected invasive component, which may significantly alter management; and (3) removes hair follicles and other adnexal structures, where melanocytes and tumor cells may extend. It is important to note, that in cases where a small partial biopsy has been performed of a larger lesion, invasive melanoma may have been missed. On the head and neck, invasive desmoplastic melanoma is known to be associated with MIS-LM. When feasible, narrow excision of most of the remaining lesion is recommended for micro-staging, before proceeding with definitive resection. Appropriate micro-staging may alter management, including an indication of nodal staging by sentinel lymph node biopsy (SLNB).[15]

Several surgical approaches can be used to treat MIS. Standard excision with 0.5-cm margin is considered an adequate approach for most MIS located on the trunk and extremities. For lesions on the head and neck, particularly MIS-LM type, techniques with more exhaustive histologic assessment of peripheral margins may be considered.

In contrast to invasive melanoma, there are limited data and no randomized controlled trials addressing surgical margins for MIS. Based on the best available evidence, the National Comprehensive Cancer Network and the American Academy of Dermatology guidelines of care recommend a 0.5-cm to 1.0-cm margin, recognizing that a 0.5-cm margin is generally associated with low rates of local recurrence for MIS, non-LM type, and for most MIS on the trunk and extremities.[11,16–18] The depth of excision should extend to the deep subcutaneous adipose tissue, due to the frequent extension of tumor cells down the follicular epithelium and the potential for occult invasive melanoma.[10]

For MIS-LM type on the head and neck, it has been demonstrated that surgical margins greater than 0.5 cm are often needed to obtain clear margins.[13,18] A prospective study of 1072 patients with 1120 MIS (without distinction between subtypes) found that a surgical margin of 9 mm removed 98.9% of tumors, whereas a margin of 6 mm removed only 86% of lesions.[19] An earlier study reported that a 1.5-cm margin was needed to excise 97% of 231 LMs and LMMs, respectively, in the head and neck region.[20] Similarly, a retrospective study of 117 patients treated with staged margin-controlled excision with rush paraffin-embedded sections, found that surgical margins of 7.1 mm and 10.3 mm were required to clear LM and LMM, respectively.[21] These findings confirm the subclinical extension frequently associated with MIS, LM type and suggest that wider surgical margins and exhaustive peripheral histologic margin assessment may be warranted.

Histopathologic evaluation of standard excision specimens, which are processed in a "breadloaf" manner, in effect only allow evaluation of approximately 2% of the true peripheral margin. In contrast, various comprehensive margin control techniques have been described for MIS-LM type, which achieve complete histologic evaluation of all peripheral margins. These exhaustive margin control methods include staged excision techniques with paraffin-embedded permanent sections, and Mohs micrographic surgery (MMS), which is performed with the use of intraoperative frozen sections. Both modalities provide the additional benefit of tissue sparing, which is particularly relevant on the head and neck, where MIS-LM type most often arises.

Staged excision techniques have been developed with the goal of achieving total margin control for complete excision of MIS-LM type before reconstruction. They differ from MMS in that all tissue analysis is performed with paraffin-embedded permanent sections. Similar to MMS, all techniques provide visualization of 100% of the peripheral margin with precise mapping in a tissue-sparing manner. There are multiple variations of staged excisions, which have not been studied comparatively. These variations include the "square" procedure, "slow Mohs" (MMS performed with permanent sections), staged radial sections, mapped serial excisions, and staged excisions with radial vertical sections, among others.

The "square" procedure is one such technique, originally described by Johnson and colleagues[22] in 1997. This technique consists of the removal of a thin, 2-mm strip of tissue in a square pattern at an initial 5-mm margin from the central lesion or scar. Subsequent en face paraffin-embedded permanent sections of the surgical margin in a vertical orientation are generated for analysis by a dermatopathologist. Positive areas within the marginal skin are identified, and repeat excisions of 2-

mm strips with additional 5-mm margins around the positive areas are performed (**Fig. 2**). The central lesion remains intact until the margins are negative, after which reconstruction can be planned at the same time as the removal of the central island. A recently published study by Moyer and colleagues[13] investigated the efficacy of staged excision with the square procedure in cutaneous head and neck melanoma with long-term follow-up. In this observational cohort study, 806 patients with head and neck melanoma were followed for a median of 9.3 years following excision of melanoma (LM or LMM) via the square technique. The estimated local recurrence rates were 1.4% and 2.2% at 5 and 10 years, respectively. The mean margin required for clearance of MIS-LM was 9.3 mm and 13.7 mm for LMM. Numerous alternative staged excision techniques have been described, which differ from the "square" procedure in certain technical considerations, but share the mutual goal of achieving exhaustive peripheral margin control with paraffin-embedded permanent sections evaluated by a dermatopathologist. Mahoney and colleagues[23] use a 5-mm initial margin of excision by removing a 2-mm strip specimen in a circumferential configuration, via the use of any of several geometric shapes. Hazan and colleagues[21] combine mapping biopsies with tumor debulking, processed in a vertical "breadloaf" manner for pathologic evaluation.

MMS is a technique traditionally used for nonmelanoma skin cancer. In this procedure, the lesion is initially debulked, then excised with a margin of normal-appearing skin and processed into horizontal frozen sections across the bottom of the specimen. This allows for microscopic evaluation of 100% of the deep and peripheral margins. The slides are reviewed by the Mohs surgeon, who marks any residual tumor on an anatomic map. Subsequently, areas of positivity are reexcised and processed in the same manner, until negative margins are achieved. The accuracy of the interpretation of frozen MMS sections is operator-dependent and relies on both the expertise of the Mohs surgeon, and the quality of the sides. Frozen sections are more susceptible to artifactual change than paraffin-embedded permanent sections, making accurate interpretation potentially more challenging. As previously noted, the distinction between atypical junctional melanocytic hyperplasia in association with LM and benign background actinic melanocytic hyperplasia, is challenging and may be more reliably made with permanent sections. In the literature, false-positive and false-negative rates for frozen section evaluation of melanocytic lesions are close to 20% and 50%, respectively.[24,25] Indeed, paraffin-embedded permanent sections remain the gold standard in the evaluation of melanocytic lesions in general.[24]

Two main variations of MMS have been described to treat MIS, traditional and modified,

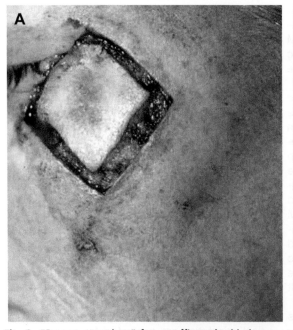 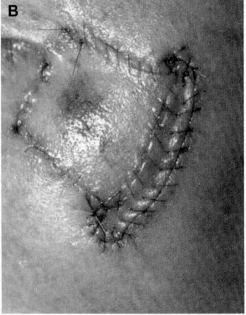

Fig. 2. "Square procedure" for paraffin-embedded permanent section complete peripheral margin control of MIS, LM type. (*A*) Stage 1, before simple repair. (*B*) Stage 2, following removal of additional 5-mm margin for the positivity at the lateral margin, followed by simple repair.

which differ in the design of the excision and the use of either frozen or permanent sections. Modified, or "slow Mohs" consists of MMS with the use of permanent sections. In addition, some Mohs surgeons use immunohistochemical stains, such as melanoma antigen recognized by T-cells 1 (MART-1, or melan-A), which may improve the detection of melanoma cells on frozen sections.[26] Regardless of the particular technique of MMS used in the treatment of melanoma, it is recommended that permanent section analysis of the central debulking specimen be performed to rule out an invasive and possibly desmoplastic component, which would upstage the patient and may alter management. Several recent studies have compared MMS with standard wide local excision (WLE) as a treatment modality for MIS. A retrospective study of 277 patients with MIS treated with MMS and 385 patients treated with standard WLE, showed no significant difference in rates of local recurrence, overall survival, or melanoma-specific survival at a median follow-up of 8.6 years.[27] Other studies, both retrospective and prospective, have shown lower rates of local recurrence for MIS on the face and ears treated with MMS compared with WLE.[28,29] It is important to note that MMS is not recommended for MIS on the trunk or extremities, nor is its use supported in the treatment of invasive melanoma in any anatomic location.

Nonsurgical treatment

Although surgery remains the gold standard of treatment for melanoma, nonsurgical treatment modalities have been studied for MIS, LM type, and may be considered as second-line therapy in patients who are not surgical candidates or when surgery would lead to unacceptable morbidity based on patient and/or tumor characteristics. In MIS, LM type, destructive modalities including liquid nitrogen cryotherapy, electrodesiccation and curettage, laser surgery, radiotherapy, and fluorouracil 5% cream are associated with high recurrence rates of 20% to 100% and are not recommended.[30,31] Imiquimod 5% cream has been used off-label for treatment of MIS, LM type, both as primary and adjuvant therapy, with different regimens and highly variable clearance rates reported in the literature. Imiquimod is a topical immune-response modifier that causes a localized immune reaction at the targeted site. Various studies have shown clearance rates between 37% and 75% when used as primary treatment, and more than 94% in the adjuvant setting after excision with narrowly clear or positive margins. The interpretation of published data is limited by variable designs, application regimens

(frequency of application and treatment duration), and treatment margins between studies. Most studies evaluating imiquimod as either primary or adjuvant therapy for MIS, LM type show lower rates of recurrence when a 2-cm margin of normal-appearing skin is treated for a minimum of 12 weeks with a total of more than 60 applications, and when a significant inflammatory response occurs.[32] No prospective, randomized trials have evaluated the long-term efficacy of imiquimod for treatment of MIS. It should be noted that when considering this option as primary treatment of MIS, LM type, there is a risk of undertreating follicular extension of melanoma or underlying invasive melanoma, especially if the latter has not been ruled out with complete histologic evaluation.[10] Thus, this treatment option should be used cautiously and in a setting where close follow-up is possible, to monitor for recurrence.

Finally, radiation therapy (RT) may be considered as second-line treatment for MIS, LM type when complete surgical removal is not possible. This treatment modality is used more commonly outside the United States. A review of primary RT for MIS, LM type from 2014, which included 9 clinical studies involving 537 patients with a median follow-up of 3 years, demonstrated a 5% recurrence rate, with progression to invasive melanoma in 1.4% of patients. Unfortunately, specific recommendations regarding primary RT for MIS could not be optimally derived from these data due to the lack of standardization in the studies.[33]

Superficially Invasive Melanoma

Sentinel lymph node biopsy

Before determining a treatment plan for invasive melanoma, the potential risk of metastasis must be assessed. SLNB allows accurate staging of patients with invasive melanoma through pathologic assessment of the regional lymph node basin. SLNB is widely considered the most important prognostic factor and staging tool for invasive melanoma, and the strongest predictor of survival.[34] Although the survival benefit of SLNB is unclear, its accuracy as a staging tool is not.[9,35] Despite more complex anatomy and lymphatic drainage pattern, it has been demonstrated that SLNB can be performed on the head and neck with safety and accuracy similar to non–head and neck locations.[36] Sentinel lymph node (SLN) status is a major consideration in the management of patients with melanoma with regard to the need for adjuvant treatment, including surgery and systemic therapy, or enrollment in a clinical trial. Importantly, a meta-analysis of 71 studies with 25,240 patients estimated a risk of ≤5% of regional nodal recurrence following a *negative* SLNB.[37]

Various guidelines have established recommendations for SLNB based on risk[11,16] (**Table 1**). Overall, SLN metastases are infrequent (<5%) in melanomas less than 0.8 mm in thickness, but occur in 5% to 12% of primary melanomas between 0.8 and 1 mm in thickness. Therefore, in patients with (clinical) stage IA melanoma (T1a: <0.8 mm Breslow thickness, nonulcerated), in whom the risk of occult nodal metastasis is less than 5%, SLNB is generally not recommended. When other adverse prognostic features are present, including a high mitotic rate ($\geq 2/mm^2$), young age, lymphovascular invasion, or a combination thereof, the risk of occult nodal disease may be increased and SLNB may be considered.[16] In patients with stage IB, with a T1b tumor (Breslow thickness 0.8–1.0 mm regardless of ulceration status, or <0.8 mm with ulceration), the risk of nodal disease is approximately 5% to 10%, and

guidelines recommend that SLNB be discussed and considered. When Breslow thickness is greater than 1 mm (stage IB with a T2a tumor, or stage II disease), the risk of occult nodal metastasis exceeds 10% and it is recommended that SLNB be discussed and offered. If SLNB is indicated, it is best performed concurrently with excision of the primary tumor. Although it may require more extensive surgery and morbidity, the SLN may still be accurately identified following prior wide excision in select patients[38] (see **Table 1**).

Currently, great interest exists in gene expression profiling tests of the primary tumor as a prognostic tool. However, there are insufficient data at this time to support the use of such tests in routine clinical practice.

Surgical treatment

Treatment of invasive melanoma includes surgical excision with appropriate margins, with or without SLNB, as discussed previously. Current surgical margin recommendations for wide excision of primary cutaneous melanoma, per National Comprehensive Cancer Network Clinical Practice Guidelines for Melanoma, are as follows: 0.5 to 1.0 cm for MIS, 1 cm for invasive melanoma ≤1.0 mm thickness, 1 to 2 cm for melanoma more than 1.0 and less than 2.0 mm thickness, and 2-cm margin for melanoma more than 2.0 mm in thickness.[16] Importantly, surgical margin recommendations are based on clinical measurement at the time of surgery, not gross or pathologic margins measured by the pathologist. Comprehensive peripheral margin control (with staged excision or MMS as described previously) may be considered on the head and neck for residual MIS, following excision of invasive LMM and paraffin-embedded permanent section evaluation of all invasive disease. For all patients with a positive SLN, multidisciplinary consultation is recommended to discuss further management, including additional surgery, adjuvant systemic therapy and/or enrollment in a clinical trial.

FOLLOW-UP

Follow-up of patients with melanoma is recommended to monitor for potential recurrence or any new primary melanomas. For patients with MIS, yearly skin examinations are recommended for life, whereas for those with stage I melanoma, follow-up visits are recommended every 6 to 12 months for 5 years, and yearly thereafter.

Table 1
Indications for sentinel lymph node biopsy (SLNB) for melanoma

Primary Invasive Melanoma	Risk of Positive SLN, %	SLNB Recommendation
T1a melanoma (<0.8 mm without ulceration) without adverse features[a]	<5	Not recommended
T1a melanoma (<0.8 mm without ulceration) with adverse features[a] T1b melanoma (0.8–1.0 mm with or without ulceration, or <0.8 mm with ulceration)	5–10	Discuss and consider
T2a melanoma (>1 mm) melanoma and higher	>10	Discuss and offer

[a] High mitotic rate, young age, lymphovascular invasion, positive deep margin.

Data from NCCN guidelines for patients – Melanoma 2018 – PAT – N – 1027 - 1217. National Comprehensive Cancer Network. Available at: https://www.nccn.org/patients/guidelines/melanoma/files/assets/common/downloads/files/melanoma.pdf. Accessed February 21, 2018.

REFERENCES

1. Guy GP Jr, Thomas CC, Thompson T, et al. Vital signs: melanoma incidence and mortality trends

and projections—United States, 1982-2030. MMWR Morb Mortal Wkly Rep 2015;64:591–6.

2. National Cancer Institute. Surveillance, epidemiology, and end results (SEER) program. Available at: https://seer.cancer.gov/. Accessed March 26, 2018.

3. American Cancer Society Cancer Facts & Figures 2018. Available at: https://www.cancer.org/research/cancer-facts-statistics/all-cancer-facts-figures/cancer-facts-figures-2018.html. Accessed February 21, 2018.

4. Whiteman DC, Whiteman CA, Green AC. Childhood sun exposure as a risk factor for melanoma: a systematic review of epidemiologic studies. Cancer Causes Control 2001;12:69–82.

5. Caini S, Gandini S, Sera F, et al. Meta-analysis of risk factors for cutaneous melanoma according to anatomical site and clinico-pathological variant. Eur J Cancer 2009;45:3054–63.

6. Boniol M, Autier P, Boyle P, et al. Cutaneous melanoma attributable to sunbed use: systematic review and meta-analysis. BMJ 2012;345:e4757.

7. Lazovich D, Isaksson Vogel R, Weinstock MA, et al. Association between indoor tanning and melanoma in younger men and women. JAMA Dermatol 2016; 152:268–75.

8. Indoor tanning restrictions for minors a state-by-state comparison. Available at: http://www.ncsl.org/research/health/indoor-tanning-restrictions.aspx. Accessed March 2, 2018.

9. Gershenwald JE, Scolyer RA, Hess KR, et al. Melanoma staging: evidence-based changes in the American Joint Committee on Cancer eighth edition cancer staging manual. CA Cancer J Clin 2017;67: 472–92.

10. Bax MJ, Johnson TM, Harms PW, et al. Detection of occult invasion in melanoma in situ. JAMA Dermatol 2016;152:1201–8.

11. Bichakjian CK, Halpern AC, Johnson TM, et al. Guidelines of care for the management of primary cutaneous melanoma. American Academy of Dermatology. J Am Acad Dermatol 2011;65: 1032–47.

12. Tannous ZS, Lerner LH, Duncan LM, et al. Progression to invasive melanoma from malignant melanoma in situ, lentigo maligna type. Hum Pathol 2000;31:705–8.

13. Moyer JS, Rudy S, Boonstra PS, et al. Efficacy of staged excision with permanent section margin control for cutaneous head and neck melanoma. JAMA Dermatol 2017;153:282–8.

14. Weyers W, Bonczkowitz M, Weyers I, et al. Melanoma in situ versus melanocytic hyperplasia in sun-damaged skin. Assessment of the significance of histopathologic criteria for differential diagnosis. Am J Dermatopathol 1996;18:560–6.

15. Karimipour DJ, Schwartz JL, Wang TS, et al. Microstaging accuracy after subtotal incisional biopsy of cutaneous melanoma. J Am Acad Dermatol 2005; 52:798–802.

16. National Comprehensive Cancer Network. Available at: https://www.nccn.org/. Accessed February 21, 2018.

17. Tzellos T, Kyrgidis A, Mocellin S, et al. Interventions for melanoma in situ, including lentigo maligna. Cochrane Database Syst Rev 2014;(12): CD010308.

18. Duffy KL, Truong A, Bowen GM, et al. Adequacy of 5-mm surgical excision margins for non-lentiginous melanoma in situ. J Am Acad Dermatol 2014;71: 835–8.

19. Kunishige JH, Brodland DG, Zitelli JA. Surgical margins for melanoma in situ. J Am Acad Dermatol 2012;66:438–44.

20. Zitelli JA, Brown C, Hanusa BH. Mohs micrographic surgery for the treatment of primary cutaneous melanoma. J Am Acad Dermatol 1997;37:236–45.

21. Hazan C, Dusza SW, Delgado R, et al. Staged excision for lentigo maligna and lentigo maligna melanoma: a retrospective analysis of 117 cases. J Am Acad Dermatol 2008;58:142–8.

22. Johnson TM, Headington JT, Baker SR, et al. Usefulness of the staged excision for lentigo maligna and lentigo maligna melanoma: the "square" procedure. J Am Acad Dermatol 1997;37:758–64.

23. Mahoney MH, Joseph M, Temple CL. The perimeter technique for lentigo maligna: an alternative to Mohs micrographic surgery. J Surg Oncol 2005; 91:120–5.

24. Prieto VG, Argenyi ZB, Barnhill RL, et al. Are en face frozen sections accurate for diagnosing margin status in melanocytic lesions? Am J Clin Pathol 2003; 120:203–8.

25. Barlow RJ, White CR, Swanson NA. Mohs' micrographic surgery using frozen sections alone may be unsuitable for detecting single atypical melanocytes at the margins of melanoma in situ. Br J Dermatol 2002;146:290–4.

26. Zalla MJ, Lim KK, Dicaudo DJ, et al. Mohs micrographic excision of melanoma using immunostains. Dermatol Surg 2000;26:771–84.

27. Nosrati A, Berliner JG, Goel S, et al. Outcomes of melanoma in situ treated with Mohs micrographic surgery compared with wide local excision. JAMA Dermatol 2017;153:436–41.

28. Bricca GM, Brodland DG, Ren D, et al. Cutaneous head and neck melanoma treated with Mohs micrographic surgery. J Am Acad Dermatol 2005;52: 92–100.

29. Bene NI, Healy C, Coldiron BM. Mohs micrographic surgery is accurate 95.1% of the time for melanoma in situ: a prospective study of 167 cases. Dermatol Surg 2008;34:660–4.

30. Cohen LM. Lentigo maligna and lentigo maligna melanoma. J Am Acad Dermatol 1997;36:913.

31. Kuflik EG, Gage AA. Cryosurgery for lentigo maligna. J Am Acad Dermatol 1994;31:75–8.

32. Swetter SM, Chen FW, Kim DD, et al. Imiquimod 5% cream as primary or adjuvant therapy for melanoma in situ, lentigo maligna type. J Am Acad Dermatol 2015;72:1047–53.

33. Fogarty GB, Hong A, Scolyer RA, et al. Radiotherapy for lentigo maligna: a literature review and recommendations for treatment. Br J Dermatol 2014;170:52–8.

34. Morton DL, Thompson JF, Cochran AJ, et al. Final trial report of sentinel-node biopsy versus nodal observation in melanoma. N Engl J Med 2014;370:599–609.

35. Faries MB, Thompson JF, Cochran AJ, et al. Completion dissection or observation for sentinel-node metastasis in melanoma. N Engl J Med 2017;376:2211–22.

36. Schmalbach CE, Nussenbaum B, Rees RS, et al. Reliability of sentinel lymph node mapping with biopsy for head and neck cutaneous melanoma. Arch Otolaryngol Head Neck Surg 2003;129:61–5.

37. Valsecchi ME, Silbermins D, de Rosa N, et al. Lymphatic mapping and sentinel lymph node biopsy in patients with melanoma: a meta-analysis. J Clin Oncol 2011;29:1479–87.

38. Gannon CJ, Rousseau DL Jr, Ross MI, et al. Accuracy of lymphatic mapping and sentinel lymph node biopsy after previous wide local excision in patients with primary melanoma. Cancer 2006;107:2647–52.

Reconstruction of the Nose

Andrew W. Joseph, MD, MPH*, Carl Truesdale, MD, Shan R. Baker, MD

KEYWORDS

- Nasal reconstruction • Facial plastic surgery • Head and neck reconstruction • Skin cancer
- Mohs excision

KEY POINTS

- Reconstruction of cutaneous nasal defects has evolved significantly over the past 50 years.
- Modern reconstructive techniques often allow for inconspicuous scars and overall nondeforming surgical results.
- Cutaneous nasal defect reconstruction should be considered within the context of nasal aesthetic subunits.
- Nasal lining, structural framework, and cutaneous covering should be independently considered; reconstruction should address all 3 components when they are involved.

INTRODUCTION

The nose occupies a central portion of the face and plays a functional role in breathing and sense of smell. Furthermore, due to its central location in the face, the aesthetics of a person's nose can profoundly impact the way he or she is perceived by the outside world. Recent research has shown that patients who exhibit a cutaneous deformity in the central portion of their face are much more likely to be perceived as less attractive by lay observers compared with those with facial deformity located elsewhere.[1–4] This finding is important because patients who are perceived negatively as a result of nasal deformity can have increased difficulty interacting with others in social situations or in the workplace.[3]

Nasal reconstruction has a history dating back thousands of years to first descriptions by physicians in India.[5] Since then, many refinements have been made to these early techniques. There are numerous textbooks dedicated to the topic, and the authors direct the interested reader to several of these excellent texts.[6–8] The current focus is to highlight some of the more common techniques used to reconstruct cutaneous defects of the nose. The authors attempt to identify common pitfalls and offer practical suggestions that they have found helpful in their clinical experience.

SURGICAL ANATOMY OF THE NOSE

Surgeons who perform nasal reconstruction should be intimately familiar with the surgical anatomy of the nose. The nose has a rigid bony and cartilaginous structural support system, which is lined on the inner surface by an epithelial layer, and covered on the outer surface by soft tissue. The latter are commonly referred to as the skin and soft tissue envelope (SSTE). The SSTE itself, from superficial to deep, is made up of the skin and 4 additional layers: superficial subcutaneous layer (fatty panniculus), the nasal superficial musculoaponeurotic system (SMAS), a deep fatty layer, and the perichondrium (or periostium), which overlies the structural framework.[9]

Skin

There are substantial variations in skin thickness and sebaceous glands density among the various subunits of the nose (see overview of the subunits

Disclosure Statement: None.
Department of Otolaryngology–Head and Neck Surgery, University of Michigan Medical School, 1904 Taubman Center, Ann Arbor, MI 48109-5312, USA
* Corresponding author.
E-mail address: josephan@umich.edu

Facial Plast Surg Clin N Am 27 (2019) 43–54
https://doi.org/10.1016/j.fsc.2018.08.006
1064-7406/19/© 2018 Elsevier Inc. All rights reserved.

in later discussion). On average, skin is thickest at the radix and supratip area, and thinnest at the rhinion and columella[10,11] (**Fig. 1**). The cephalic half of the nose is composed of smaller and less densely populated sebaceous glands compared with the caudal half.[12] Skin with higher density of sebaceous glands, such as that on the caudal aspect of the nose, tends to be less pliable and more likely to develop trapdoor deformities following surgical procedures. Surgeons should be mindful of these differences when planning local flap reconstructions, because skin recruited from an area of skin with different thickness or density of sebaceous glands may result in a more conspicuous scar.

Subcutaneous Tissues and Superficial Musculoaponeurotic Layer

The superficial subcutaneous layer located just deep to the skin has fibrous connective tissue ligaments that transit the layer and anchor the underlying SMAS to the overlying dermis. The SMAS layer contains the encapsulated facial mimetic muscles of the nose, including the transverse nasalis, anomalous nasi, levator labii superioris alaeque nasi, dilator naris, compressor narium minor, and the depressor septi, and alar nasalis. These muscles were well described more than 70 years ago and serve a role in both facial expression as well as a functional role in preventing collapse of the nasal airway with respiration.[13]

Bony and Cartilaginous Framework

The underlying skeletal support of the nose differs among the upper, middle, and lower thirds of the

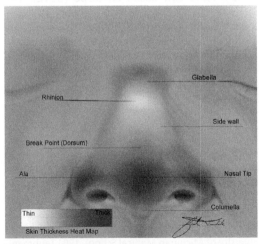

Fig. 1. Average changes in nasal skin thickness by anatomic subunit. In general, nasal skin thickness increases as one proceeds caudally along the nasal sidewalls and dorsum. (*Courtesy of* Carl Truesdale, MD, Ann Arbor, MI.)

nose. The structural support of the upper third of the nose is provided by the paired nasal bones, which articulate with the nasal (ascending) process of the maxilla. The nasal bones are thinner at their caudal aspects and become progressively thicker in the cephalic portions. The middle third and lower third of the nose derive structural support primarily from cartilaginous structures and their fibrous attachments. The structure of the middle third of the nose results from paired upper lateral cartilages, which join the cartilaginous nasal septum at the midline. The lower third of the nose, namely the tip and portions of the nasal alae, receives its support from the lower lateral nasal cartilages and the caudal cartilaginous nasal septum.

Nasal Lining

The lining of the inner surface of the nose changes in its composition depending on the proximity to the nasal vestibule. Within the nasal vestibule, the inner surface of the nose is lined by keratinized stratified squamous epithelium. As one proceeds deeper into the nose, this epithelium transitions into pseudostratified columnar ciliated epithelium (nasal mucosa), which often takes a glistening appearance.

Aesthetic Subunits of the Nose

Early twentieth century approaches to facial reconstruction focused on obliteration of soft tissue defects without attention to whether donor tissue possessed similar qualities. Since then, surgeons have begun to discuss and implement notions of the facial aesthetic subunits.[14] Reconstructions that respect facial aesthetic subunits allow resultant scars to be situated along natural boundaries and to mimic natural shadows or lighted ridges.

The nose was originally considered a single aesthetic subunit of the face, despite an appreciation that there was differing thickness of nasal skin.[14] However, the pioneering work by Burget and Menick[15] recognized the topographic nature of the nose and described the following nasal subunits: nasal tip, dorsum, sidewalls, alar lobules, and soft tissue triangles. Most reconstructive surgeons now also consider the nasal columella to be a separate subunit. There have been several proposed additions or modifications to the original nasal aesthetic subunits, including consideration of the nasal dorsum and nasal tip as one subunit. Others have proposed consideration of the nasal tip as 2 independent hemitip subunits.[16] **Fig. 2** details the currently recognized nasal aesthetic subunits.

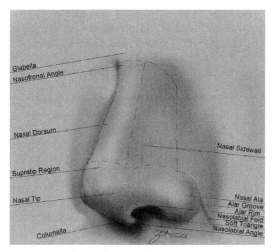

Fig. 2. Nasal aesthetic subunits and important external landmarks. (*Courtesy of* Carl Truesdale, MD, Ann Arbor, MI.)

The subunits differ in skin qualities (texture, thickness, pilosebaceous structures) and underlying structural framework, the latter of which contributes to differing contour. With regard to skin characteristics, the nasal tip, nasal alae, and radix have the thickest skin with more pilosebaceous units. Conversely, the skin of the rhinion, which overlies the osseocartilaginous junction along the dorsum, is usually the thinnest. The upper nasal sidewall skin is thin, which progressively becomes thicker along the more caudal aspect (see **Fig. 1**). Reconstructive surgeons should be mindful of these differences, because recruitment of skin of differing thickness for repair may lead to suboptimal results.

OVERVIEW OF THE MANAGEMENT OF NASAL DEFECTS
Individualized Treatment Planning

Planning of nasal reconstruction is a highly individualized process, and there is a multitude of factors to consider. Patient goals are at the forefront of these considerations. An elderly patient with multiple medical comorbidities may desire the most expeditious reconstruction rather than one requiring a staged procedure. It is imperative to have a frank discussion with patients when discussing multiple treatment options. A photograph book of typical reconstructive results observed with each technique is often helpful to facilitate these discussions.

From a medical perspective, tobacco use is one of the most important risk factors for complications and should play a central role in treatment planning. Beyond anesthesia-related complications, tobacco use has been strongly associated with higher risk for skin graft and local flap failure.[17] In patients who are active smokers or have only recently quit, it may be beneficial to avoid skin grafts when possible. Likewise, in tobacco users who undergo local flap reconstructions, it is advisable to maintain an ample base of the flap and perform minimal thinning of the skin flap. These patients should be counseled about their increased risk for complications.

MANAGEMENT OF DEFECT BY NASAL AESTHETIC SUBUNIT

Defects of the nose may be classified by various characteristics, including size, location, and affected tissues. Although the full gamut of the reconstructive ladder may be used and should be considered, most nasal cutaneous defects can be reconstructed by granulation, full-thickness skin grafts, or a variety of local flaps. However, defects that involve the loss of structural support require significantly more complex reconstructive procedures. In this article, the authors focus on the reconstruction of cutaneous defects by anatomic location.

Nasal Dorsum and Sidewall

The nasal dorsum and nasal sidewall are 2 of the major nasal aesthetic subunits. Because reconstructions of these areas often require similar approaches, the authors discuss them together. The nasal dorsum and the nasal sidewall are often considered the least complicated areas to reconstruct. The dorsal nasal skin is frequently mobile, facilitating recruitment into deficient areas. In contrast to the nasal tip and glabella, the skin of the dorsum and sidewalls is less sebaceous.[18] Reconstruction of caudal nasal dorsum defects is often best accomplished with a paramedian forehead flap (PMFF). Similarly, large nasal sidewall defects are ideally resurfaced with forehead skin. However, numerous reconstructive approaches are available to surgeons, as discussed later.

Primary closure of nasal dorsum and sidewall defects
Small cutaneous defects (<1 cm) of the caudal third of the dorsum and sidewall may in some situations be repaired with local advancement flaps and primary closure. For nasal dorsum defects, a fusiform closure may be oriented in the transverse or vertical (craniocaudal) dimension, which is in part related to the size and shape of the cutaneous defect. Vertically oriented closures are generally reserved for defects in the midline or along the

dorsum-sidewall junction (**Fig. 3**). Transverse primary closures are well suited for defects situated in the supratip area. However, it should be noted that primary transverse closure of even small defects can result in nasal tip rotation (sometimes desirable in the elderly patient with senile nasal tip ptosis). In cases whereby a patient has a significant bony or cartilaginous dorsal convexity, reduction of the dorsal hump can be performed simultaneously to facilitate closure, by lessening wound closure tension.

Transposition flaps

A variety of simple transposition flaps may be used in reconstruction of nasal dorsum and cephalic nasal sidewall defects. Use of these flaps is limited in areas with thicker sebaceous skin (nasal tip, nasal ala), due to limited mobility of these tissues and propensity to form a trapdoor deformity.

The note flap, so named because it takes the shape of a musical eighth note, is a transposition flap commonly used for reconstruction of dorsum and sidewall defects that are round and less than 1.5 cm in diameter.[19] The donor site for this flap is designed by drawing a tangent to the defect that is 1.5 times the defect diameter, while a second line is drawn from the end of the tangent line at an angle of 50° to 60° to form a triangular flap (**Fig. 4**). After performing skin incisions for the flap, wide undermining of the nasal skin in the subfascial plane is necessary to facilitate transposition of tissue and limit tension on closure. The donor site is closed first, and the triangular flap is then fixated into position. It is often necessary to trim or deepithelialize the distal end of the triangular flap so that it fits properly into the circular defect. A standing cone is next excised at the base of the defect.

The Z-plasty is another transposition flap that can be useful in nasal reconstruction. These flaps can be designed to transpose skin in a horizontal fashion in order to close midline defects.

Dorsal nasal flap

The dorsal nasal flap may also be used to reconstruct nasal dorsum or upper lateral sidewall defects that are up to 2.5 cm in size. Defects reconstructed using this flap are ideally situated within the middle and lower third of the nose. The dorsal nasal flap recruits skin from the glabella, and the secondary defect is closed in a V-to-Y fashion. The dorsal nasal flap design is

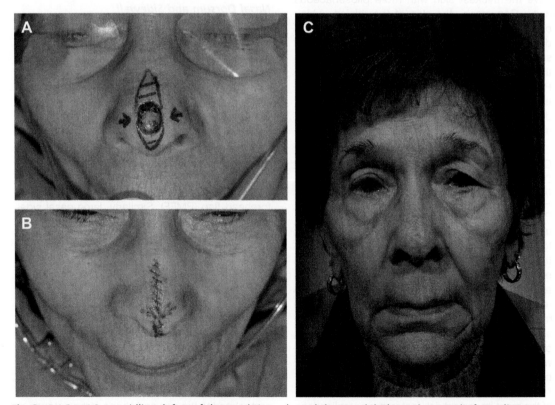

Fig. 3. A 1.2 × 1.0-cm midline defect of the nasal tip and nasal dorsum. (*A*) Planned removal of standing cutaneous deformities and bilateral cutaneous advancement flaps. (*B*) Completed closure of defect. (*C*) Two-month postoperative result.

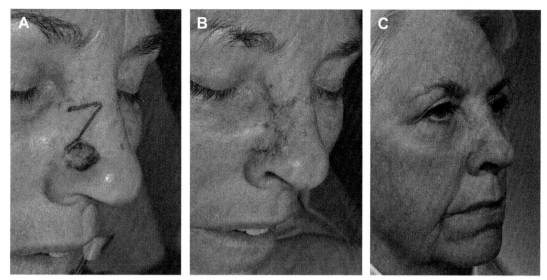

Fig. 4. A 1.2 × 1.2-cm defect of the right lower nasal sidewall and nasal ala. (*A*) Design of "note flap" used for closure. (*B*) Completed closure of defect. (*C*) One-year postoperative result.

begun by drawing a triangularly shaped flap over the glabella, and a line is extended from the base of one side of the triangle along the sidewall-cheek junction until it reaches the site of the defect. For smaller defects of the dorsum (<2 cm), the lateral incision for the flap may be designed along the dorsum-sidewall junction. After injection of local anesthetic, incisions are made around the planned periphery of the flap. The glabella is underlined in the subcutaneous plane while the nasal skin is undermined in the subfascial plane. The flap is rotated and advanced into position, and the secondary defect is closed in a V-to-Y fashion. The last step is removal of the standing cutaneous deformity from the skin adjacent to the defect.

When the dorsal nasal flap is used for nasal reconstruction, thick sebaceous skin of the glabella is advanced onto the normally thin skin of the dorsum or sidewalls (**Fig. 5**). Unfortunately, this often results in a postoperative mismatch in skin thickness and contour irregularity. Given the abundance of other reconstructive options that allow for better aesthetic outcomes, this flap is not often favored by the authors.

Skin grafting

In select patients, full-thickness skin grafts may be used to repair cutaneous defects of the nasal dorsum and nasal sidewalls. Although local flap reconstructions are generally favored over skin grafts, the latter can be useful in patients with significant medical comorbidities, superficial defects, and large defects in patients who do not wish to undergo a PMFF. Skin grafts often have

suboptimal outcomes in patients with thicker sebaceous skin or darker complexion. Conversely, patients with thin atrophic skin and solar damage are generally better candidates for skin grafting because the grafts tend to blend better in these situations. Donor site scars resulting from harvest of preauricular, postauricular, supraclavicular, and pretrichial skin grafts can be well hidden. The donor skin harvested from these areas is well suited for reconstruction of nasal defects.

Dermabrasion can serve as an invaluable technique for improving the ultimate outcome in patients with full-thickness skin grafts as well as in cases whereby a smooth transition is desired between local flap and surrounding native tissue. In these cases, dermabrasion with medium-grit drywall sandpaper, bovie scratch pad, or a powered rotatory dermabrader can help smoothen areas with uneven texture or subtle irregularities in contour, as well as those with color mismatch. When necessary, dermabrasion is generally performed 2 to 3 months after a skin graft or local flap procedure, although it may be performed as soon as 6 weeks after the initial surgery.

Nasal Tip Reconstruction

The reconstruction of nasal tip defects can be challenging due to the convexity of this subunit. Burget and Menick[15] has advocated that for cases in which a defect comprises greater than 50% of a convex nasal aesthetic subunit (the nasal ala and the nasal tip), the remaining portion of the subunit should also be excised and resurfaced with the original defect.[15] In these cases, because the

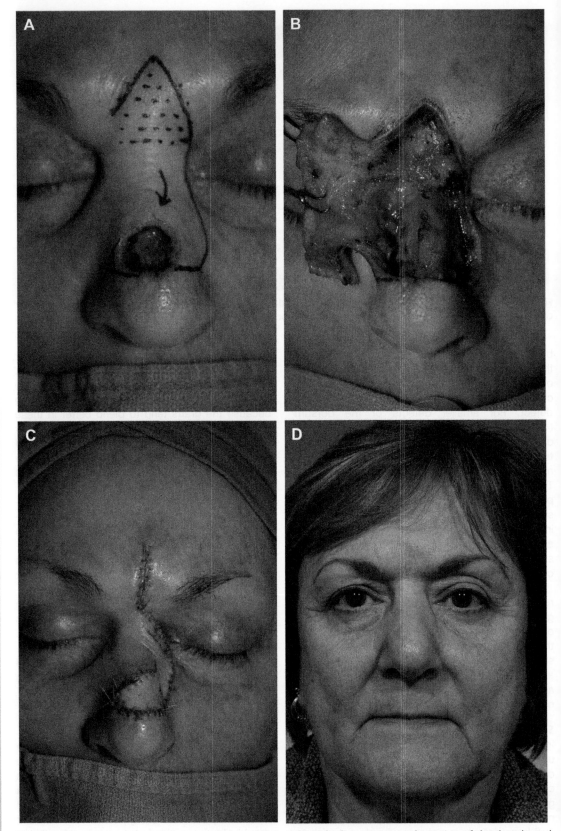

Fig. 5. A 1.5 × 1.2-cm defect of the nasal dorsum. (*A*) Anticipated advancement and rotation of the dorsal nasal flap. (*B*) Wide undermining is performed in the subfascial plane. (*C*) Completed closure of defect. (*D*) Postoperative result 7 months following glabellar flap and 2 months following dermabrasion.

scars are situated at the periphery of the subunit, slight wound contraction does not result in an unfavorable aesthetic outcome, because it contributes to natural convexity within the subunit.

There are several reconstructive approaches that may be considered and are discussed later. The final reconstruction plan should be determined based on patient preference as well as individual patient factors.

Nasal bilobe flap

The bilobe flap is a local flap that is oftentimes considered a workhorse for nasal defect reconstruction. Generally, the bilobe flap is selected for defects that are less than or equal to 1.5 cm in size, although this can vary somewhat depending on the quantity of nasal skin available for recruitment.

The modification of the bilobe flap as described by Zitelli[20] is the most common modern technique used for reconstruction of nasal defects. With the Zitelli technique, the angle formed between the axis of the primary defect and the axis of the secondary lobe is approximately 90°, which results in a smaller standing cutaneous cone when compared with the classic design.[20] The base of the bilobe flap may be positioned either laterally or medially depending on the reconstructive need.

The surgical technique begins with measuring the radius of the defect.[8] A point is then marked with a fine skin pen near the alar groove approximately one radius from the periphery of the defect. This point forms the axis of rotation. Alternatively, the flap may be designed as a medially based

bilobe flap (**Fig. 6**). Next, a suture is passed full thickness from the alar vestibular mucosa through the external skin at the previously marked point. The suture is then used to precisely draw greater and lesser arcs from the far periphery and the center of the defect, respectively. The distance between the lesser and greater arcs is rechecked using a caliper, which should be equal to the radius. Attention is next focused on marking the primary and secondary lobes of the flap. The primary lobe width is equal to the diameter of the defect, whereas the secondary lobe is generally slightly smaller. The primary and secondary lobes may be drawn with either squared or curved edges. The primary lobe height fits within the greater and lesser arcs, whereas the secondary lobe extends to be approximately twice this height. The axis of the primary and secondary lobes of the flap should form an approximately 45° angle. The axis of the secondary lobe and the center of the defect should form an approximately 90° angle. A standing cutaneous cone may be anticipated along the base of the defect.

Local anesthetic is infiltrated into the entire nasal soft tissue envelope. After performing the skin incisions along the previously outlined flap, wide undermining of the flap is performed deep to the nasal musculoaponeurotic layer, superficial to the perichondrium of the nasal cartilages and the periosteum of the nasal bones. Because the area of the greatest tension is along the secondary lobe, the secondary defect is first closed with a 5-0 monofilament absorbable deep dermal suture. The primary lobe is next transposed into position

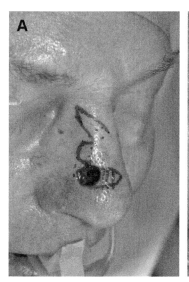 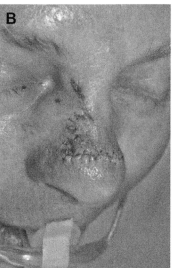 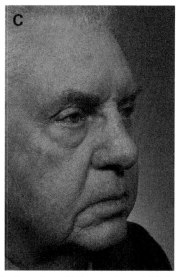

Fig. 6. A 1.2 × 1.3-cm defect of the right nasal tip and lower sidewall. (*A*) Design of medially based nasal bilobe flap. (*B*) Completed closure of defect. (*C*) Postoperative result 5 months following bilobe flap and 2 months following dermabrasion.

and fixated into position with 1 or 2 deep dermal sutures. The skin closure is next accomplished with a combination of vertical mattress sutures and simple interrupted sutures. The standing cutaneous cone is addressed last and excised with close attention to the position of the ipsilateral nasal ala, which can be easily distorted.

Paramedian forehead flap

The PMFF is commonly used for reconstruction of large nasal tip defects, nasal dorsum or sidewall defects, nasal ala defects, or defects that involve multiple subunits (**Fig. 7**). The PMFF is designed based on the supratrochlear artery and vein, which emerge from the orbit near the median brow, at a point that is approximately 2.0 cm lateral from the midline.[7] Some investigators may choose to locate the vascular pedicle with the aid of a Doppler probe, although this is not required.

The surgical technique of reconstruction with the PMFF begins first with preparation of the flap recipient site. The margins of the defect may be converted from curvilinear to a squarer configuration to reduce a trapdoor deformity. If a nasal tip defect encompasses greater than 50% of the surface area of the subunit, the remaining nasal tip skin is generally excised as well. When a defect involves less than 50% of the nasal tip surface area and is situated on one side of midline, heminasal reconstruction may be considered with excision of the remaining half of the nasal tip skin.[7,16]

After the defect is prepared, an exact template of the defect is made using flexible material such as foam or nonabsorbent dressing material. Once the template is created, it is transposed onto the forehead ipsilateral to the side where most of the nasal defect is situated. The template is centered along a line drawn vertically through the medial brow (2 cm from midline) and positioned with the distal aspect of the flap drawn just anterior to the start of the hairline. A skin pen is used to outline the template on the forehead skin. In order to confirm adequate length of the pedicle, a free suture tie is extended from the medial brow to the distal aspect of the template and then rotated to the furthest portion of the nasal tip defect. If the pedicle is suspected to be too short, the template may be moved further into the hair-bearing skin of the scalp, or the pedicle itself may be extended slightly inferior to the brow. After the template is marked, the anticipated pedicle position is marked as an extension from the inferior aspect of the outlined template. The pedicle should be approximately 15 mm wide, which allows for sufficient arterial and venous flow, as well as appropriate movement along the pedicle.

The entire forehead is infiltrated with local anesthetic. Next, the margins of the flap are incised beginning at the distal aspect of the flap. Incisions are carried down to the subfascial plane while preserving the frontal bone pericranium. The flap may be rapidly elevated from superior to inferior in the subfascial plane until the level of the corrugator supercilii. It is often necessary to divide the corrugator muscle in order to achieve sufficient release. Care must be taken to avoid injury to the vascular pedicle inferior to the level of the brow, and any skin incisions should not be carried into the subcutaneous tissue at this level. After elevation of the forehead flap, the adjacent forehead tissue is undermined in the subfascial plane and the donor site is closed in a layered fashion for small to medium-sized defects. Standing cutaneous cones are removed, often with their extension into the hair-bearing scalp. Large secondary forehead defects are not always able to be completely closed, but these defects often heal well with secondary intention. Defects that are left to heal by secondary intention can be further addressed with scar revision at a later time.

After closure of the forehead site, the forehead flap is very carefully thinned of galea along the distal aspect that is intended for inset. Care is taken to preserve the subdermal vascular plexus, which provides perfusion to this portion of the flap.[7] It is important to note that in patients who are active smokers, thinning of the flap should be very conservative or deferred until a subsequent stage. After the flap has been thinned, it is rotated toward the midline into position. The flap is fixated into position along the distal aspect with a series of vertical mattress skin sutures. Deep dermal sutures are generally not used. A running absorbable suture may be used along the periphery to meticulously approximate the wound edges. Pedicle division is performed approximately 3 weeks after the first stage surgery. The procedure for pedicle division is outlined elsewhere.[7]

Full-thickness skin graft

Full-thickness skin grafts are commonly used for nasal tip reconstruction in patients with large defects when the patient does not wish to undergo the PMFF. In contrast to skin grafts for defects of the nasal sidewall and dorsum, skin grafts used for nasal tip defects are thinned minimally because the native nasal tip skin is much thicker.

Nasal Ala

Reconstruction of the nasal ala is complex. Cicatricial forces can result from even small defects in the nasal ala, which may cause both functional sequelae (nasal obstruction) as well as alar notching. These sequelae likely result from the fact that

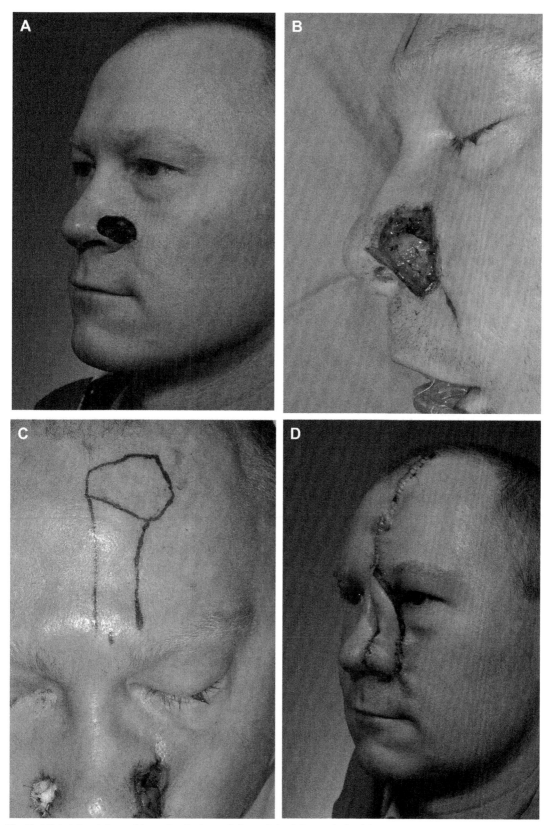

Fig. 7. (*A*) A 1.9 × 1.4-cm skin and soft tissue defect of the left nasal ala. (*B*) Auricular cartilage graft is used for structural support. (*C*) Anticipated design of left PMFF. (*D*) One week following inset of left PMFF.

the lateral nasal ala is predominantly comprised of fibrofatty tissue without any rigid structural support. In order to avoid these suboptimal outcomes, reinforcing the structural support of the lateral nasal ala through the use of cartilage grafting is often necessary when defects approach within 5 mm of the margin. Cartilage framework grafts taken from the concha cavum (often contralateral) and concha cymba are generally preferred due to their desirable contour, ease of harvest, and relative lack of donor site morbidity.

For nasal ala defects, the best outcomes are often observed after the entire subunit is reconstructed. It should be noted that it is advantageous to preserve a 1- to 2-mm strip of skin situated along the alar-facial junction. Preservation of this strip of tissue at the alar-facial junction avoids the difficult reconstruction of this aesthetic boundary, because this area often forms depressed scar tissue when disturbed.

For most patients, the reconstructive method of choice for large deep skin defects limited to the nasal ala without significant extension to the nasal tip or nasal sidewall is an interpolated melolabial flap. However, it should be noted that younger patients without deepened nasolabial folds will typically have a better result with a PMFF. Although superiorly based transposition flaps situated along nose-cheek junction are easy to perform and may also be used, they have the distinct disadvantage of causing effacement to the supra-alar groove, an important aesthetic landmark. Therefore, the authors find transposition flaps to be less than ideal for reconstruction of the nasal ala.

Interpolated melolabial flaps

The interpolated melolabial flap may be designed with either a cutaneous pedical or a subcutaneous island pedicle. Each has distinct advantages and disadvantages. The cutaneous interpolated melolabial flap is a peninsular flap with a superiorly based pedicle. The flap is designed such that the skin recruited for the flap originates from the cutaneous tissue adjacent to the melolabial fold. The advantage to the cutaneous pedicle design is the relative ease of harvest, because the flap is raised in a similar fashion as other cutaneous flaps based on the skin pedicle. Furthermore, this flap avoids blunting of the alar groove that can occur with transposition flaps used in this area. Nonetheless, a noteworthy disadvantage to this approach is that a greater amount of the medial cheek skin abutting the melolabial crease is disturbed, which can result in potential effacement of the melolabial fold when the cutaneous pedicle is ultimately excised.

The approach generally favored by the authors is to design the melolabial flap as a subcutaneous pedicled island flap. In this technique, a template of the alar defect is created from the contralateral nasal ala. The template is then reversed and transposed onto the medial cheek skin lateral to the melolabial crease, just superior to the position of the oral commissure. The outline of the template is drawn such that it is incorporated into a crescentic-shaped skin flap, with the superior aspect tapering to a point near the alar-facial junction, while the inferior portion can taper into the labiomandibular crease (**Fig. 8**). Following flap design, planned incisions are made with a scalpel,

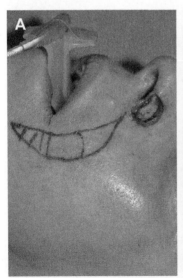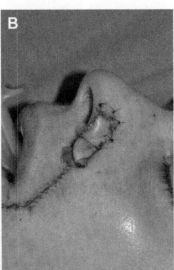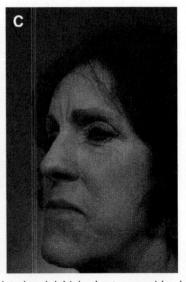

Fig. 8. A 1.3 × 1.4-cm defect of the left nasal ala. (*A*) Design of interpolated melolabial subcutaneous island pedicle flap. Note auricular cartilage graft that has already been placed into position. (*B*) Completed inset of flap. (*C*) Three months postoperative result following debulking procedure.

and the distal portion of the flap is elevated, leaving only 1 to 2 mm of subcutaneous tissue on the flap. As the dissection proceeds superiorly, greater subcutaneous tissue is preserved on the flap and a deeper plane of dissection is required to sufficiently free the subcutaneous pedicle from the zygomaticus muscles. Gentle blunt dissection is used to free the tissue surrounding the pedicle from adjacent attachments. After the pedicle is sufficiently freed, the flap is rotated toward the midline and into position such that the inferior portion of the flap becomes the medial portion of the reconstructed ala, while the lateral portion of the flap becomes the caudal margin of the reconstructed ala. Vertical mattress and simple interrupted skin sutures are used to fixate the interpolated flap into position. Division of the subcutaneous pedicle of the flap is performed approximately 3 weeks after the initial procedure. It is often advantageous to counsel patients that a third procedure for contouring may be required 2 to 3 months after pedicle division.

Nasal Lining Defects

Defects in the nasal mucosal lining should be reconstructed separately from the framework and cutaneous defects of the nose. Numerous nasal mucosal reconstructive techniques have been described.

The reconstructive surgeon is most commonly faced with the challenge of reconstructing nasal ala lining defects. One of the simplest lining flaps is a bipedicled vestibular skin advancement based medially on the septum and laterally from the nasal floor. This flap may be used for lining defects of the ala that are smaller than 1 cm in a craniocaudal dimension. After measuring the dimensions of the defect, local anesthetic with epinephrine is used to hydrodissect the vestibular skin from its attachments. A transverse incision is then made through the vestibular skin near where an intercartilaginous incision would be placed for rhinoplasty. Sharp scissors are used to meticulously dissect the vestibular skin flap free from deep attachments. The bipedicled flap is then advanced caudally and suture-fixated into position. The secondary defect created from advancement of the nasal vestibular skin may be reconstructed with a full-thickness skin graft (which is often harvested from standing cutaneous deformities when performed in conjunction with an interpolated flap), a composite chondrocutaneous graft taken from the ear, or with a separate septal mucoperichondrial flap.[21]

For alar lining defects greater than 1 cm in size, the nasal septal mucoperichondrial hinge flap is a frequently used technique. With this procedure,

parallel mucoperichondrial incisions are made in a longitudinal manner along the nasal septum, 1.5 cm inferior to the dorsum and parallel to the nasal floor. A posterior vertical incision joins the longitudinal incisions, and the mucoperichondrial flap is elevated in a subperichondrial plane from posterior to anterior. During elevation, care is taken to preserve attachment of the flap to the caudal 1 cm of the septum in order to maintain vascularity from the septal branch of the superior labial artery. Following elevation, the flap is then reflected into the vestibular lining defect and suture-fixated into position. The pedicle of the flap may be divided 3 weeks later, whereas the secondary septal mucosal defect may be left to remucosalize on its own.

It should be noted that the vascularity of the above flaps may be especially tenuous in active smokers. In these situations, the surgeon should consider additional techniques, including chondromucosal pivotal flaps, prelaminated PMFFs, and folded or extended PMFFs.[6,7] The folded PMFF is a commonly used technique, and the procedure involves 3 principal stages.[22] In the first stage, a lining flap is designed adjacent to the distal portion of the PMFF. During inset of the flap, the distal lining portion of the flap is inset into the lining defect of the ala and the flap is then folded back upon itself.[22] During an intermediate stage performed 3 weeks after the initial surgery, the distal forehead flap is incised at the folded junction between the vestibular lining and the ala margin. The forehead flap is then tinned, any necessary structural cartilage grafts positioned into the defect, and the flap is reinset to resurface the remaining cutaneous defect. In a final stage, the pedicle is divided 3 weeks after the intermediate stage. The folded PMFF can allow for excellent functional and aesthetic outcomes. However, the technique does necessitate patients' willingness to allow the forehead flap pedicle to remain in place for 6 weeks.

SUMMARY

Nasal reconstruction is a challenging endeavor. Reconstructive techniques that have been refined over the past 50 years now allow patients to experience excellent outcomes in most cases. Modern nasal reconstruction relies heavily on the nasal subunit principle, and the reconstructive surgeon must consider differences in tissue qualities across these subunits when formulating reconstructive plans. Structural or internal lining defects require more complex reconstruction, often mandating a variety of approaches including cartilage or bone grafting, as well as nasal septal or turbinate flaps.

REFERENCES

1. Dey JK, Ishii M, Boahene KDO, et al. Impact of facial defect reconstruction on attractiveness and negative facial perception. Laryngoscope 2015. https://doi.org/10.1002/lary.25130.

2. Godoy A, Ishii M, Dey J, et al. Facial lesions negatively impact affect display. Otolaryngol Head Neck Surg 2013;149(3):377–83.

3. Godoy A, Ishii M, Byrne PJ, et al. How facial lesions impact attractiveness and perception: differential effects of size and location. Laryngoscope 2011; 121(12):2542–7.

4. Roxbury C, Ishii M, Godoy A, et al. Impact of crooked nose rhinoplasty on observer perceptions of attractiveness. Laryngoscope 2012;122(4):773–8.

5. Sorta-Bilajac I, Muzur A. The nose between ethics and aesthetics: sushruta's legacy. Otolaryngol Head Neck Surg 2007;137(5):707–10.

6. Menick FJ. Nasal reconstruction art and practice. Edinburgh (Scotland): Mosby/Elsevier; 2009. Available at: https://www.clinicalkey.com/dura/browse/bookChapter/3-s2.0-C20090375169. Accessed March 17, 2018.

7. Baker SR. SpringerLink (Online service). Principles of nasal reconstruction. New York: Springer Science+Business Media, LLC; 2011. Available at: https://doi.org/10.1007/978-0-387-89028-9. Accessed February 5, 2018.

8. Baker SR. Local flaps in facial reconstruction. Philadelphia: Elsevier/Saunders; 2014. Available at: https://www.clinicalkey.com/dura/browse/bookChapter/3-s2.0-C20120004012. Accessed February 5, 2018.

9. Oneal RM, Beil RJ, Schlesinger J. Surgical anatomy of the nose. Clin Plast Surg 1996;23(2):195–222.

10. Cho GS, Kim JH, Yeo N-K, et al. Nasal skin thickness measured using computed tomography and its effect on tip surgery outcomes. Otolaryngol Head Neck Surg 2011;144(4):522–7.

11. Lessard M-L, Daniel RK. Surgical anatomy of septorhinoplasty. Arch Otolaryngol 1985;111(1):25–9.

12. Michelson LN, Peck GC, Kuo H-R, et al. The quantification and distribution of nasal sebaceous glands using image analysis. Aesthetic Plast Surg 1996; 20(4):303–9.

13. Griesman B. Muscles and cartilages of the nose from the standpoint of a typical rhinoplasty. Arch Otolaryngol 1944;39(4):334–41.

14. Gonzalez-Ulloa M, Castillo A, Stevens E, et al. Preliminary study of the total restoration of the facial skin. Plast Reconstr Surg (1946) 1954;13(3):151–61.

15. Burget GC, Menick FJ. The subunit principle in nasal reconstruction. Plast Reconstr Surg 1985;76(2): 239–47.

16. Noel W, Duron JB, Jabbour S, et al. Should we consider the hemi-tip as a proper aesthetic subunit in a nasal reconstruction? J Plast Reconstr Aesthet Surg 2017;70(8):1112–7.

17. Goldminz D, Bennett RG. Cigarette smoking and flap and full-thickness graft necrosis. Arch Dermatol 1991;127(7):1012–5.

18. Burget GC. Modification of the subunit principle. Arch Facial Plast Surg 1999;1(1):16–8.

19. Walike JW, Larrabee WF. The "note flap". Arch Otolaryngol 1985;111(7):430–3.

20. Zitelli JA. The bilobed flap for nasal reconstruction. Arch Dermatol 1989;125(7):957.

21. Burget GC, Menick FJ. Nasal support and lining: the marriage of beauty and blood supply. Plast Reconstr Surg 1989;84(2):189–202.

22. Menick FJ. A new modified method for nasal lining: the Menick technique for folded lining. J Surg Oncol 2006;94(6):509–14.

Reconstruction of the Cheek

Nathan D. Cass, MD, Adam M. Terella, MD*

KEYWORDS

- Cheek reconstruction • Cheek rotation advancement flap • Cervicofacial flap
- Facial plastic surgery

KEY POINTS

- The cheek possesses unique characteristics that lend advantages and challenges to the reconstruction of defects.
- Achieving normality of the cheek requires attention to symmetry, contour, color, and texture.
- A well-planned cheek reconstruction takes into account many factors: orientation of relaxed skin tension lines, lines of maximum extensibility, surface contour, subcutaneous anatomy, patient age, comorbidities, prior surgery or radiation, wound size, depth, and location relative to central face subunits.

INTRODUCTION

The cheek possesses unique characteristics that lend advantages and challenges to the reconstruction of defects. The cheek is a peripheral facial unit,[1] and primary gaze is more often drawn to the central facial units—eyes, nose, and lips. As such, its normal role is as a "backdrop" for these central facial units, framing and supporting those more intricate features.

Achieving normality of the cheek requires attention to symmetry, contour, color, and texture.

A well-planned cheek reconstruction takes into account many factors: orientation of relaxed skin tension lines (RSTLs), lines of maximum extensibility (LME), surface contour, subcutaneous anatomy, patient age, comorbidities, prior surgery or radiation, wound size, depth, and location relative to central face subunits.

As the largest aesthetic facial unit, the cheek's substantial surface area as well as its smooth and slightly convex contour can create significant difficulty in camouflaging incisions and irregularities. The cheek has relatively few shadows and depressions in which to hide incisions. Also, because the cheek is highly involved in expressing emotion, dynamic facial movement often further highlights deficits.

Anatomy of the Cheek

The cheek can be divided into 4 anatomic subunits—medial, lateral, zygomatic, and buccal[2,3] (Fig. 1). Laterally and inferiorly, the cheek abuts the preauricular crease, temporal hairline, and inferior border of the mandible. Aesthetically sensitive central facial subunits mark its superior and medial boundaries: the lower eyelid, nasal sidewall and ala, nasolabial fold, and the lip and oral commissure. Ideally, any closure or flap is placed at these peripheral boundaries to optimize scar camouflage.

The cheek is composed of epidermis, dermis, and a relatively thick subcutaneous layer. The superficial musculoaponeurotic system (SMAS) sits deep to subcutaneous fat and is continuous with the platysma inferiorly and the temporoparietal fascia superiorly. The SMAS overlies the parotid

Disclosure Statement: The authors have no conflicts of interest to disclose.
Department of Otolaryngology, University of Colorado School of Medicine, 12631 East 17th Avenue, B205, Aurora, CO 80045–2527, USA
* Corresponding author.
E-mail address: adam.terella@ucdenver.edu

facialplastic.theclinics.com

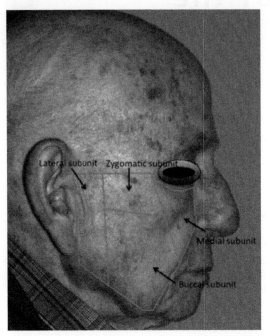

Fig. 1. The cheek aesthetic unit is commonly divided into 4 subunits—medial, lateral, zygomatic, and buccal. These subunits correspond to soft tissue and underlying bony anatomy.

gland, facial mimetic musculature, and the facial nerve. Anterior to the parotid, branches of the facial nerve become closely related to the deep layer of the SMAS; thus, dissection deep to this layer requires care to prevent facial nerve injury.

The retaining ligaments of the face are strong and fibrous attachments that originate from the periosteum and travel through facial layers to insert into the dermis. Pertinent to cheek reconstruction are the zygomatic and masseteric retaining ligaments[4]; release of these structures in the subcutaneous plane should improve tissue mobility.

The cheek derives its vascular supply from the infraorbital artery, transverse facial artery, and the facial artery's terminal branch, the angular artery. Most cheek reconstructions use random flaps that are perfused through the subdermal plexus.

Patient Characteristics

In most cases, an intact contralateral cheek will be available for comparison and as a reconstructive goal. Skin quality, mobility, and laxity should be given special attention, because this plays a major role in determining reconstructive options—elastic or lax skin may allow more local tissue advancement and limit distortion of surrounding facial

structure, whereas thick, tight, scarred, or irradiated skin may limit the surgeon to larger or more distant flaps.

Comorbid conditions that have been shown to impact local and regional flap outcomes include cardiac and vascular comorbidities, systemic comorbidities such as diabetes mellitus, active tobacco consumption, and immunosuppression.[5] These factors must be taken into consideration when choosing an appropriate reconstructive technique and while counseling patients on the challenges of the reconstruction.

Defect Analysis

The size, shape, and subunit location of the defect should be considered. Reconstructive options vary by subunit based on the availability of adjacent tissue, and proximity to central facial units (lower eyelid, nasal sidewall or ala, lip or commissure). A common clinical scenario is a "composite defect" involving cheek and adjacent critical central facial units. A composite defect certainly constitutes a more difficult reconstruction than those confined to the cheek and are discussed later in further detail. Briefly, these "composite defects" are best conceptualized as 2 defects, that is, a cheek defect and a nose defect, or a cheek defect and an eyelid defect.

Wound depth is also important to gauge. Ideally, the reconstruction restores an appropriate tissue mass and volume to the defect. Random flaps have a minimum thickness and must include the subdermal plexus that travels superficially in the subcutaneous tissue. In the case of a very superficial defect, the wound may require deepening instead of the flap being further thinned. Similarly, deep defects will require a thick flap.

When evaluating a defect, it is important to see not only the defect but also ways in which the defect can be strategically changed—one must see not only what is missing, but also what could be additionally removed en route to the most functional and aesthetically pleasing reconstruction.

Finally, the defect's cause should be taken into account—specifically, whether ongoing surveillance of the wound bed is necessary. As reconstructive surgeons, it is critical to apply oncologically sound principles and to devise treatment plans that make allowance for future cancer care needs.

Donor Site Analysis

Potential donor sites should be assessed for color, thickness, and quality match with the defect site. Skin of the cheek is not as sebaceous as nose, but more than that of neck, which can pose challenges in creating a seamless transition between donor and native skin. Color differential may also be present if the patient is light-skinned but tans, as the native cheek skin may be darker than neck or jawline. Finally, skin and subcutaneous fat of the neck are often thinner than that of the cheek, occasionally creating a depth mismatch for large cervicofacial flaps.

RECONSTRUCTION TECHNIQUES
Small Defects

Secondary intention
Healing by secondary intention is the lowest rung on the reconstructive ladder, but has limited utility on the cheek. Small defects, especially in concave areas, may heal quite nicely by secondary intention. On convex surfaces such as the central expanse of the cheek, this option is rarely favorable and will lead to an unaesthetic scar. One exception is the preauricular area, where even relatively large defects can be left to granulate with acceptable cosmesis. The nasofacial groove is also an appropriate location in which to hide wounds healed by secondary intention due to its concave surface and the smooth transition between the lateral nasal wall and the medial border of the cheek. This technique should be avoided in proximity to the lower eyelid because scar contracture will often lead to ectropion. In general, a wound healing by secondary intention should be kept moist with ointment, to promote healing of the wound from deep to superficial. The goal is to prevent drying and crust formation by providing a semiocclusive environment. If crusts form, they can be softened with 3% hydrogen peroxide. Petrolatum ointment is applied to the wound surface and then covered with a semiocclusive dressing; this should be repeated daily until the wound has healed.

Primary closure (fusiform, M-plasty)
Because of significant elasticity and laxity inherent to cheek skin, as well as extensive subcutaneous fatty tissue and a lack of deep bony support, even moderately large wounds of the cheek can be nicely repaired by primary closure. The overall quality, elasticity, and thickness of the skin dictate the size of defect that may be closed in an individual patient. Elderly patients with excess or lax skin may tolerate primary closure of defects up to 4 cm.

Whenever possible, the closure should be placed in peripheral subunit borders of the cheek or in RSTLs. Medially, repairs often parallel the nasofacial sulcus or melolabial fold. Laterally, repairs more ideally follow RSTLs. Long, linear repairs of the cheek are ideally oriented coursing superomedial to inferolateral, which parallel both the melolabial fold and RSTLs[6] (**Fig. 2**). Adequate undermining of the skin and subcutaneous tissue is essential for obtaining a tension-free closure.

Converting a circular or irregular defect into a fusiform shape with equal angles of 30° helps facilitate primary closure and minimizes the standing cone deformity. In larger defects, and those crossing prominent convexity, a lazy S-shaped closure produces a more favorable scar.

Last, adding an M-plasty can help shorten the scar produced from a standard fusiform defect. In this way it can be useful to prevent an incision from extending across an aesthetic subunit.

FLAPS BY CHEEK REGION

Clearly, no one method of reconstruction is ideal for all defects, and the unique characteristics intrinsic to each patient and defect must be weighed. However, there are reconstructive techniques that better lend themselves to a specific aesthetic subunit of the cheek. The authors

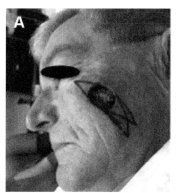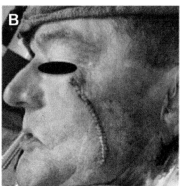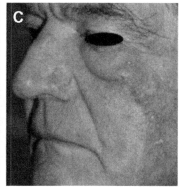

Fig. 2. (*A*) A 2 × 2-cm skin defect of the buccal/zygomatic aesthetic subunit. Fusiform excision planned parallel to RSTLs. (*B*) Wound closed primarily. (*C*) 3 months postoperatively. Scar approximates RSTL. No revision surgery performed. (*Courtesy of* Mariah Brown, MD, Aurora, CO.)

discuss various techniques available and highlight those that have been most commonly used by the authors (**Table 1**); it is not their intention to provide a comprehensive list of all available reconstructive options.

Medial Defects

The medial cheek aesthetic subunit borders the medial canthus and lower eyelid superiorly, the nasofacial groove medially, and the melolabial fold inferomedially. Whenever possible, medial cheek repair should use the melolabial fold, and to a lesser extent the nasofacial groove, as a means for incision camouflage. Hiding incisions within the nasofacial groove may be advantageous when a defect does not cross into the lateral nasal sidewall. However, for the common clinical scenario in which the defect involves the cheek and lateral nasal sidewall, it is important to recognize that this transition is usually a very smooth and gradual transition. Furthermore, the sebaceous quality of medial cheek skin closely mirrors that of the lateral nasal sidewall. Although this is a departure from the subunit principle, the authors will often consider a cheek advancement flap to resurface the medial cheek in continuity with a lateral nasal sidewall defect.

Small and medium-sized wounds, vertically oriented in the medial cheek, can most often be closed in a linear fashion via primary closure technique, using the significant skin laxity in the region and using techniques discussed earlier. If a linear closure would result in undue tension on the lower eyelid or upper lip, the authors prefer to use a cheek rotation-advancement flap, or a laterally based cervicofacial rotation-advancement flap.

The cheek rotation-advancement flap is a workhorse for medium-sized medial cheek defects. Classically, it has an inferomedial base and is rotated anteriorly, and/or superiorly. The flap is designed horizontally and laterally from the medial defect, extending across the inferior orbital rim, curving gently above the zygomatic arch and just above the lateral canthus. In this way, the resultant scars are at the borders of aesthetic subunits (**Fig. 3**). A standing cone of tissue is anticipated and excised within the melolabial crease. The degree of rotation versus advancement largely depends on the specific defect. **Fig. 3**A, B uses a significant rotation component, whereas **Fig. 3**C, D uses a greater advancement component.

Preventing lower eyelid retraction and ectropion is paramount. In the case of medium-sized medial defects, combining the following techniques is usually adequate. First, the horizontal incision (and thus the flap) must be brought *above* the level of the lateral canthus, allowing the flap to support rather than weigh down the lower eyelid (**Fig. 4**). Second, supporting sutures should be placed from the flap to the periosteum of the inferior orbital rim. Together, these maneuvers will ensure stable suspension of the soft tissue and prevent ectropion.

For larger defects of the medial cheek, which may encompass the medial, buccal, and/or zygomatic cheek subunits, the cheek rotation advancement flap can be extended into a classic cervicofacial rotation-advancement flap. Similar to the cheek rotation advancement flap, the incision follows the infraorbital rim, then gently swings above the level of the lateral canthus, proceeds down the temporal hairline and then into the preauricular crease. The incision is then continued around the lobule and posteriorly

Table 1
Cheek reconstruction considerations

| Location | Defect Size | | |
	Small	Medium	Large
Lateral	Primary closure	Interiorly based advancement flap postauricular Transposition or bilobed flap	Cervicofacial rotation advancement flap
Medial	Primary closure	Primary closure Cheek rotation advancement flap	Cervicofacial rotation advancement flap
Buccal	Primary closure	Transposition flap Bilobed flap Island pedicle flap	Large bilobed flap Cheek rotation advancement flap
Zygomatic	Primary closure	Transposition flaps	Cheek rotation- advancement flap Cervicofacial rotation advancement flap

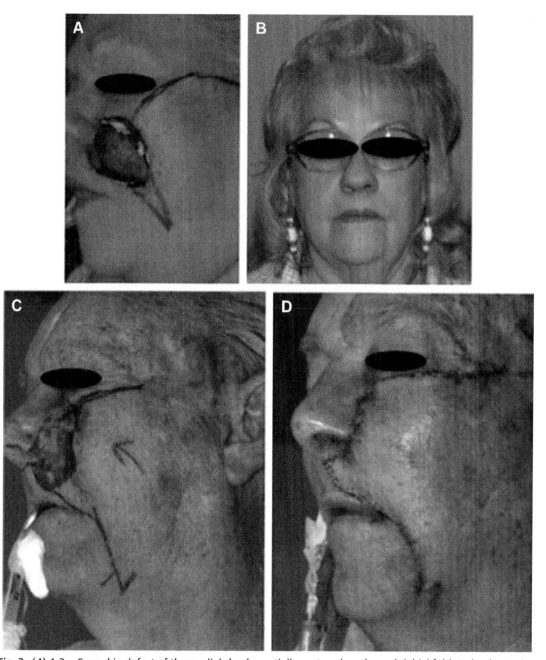

Fig. 3. (*A*) A 3 × 5-cm skin defect of the medial cheek, partially centered on the melolabial fold. A cheek rotation advancement flap is planned. Standing cone deformity excised at time of primary surgery. (*B*) 6 months postoperatively. Medial component of scar camouflaged within melolabial crease. (*C, D*) A 3 × 4.5-cm skin defect of medial cheek and lateral upper lip. Cheek advancement flap planned. Where possible, incisions are placed at borders of cheek aesthetic subunits.

behind the ear, along the lateral inferior hairline. The inferior extent of the flap is placed in a transverse cervical crease and may be thought of a "back-cut" of sorts; as it is carried progressively anteriorly, the flap's superior advancement is increased. Inferior extension may end in the neck or, depending on defect size, may extend over the clavicle into the pectoral region (**Fig. 5**). An inferomedial standing cone within the melolabial fold is expected and can be excised at the time of surgery or, if vascular compromise is of concern, in a delayed fashion.

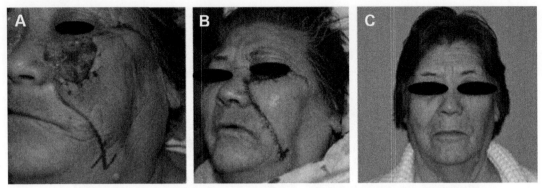

Fig. 4. (*A*) A 4 × 3-cm defect of the medial cheek. Cheek advancement flap planned. Lateral incision extending above the lateral commissure and medial incision within the melolabial fold. (*B*) Z-plasty designed at base of flap to improve mobility and prevent need for Burow triangle excision. Supporting sutures used to prevent ectropion (*C*) 3 months postoperatively.

Generally, cheek rotation-advancement and cervicofacial flaps are dissected in a subcutaneous, supra-SMAS plane in the face. However, for larger flaps, a sub-SMAS dissection can be used lateral to the zygomaticus major and inferior to the zygomatic arch. For flaps extending into the neck, transitioning to a subplatysmal plane inferior to marginal mandibular nerve may further improve blood flow to the flap. As these flaps cross the infraorbital region, incisions can be placed in a subciliary crease or at the infraorbital rim in the lower lid crease. The authors prefer to decrease

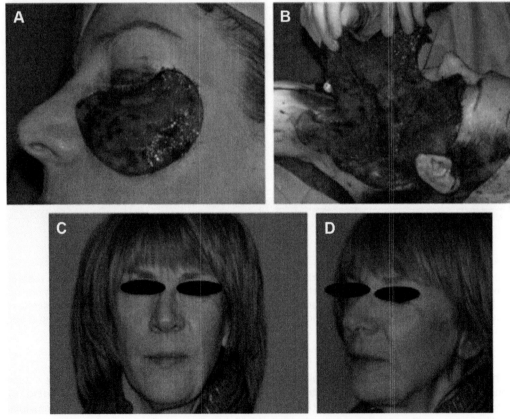

Fig. 5. (*A*) Large superficial defect involving medial and zygomatic aesthetic subunits. (*B*) Cervicofacial flap reconstruction with subplatysmal dissection in the neck. Full thickness skin graft to lower eyelid anterior lamella defect. (*C, D*) 6 months after delayed excision of standing cone deformity.

the risk of ectropion by avoiding disruption of pretarsal skin and placing incisions in the lower lid crease, although it should be noted that this might produce prolonged lower eyelid lymphedema.

As previously discussed, flaps approaching the lower eyelid should be secured to the periosteum of the infraorbital rim to ensure stable suspension of the soft tissue and prevent ectropion. In patients with significant lower lid laxity and mobility, a concomitant canthopexy can be completed to further mitigate the risk of lower eyelid ectropion.

Lateral Defects

The lateral cheek aesthetic subunit borders the tragus and lobule of the ear posteriorly, temporal hairline superiorly, and the mandibular margin or jawline inferiorly. The lateral cheek unit is less prominent than the medial portions, so irregularities draw viewer gaze less frequently. The preauricular crease hides incisions very well. When possible, small and medium-sized defects in this region are closed in vertical linear fashion and ideally within the preauricular crease. Even in young adults, lateral neck skin is often lax and may be widely undermined in order to facilitate an inferiorly based advancement flap. Removal of Burow triangle inferior to the ear lobule facilitates the superior advancement.

The postauricular transposition flap is useful for defects that are very lateral on the cheek, just anterior to the tragus. An inferiorly based postauricular transposition flap is created by placing incisions in the postauricular sulcus and along the lateral posterior hairline. The flap is elevated off the mastoid fascia and transposed to the preauricular defect.[7] For slightly more anterior defects, a bilobed flap can be used to borrow tissue from the posterior portion of the cheekneck border, when the laxity is abundant, as seen in **Fig. 6**.

For defects greater than 3 cm, a cervicofacial rotation advancement flap as previously described is most useful.

Zygomatic Defects

Reconstruction of defects in the zygomatic cheek is influenced by several anatomic factors. Close proximity to the lateral lower eyelid and periorbital region creates an intrinsic risk of lower eyelid retraction; this risk, however, is low, because most local flaps used in zygomatic reconstruction create a lateral force vector *parallel* to the lower eyelid. The temporal branch of the facial nerve traverses the mid portion of the zygoma, as a single branch or up to as many as 4 branches, within the temporoparietal fascia[8]; its superficial course renders it prone to injury. This subunit has underlying bony support from the zygoma and malar process of the maxilla. Last, the zygomaticocutaneous suspensory ligaments can limit tissue mobility.

For small defects up to 1 cm, primary wound closure should be oriented parallel to the crow's feet wrinkles. Transposition flaps, such as the rhombic flap, are very useful for reconstructing medium-sized defects in this region. The flap design is well described by others.[9–11] In brief, RSTLs are identified, allowing for identification of LMEs that run perpendicular to RSTLs. The LMEs adjacent to the defect serve as parallel sides of the rhombus. The remaining 2 sides are marked so as to create angles approximating 60° and 120°. Next, a diagonal, bisecting a 120° angle, is extended a distance equal to the length of the side of the rhombus. The final limb is planned parallel to the LME and of equal length (**Fig. 7**).[9]

Using the above technique, 2 potential flap configurations can result; the "ideal" configuration orients tension vectors that minimize lower eyelid and upper lip distortion. The greatest wound tension is at the donor site, and the greatest tension vector runs parallel to the defect border adjacent to the flap.[10]

Similar to medial and lateral cheek defects, zygomatic defects may also be reconstructed with a cheek rotation-advancement flap, according to principles enumerated earlier (**Fig. 8**).

Buccal Defects

The buccal portion of the cheek constitutes the largest subunit. Primary closure parallel to RSTLs is preferred for defects up to 2 to 3 cm, depending on tissue laxity. Transposition flaps, such as the previously discuss rhombic flap, are also popular in this location; however, scars resulting from transposition flaps never completely fall within RSTLs. Cervical skin laxity lends itself nicely to low buccal defect reconstruction. A bilobed flap, with design similar to that used on the nose, efficiently achieves this closure. The advantage of the bilobed flap is its ability to recruit laxity from significant distance, and having a tension vector perpendicular to the closure[6] (**Fig. 9**). Last, cheek rotation-advancement flaps can be used, applying principles similar to those discussed in medial cheek reconstruction. However, in this location, incisions will by necessity often cross directly through subunits.

Island pedicle advancement flaps can have limited utility in buccal defects. The abundant

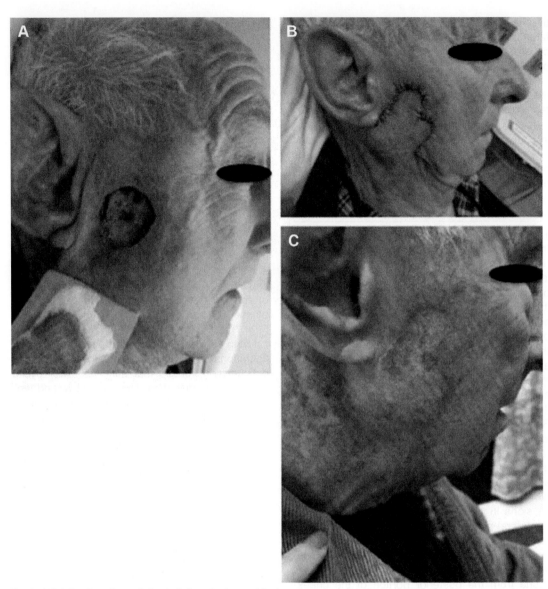

Fig. 6. (*A*) A 3 × 3-cm lateral cheek defect. Patient with abundant neck skin laxity. (*B*) Bilobed flap used to borrow tissue from posterior cheek and superior neck. (*C*) 3 month postoperatively. (*Courtesy of* Mariah Brown, MD, Aurora, CO.)

subcutaneous fat in the medial buccal region enables the mobilization of a hearty subcutaneous pedicle, and thus efficient flap mobility. The resulting triangular scar can be somewhat unaesthetic, and significant pin cushioning can occur.

For low buccal defects or "composite" buccal/upper lip defects, when jowl and upper neck laxity are sufficient, an inferiorly based island pedicle advancement flap centered in the prejowl sulcus can be a reasonable choice. In **Fig. 10**, this flap was combined with a contralateral lip advancement to reconstruct the defect.

Complex "Composite" Subunit Defects

As has been discussed earlier, one hallmark of a well-planned cheek reconstruction is avoidance of distortion of aesthetically sensitive subunits. Commonly, a cheek defect will cross peripheral subunit borders and involve the lower eyelid, nose, or lip. In this situation, it is generally best to avoid crossing this peripheral border with a single flap, and more optimal to use 2 flaps. Such is the case when reconstructing a nose and cheek defect, or a cheek and eyelid defect. Using one flap for the nose and another flap for the cheek helps reestablish the boundaries between cheek

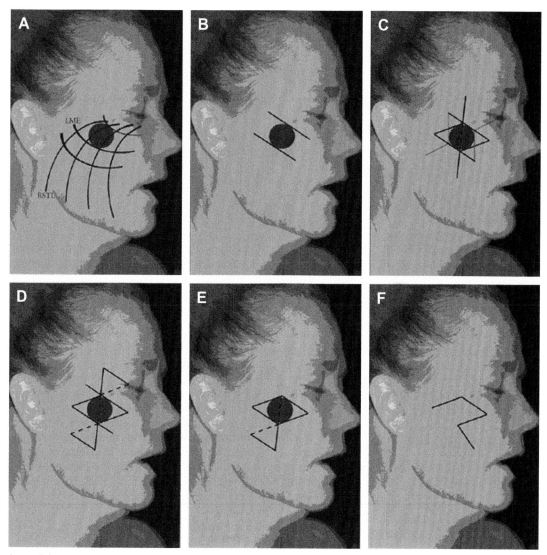

Fig. 7. (*A*) Proper orientation of RSTL and LME in the cheek, running perpendicular to each other. (*B*) The first 2 limbs of the rhombic are drawn parallel to LME. (*C*) Two possible rhombi are able to be drawn. The rhombus that maximizes the tissue distance between the defect and eye is chosen. (*D*) Again, 2 Limberg flaps are possible for each rhombus drawn, and the flap that would minimize secondary tissue movement in proximity to the eye is chosen. (*E*) Final design of Limberg flap. (*F*) Final appearance of suture lines after excision of the skin within the rhombus, transposition of the flap, and closure of both primary and secondary defects. (*From* Furr M, Wang T. Complex local flap design in cheek reconstruction. Oper Tech Otolaryngol Head Neck Surg 2011;22:53–8.)

and nose (**Fig. 11**). The surgeon should not attempt to simply fill the defect or patch the hole. It is far better to reconstruct each aesthetic subunit individually.

TECHNIQUE HIGHLIGHTS
Delayed Excision of a Standing Cone

Rotation advancement flaps result in a standing cutaneous deformity at the inferior aspect of the leading flap edge. These standing cones can be excised at the time of primary reconstruction; however, for flaps with concern for ischemia (due to size, tension, or comorbidities such as smoking) the standing cone is left in place. At approximately 2 weeks, when flap perfusion has improved and the risk of ischemia is reduced, the standing cone is easily excised (**Fig. 12**).

Supporting Sutures

Cheek flaps in proximity to the lower eyelid or alar facial sulcus benefit from supporting sutures

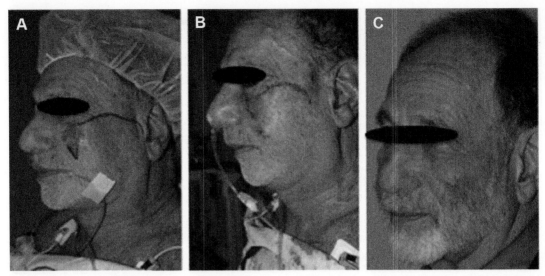

Fig. 8. (*A*) A 2.5 × 3.2-cm defect of the zygomatic/medial cheek. (*B*) Cheek rotation-advancement flap with standing cone parallel to RSTL. (*C*) 2-month postoperative result.

placed from the flap to the underlying periosteum. Without suspension, flaps can easily create lower eyelid retraction, ectropion, and/or distortion of the alar base. The zygomatic arch, infraorbital rim, and frontal process of maxilla are all useful for suspending soft tissue reconstructions.

Concurrent Canthopexy

Lower eyelid retraction following the reconstruction of medial cheek is a common complication, especially in patients with significant lower eyelid laxity. In these patients, it is often appropriate to complete a canthopexy at the time of primary cheek repair. One technique preferred by the authors is to use a double-armed 5-0 Prolene OPS to suture the tarsal plate and lateral retinaculum to the lateral orbital rim periosteum. A mattress suture is used to prevent twisting. Care is taken to place the suture along the medial aspect of the orbital rim to ensure the lid margin remains against the globe. In patients with significant preoperative lower eyelid laxity, a tarsal strip and lid shortening rather than a canthopexy should be considered.

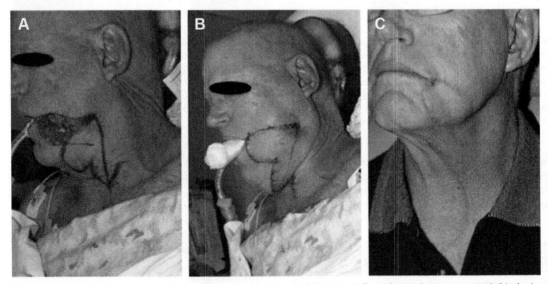

Fig. 9. (*A*) A 4.5 × 5-cm defect of the buccal aesthetic subunit. (*B*) Bilobed flap planned to use cervical skin laxity. (*C*) 2 months postoperatively. A disadvantage of this technique is that resulting scar does not parallel RSTLs and crosses aesthetic unit boundaries.

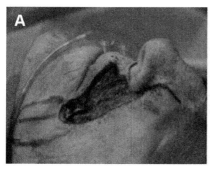
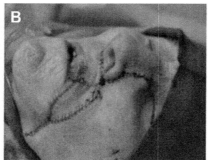
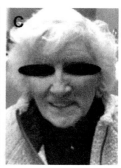

Fig. 10. (A) "Composite" defect involving buccal/medial cheek and upper lip. (B) Significant laxity of jowl soft tissue enables good mobility of island pedicle V-to-Y advancement flap. A contralateral advancement flap of the lip was also used. (C) 2 months postoperatively.

It should be noted that medial cheek reconstruction causing lower lid retraction and ectropion is often due to shortening of the anterior lamella. Horizontal tightening by a canthopexy alone will not compensate for a poorly designed reconstruction with insufficient anterior lamella height.

Z-Plasty

Z-plasty is useful in cheek reconstruction for distributing tension in a tangential fashion to the areas under most strain and for creating broken line closures. The authors often use a Z-plasty at the end of a flap incision in order to slightly assist mobilization while also decreasing the need for an equalizing Burow triangle excision (see **Fig. 4**).

COMPLICATIONS
Flap Necrosis

A feared complication in cheek reconstruction is ischemia leading to flap necrosis. Most commonly this results from both inadequate vascularity and excessive tension. Excess tension on a flap, especially across a convex bony base such as the zygoma or mandible, may lead to arterial or venous insufficiency. The subdermal vascular plexus perfuses random pattern flaps and generally on the face and cheek should have a maximum length-to-base ratio of 3:1.[12] Increasing the ratio significantly increases the risk for distal tip necrosis. These ratios serve as guidelines that must be considered in the context of patient-specific factors such as diabetes, peripheral vascular disease, and active smoking status, which can adversely affect flap perfusion. Smoking in particular causes microvascular vasoconstriction as well as chronic tissue hypoxia due to carboxyhemoglobinemia; it also increases perioperative adverse events and postoperative morbidity due to its effects on a host of organ functions.[13] If the patient is to quit smoking, the authors recommend doing so at least 2 weeks in advance of planned reconstruction.

Last, unrecognized hematoma and failure to promptly drain a hematoma under a large flap likely will lead to necrosis. Hematoma-related necrosis of flaps occurs because of the "internal pressure" and because of a toxic effect of a mass of blood on the skin flap.[14]

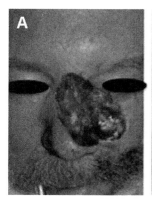
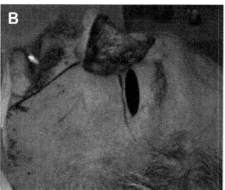
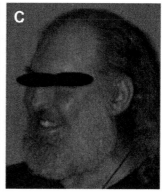

Fig. 11. (A) "Composite" defect involving nose and medial cheek aesthetic subunit. (B) Medial cheek defect reconstructed with cheek advancement flap and nose defect reconstructed with paramedian forehead flap. (C) 3 months postoperatively, nasofacial groove reestablished.

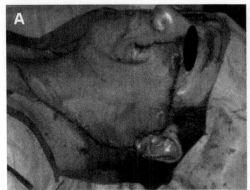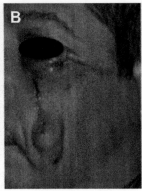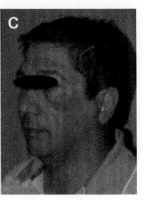

Fig. 12. (*A*) Large cervicofacial flap. (*B*) Large standing cone left in place at time of primary repair to ensure maximum distal flap perfusion. The standing cone was excised 2 weeks later. (*C*) 3 months postoperatively.

Wound Dehiscence

It is uncommon for a well-planned cheek reconstruction to dehisce. Careful attention to supporting sutures and an appropriate layered closure limits tension on skin edges and helps decrease this occurrence. In the authors' experience, extremely sebaceous skin increases the risk of dehiscence, because skin sutures more easily pull through. In this situation, using vertical mattress sutures is beneficial.

Scar Hypertrophy

Scar hypertrophy can result from increased wound tension leading to increased fibroblast proliferation, or due to patient predisposition. Appropriate anticipatory guidance should be given at the preoperative visit if the patient has a history of significant scarring from minor injuries or from prior surgeries. One or 2 injections of triamcinolone acetonide into the hypertrophic scar at concentrations between 10 and 20 mg/mL usually mitigate the scar. Pulsed-dye laser and intralesional 5-fluorouracil injection are also helpful and improve the hypertrophic scar.

Ectropion

Lower eyelid malposition may occur because of flap tension, lid laxity, or edema. Utilization of supporting sutures, using a high lateral arc above the level of the lateral canthus, concurrent canthopexy, and/or skin grafting the lower eyelid/anterior lamella all help reduce the incidence of this complication.

REFERENCES

1. Menick FJ. Artistry in aesthetic surgery. Aesthetic perception and the subunit principle. Clin Plast Surg 1987;14:723–35.

2. Dobratz EJ, Hilger PA. Cheek defects. Facial Plast Surg Clin North Am 2009;17:455–67.

3. Jowett N, Mlynarek AM. Reconstruction of cheek defects: a review of current techniques. Curr Opin Otolaryngol Head Neck Surg 2010;18:244–54.

4. Alghoul M, Codner MA. Retaining ligaments of the face: review of anatomy and clinical applications. Aesthet Surg J 2013;33:769–82.

5. Gazzalle A, Teixeira LF, Pellizzari AC, et al. Effect of side-stream smoking on random-pattern skin flap survival in rats. Ann Plast Surg 2014;72:463–6.

6. Goldman D, Dzubow L, Yelverton C. Facial flap surgery. New York: McGraw Hill; 2013.

7. Bennet RG. Cheek reconstruction. In: Rohrer TE, Cook JL, Nguyen TH, et al, editors. Flaps and grafts in dermatologic surgery. Philadelphia: Saunders/Elsevier; 2008. p. 159–77.

8. Babakurban ST, Cakmak O, Kendir S, et al. Temporal branch of the facial nerve and its relationship to fascial layers. Arch Facial Plast Surg 2010;12:16–23.

9. Furr M, Wang T. Complex local flap design in cheek reconstruction. Oper Tech Otolayngol Head Neck Surg 2011;22:53–8.

10. Park S, Little S. Rhombic flaps. In: Baker S, Swanson N, editors. Local flaps in facial reconstruction. St Louis (MO): Mosby; 1995. p. 213–30.

11. Bradley DT, Murakami CS. Reconstruction of the cheek. In: Baker SR, editor. Local flaps in facial reconstruction. Philadelphia: Mosby/Elsevier; 2007. p. 525–56.

12. Mathes S, Nahai F. The reconstructive triangle: a paradigm for surgical decision making. In: Mathes S, Nahai F, editors. Reconstructive surgery: principles, anatomy, and technique. New York: Churchill Livingston; 1998. p. 9–36.

13. Rodrigo C. The effects of cigarette smoking on anesthesia. Anesth Prog 2000;47:143–50.

14. Hillelson RL, Glowacki J, Healey NA, et al. A microangiographic study of hematoma-associated flap necrosis and salvage with isoxsuprine. Plast Reconstr Surg 1980;66(4):528–33.

Reconstruction of Defects Involving the Lip and Chin

Katie Geelan-Hansen, MD*, Joseph Madison Clark, MD, William W. Shockley, MD

KEYWORDS

- Lip reconstruction • Chin reconstruction • Oral reconstruction • Lip defects
- Local reconstructive flaps • Oral cavity defects

KEY POINTS

- The lips are specialized structures that have a vital role in oral function, speech, and animation, and they are also important aesthetic features.
- Reconstruction of lip defects should restore both aesthetics and function.
- Multiple local flaps provide reconstructive options for defects of the lip and chin.
- Secondary reconstruction follows the same principles as primary reconstruction, although hinge flaps play a role in achieving a successful outcome.

INTRODUCTION

Reconstruction of defects involving the lips and chin can present a challenge to even the most experienced surgeon. Thorough assessment of the defect, including size, location, depth, involvement of adjacent subunits, and the effect on function, is critical to the success of the reconstruction. Goals of reconstruction include restoration of normal anatomy, oral competence, lip motion, minimizing secondary deformity, and optimizing the cosmetic result.[1] Perioral and oral tissue are best matched with like tissue from local flaps. Multiple local flaps are described for reconstruction of this region and provide the versatility needed to match individual patient needs. This article focuses on reconstructive options for defects of the lips and chin.

ANATOMY OF LIP AND CHIN

Lips are the prominent feature in the lower third of the face. The lip esthetic units extend vertically from the subnasale to the mental crease and horizontally between the melolabial creases and the labiomental creases. They are composed of skin, muscle, and mucosa (**Fig. 1**). The red line marks the border of the dry vermilion surface and the wet lip mucosa.[2] The transition of the red lip and the skin is the vermilion border. The vermillion is made up of modified mucosa that lacks minor salivary glands, whereas the color of the vermilion is the result of a rich blood supply under a thin epithelial layer.[3] The white roll is the landmark corresponding to the pars marginalis of the orbicularis oris that separates the vermilion from the cutaneous lip.[4] From the oral commissure lateral to medial, the upper lip has a gentle superior medial curvature. The width of the vermilion increases from the oral commissure to the central upper lip with the widest segment present at the crest of Cupid's bow.[4] These peaks correspond to the inferior philtral ridges, and there is then a V-shaped indentation of the mucocutaneous junction, which corresponds with a prominent tubercle of the red lip inferiorly.[3,4] The philtrum is composed of 2 parallel or divergent raised ridges with a central dimple.[5] The ridges of the philtrum are thought to

Disclosures: No.
Division of Facial Plastic and Reconstructive Surgery, Department of Otolaryngology–Head and Neck Surgery, University of North Carolina at Chapel Hill, 170 Manning Drive, Campus Box 7070, Chapel Hill, NC 27599, USA
* Corresponding author.
E-mail address: kgeelanhansen@gmail.com

Facial Plast Surg Clin N Am 27 (2019) 67–83
https://doi.org/10.1016/j.fsc.2018.08.008
1064-7406/19/© 2018 Elsevier Inc. All rights reserved.

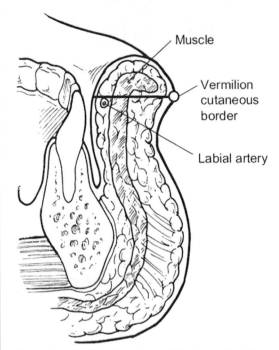

Muscle

Vermilion
cutaneous
border

Labial artery

Fig. 1. Cross-sectional anatomy of the lower lip. (*From* McCarn KE, Park SS. Lip reconstruction. Facial Plast Surg Clin North Am 2005;13:302; with permission.)

arise from dermal attachments of pars peripheralis of the orbicularis oris, although this may not be the only structure contributing to the landmark.[5] The cutaneous upper lip is divided into 3 subunits composed of 2 lateral compartments and one philtral (central) segment (**Fig. 2**). The upper lip contrasts with the lower lip, which is a single esthetic subunit.[2,6] The visible lower lip is widest in the central portion with a relative central indentation to correspond to the upper lip tubercle with tapering laterally as it ends at the oral commissure. The orbicularis oris makes up the major muscular component of the lips, which is most commonly thought of as a sphincter due to the orientation of the muscle fibers. However, this muscular compartment can also be considered as 4 independent subunits that interlace, giving the impression of a sphincter.[7] The orbicularis muscle is affixed laterally without a bony attachment but rather inserts at the muscular modiolous.[6]

The adjacent esthetic unit just inferior to the lips is the chin. This convex mound of skin and soft tissue extends from the labiomental crease to the mandibular margin and inferiorly to the submental crease. The muscles of the chin include the mentalis, the depressor labii inferioris, and the depressor angular oris.[8]

The blood supply to the lips is derived from the facial artery, branching into the inferior and superior labial arteries, which supply the upper and lower lips, respectively.[9] The upper lip is also supplied by branches of the angular artery.[9] The chin is supplied by the inferior labial artery and the mental artery, a branch of the inferior alveolar artery.[9]

Sensory innervation to the perioral area and chin comes from the maxillary and mandibular branches of the trigeminal nerve. The infraorbital nerve provides sensation to the upper lip, whereas lower lip and chin sensation is provided by the mental nerve.[2] The motor supply to the lower third of the face arises from the buccal and marginal mandibular branches of the facial nerve.[1]

DEFECTS OF THE LIPS AND CHIN: ANALYSIS

Reconstructive decision making for lip defects is commonly based on the horizontal extent of the lip defect. Most often the lip is divided into horizontal thirds in order to further characterize the size of the defect.[6] The depth of the defect in relation to the orbicularis oris is an important consideration. Detailed alignment of the orbicularis oris and the vermilion border are paramount in reconstruction of the lip.[2] In appropriate circumstances, the subunit principle can be applied: maintaining the borders of the subunits and reconstructing the entire subunit if the majority (>50%) has been affected.[6] This concept however must always be balanced with functional considerations. Other principles of wound closure apply, such as incision placement in relaxed skin tension lines as well as conservative debridement and hemostasis.[10]

Chin reconstructive procedures fall within the basic principles of incision planning and wound closure. Whenever possible, the surgeon should use esthetic boundaries when designing flaps, and sacrifice of normal skin should be kept at a minimum to preserve volume for chin projection. Preserving the contour of the chin is more important than the cutaneous scars that may arise from reconstruction.

HEALING BY SECOND INTENTION

Wound healing by second intention is a recognized treatment option in superficial wounds of the lip and chin. Secondary wound healing can be used in defects superficial to the orbicularis oris in the lip mucosa and the vermilion, even with a few millimeters of extension into the cutaneous lip.[11–13] Superficial defects of the upper lip and philtrum can also heal secondarily with

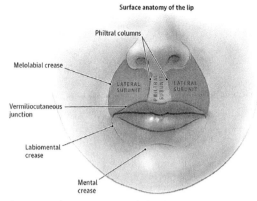

Surface anatomy of the lip

Philtral columns

Melolabial crease

LATERAL SUBUNIT   PHILTRAL SUBUNIT   LATERAL SUBUNIT

Vermiliocutaneous junction

Labiomental crease

Mental crease

Fig. 2. Surface anatomy of the lip. (*From* Pepper JP, Baker SR. Local flaps: cheek and lip reconstruction. JAMA Facial Plast Surg 2013;15(5):378; with permission.)

excellent results, but wounds with significant extension into the vermilion are more likely to heal with an unacceptable result.[11] Secondary healing of deep wounds are more likely to result in depressed or hypertrophic scars. Likewise, deep defects that extend into the vermilion often heal with distortion that may not be acceptable.[11,14] Becker and colleagues[11] further contend that Mohs defects of the chin that heal by second intention may result in a stellate scar

with dimpling; thus, these patients would benefit from primary surgical repair.

The authors seldom recommend healing by second intention and typically favor surgical repair, which provides a better and more predictable result.

MUCOSAL AND VERMILION DEFECTS
Mucosal Cross Lip Flaps

The mucosal cross lip flap is an interpolated flap that requires a 2-stage reconstruction and is designed for defects isolated to the mucosa and/or vermilion.[8] This flap may be a single pedicle, for smaller defects, or a bipedicle flap, for wider defects. Other variations include incorporation of the orbicularis oris into the flap to match the depth of the defect. The blood supply is derived from the labial artery, which can sometimes be incorporated into a larger flap.[8] The first stage is planned using the labial mucosa immediately posterior to the posterior vermilion line. The flap is elevated in a plane superficial to the orbicularis oris. This tissue is then inset to reconstruct a vermilion defect of the opposite lip. The width of the flap is determined by the defect size, but one must consider closure of the donor site. Division of the pedicle with inset of the flap is performed 3 weeks later.[15]

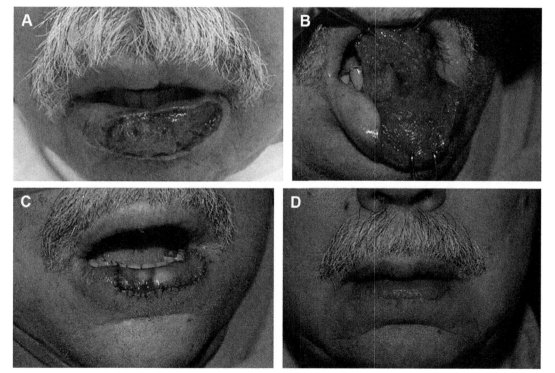

Fig. 3. Mucosal advancement flap. (*A*) Mohs defect lower lip. (*B*) Elevated mucosal advancement flap. (*C*) Immediate result following reconstruction. (*D*) Postoperative result at 1 month.

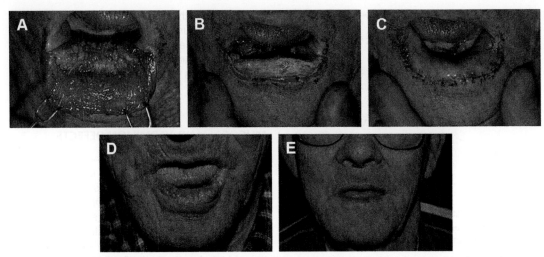

Fig. 4. Mucosal advancement flap with primary dermal fat graft. (*A*) Vermilion defect with elevated mucosal advancement flap. (*B*) Dermal-fat graft sutured to underlying orbicularis muscle. (*C*) Immediate result following closure. (*D*) Preoperative photograph with diffuse lower lip lesion (severe dysplasia). (*E*) Postoperative result at 6 months.

Mucosal Advancement Flap

The mucosal advancement flap is the preferred reconstructive technique following a vermilionectomy for precancerous lesions, carcinoma in situ, or superficially invasive lip cancers (**Fig. 3**). The mucosal advancement flap is elevated in a plane deep to the minor salivary glands and superficial to the orbicularis oris.[8] The width of the flap is designed based on the width of the defect. The flap is typically elevated to the gingivolabial sulcus. The advanced mucosa has a random blood supply but can be used with good reliability. Potential complications include scar contracture, thin lip deformity, retroversion of the lower lip, distortion of the vermilion border, mucosal retraction, decreased sensation, and color mismatch.[1] The senior author has on occasion used a primary dermal-fat graft to augment the lower lip. The dermal fat graft is harvested from the supraclavicular region. The amount of fat necessary can be tailored to the individual defect. The graft is applied as a horizontal strip of tissue over the orbicularis oris, matching the dimensions of the missing vermilion (**Fig. 4**). The graft is situated under the mucosal advancement flap in order to avoid loss of the normal fullness of the lower lip, which often occurs.

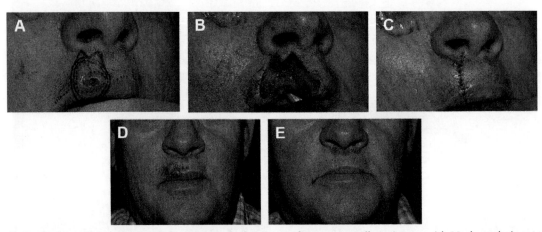

Fig. 5. Wedge excision with M-plasty. (*A*) Proposed excision of squamous cell carcinoma with M-plasty design, to avoid involvement of the nasal sill. (*B*) Defect following excision with negative frozen section margins. (*C*) Immediate result following closure. (*D*) Preoperative photograph, squamous cell carcinoma right upper lip. (*E*) Postoperative photograph at 6 months.

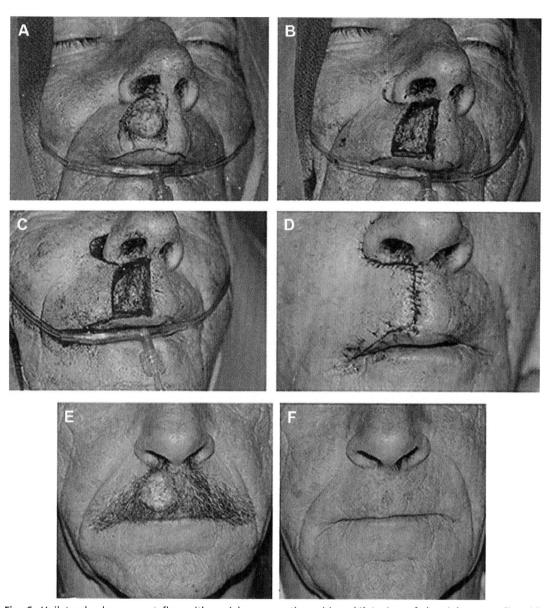

Fig. 6. Unilateral advancement flap with perialar crescentic excision. (*A*) Lesion of the right upper lip with marked margins and aesthetic unit boundaries. (*B*) Defect following excision with negative frozen sections. (*C*) Excision of the perialar tissue and elevation of advancement flap. (*D*) Immediate result following closure. (*E*) Preoperative photograph with keratoacanthoma right upper lip. (*F*) Postoperative result at 3 months.

SMALL TO MODERATE DEFECTS

Primary closure after fusiform excision for lip defects superficial to the orbicularis oris can provide excellent esthetic results. Avoidance of crossing an esthetic unit can sometimes be accomplished by using an M-plasty, creating a wider horizontal plane of excision and a shorter vertical plane of excision (**Fig. 5**). Orientation of the fusiform excision should be parallel with the long axis of the relaxed skin tension lines.[2,6,8] Partial thickness defects approaching or involving the vermilion can be

converted to full-thickness defects providing an optimal closure. Pepper and Baker[16] recommend that any defect 1.5 to 3 cm in the vermiliocutaneous central lip be converted to full-thickness defects and closed primarily.

Full-thickness defects of up to one-third of the upper lip and one-half of the lower lip can often be closed primarily.[1] The size of the defect that can be closed varies with each patient, but in general, there is more extensibility in older patients, in whom defects up to one-half of the lower lip can

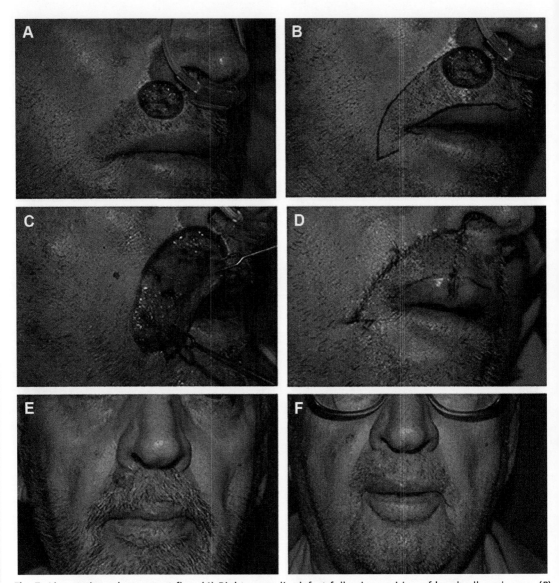

Fig. 7. Lip rotation-advancement flap. (*A*) Right upper lip defect following excision of basal cell carcinoma. (*B*) Proposed advancement-rotation flap with marked vermilion border. (*C*) Elevation of flap in supramuscular plane. (*D*) Immediate result following closure. (*E*) Preoperative photograph with basal cell carcinoma. (*F*) Postoperative result at 2 months.

be closed. The advisability of this reconstructive option still lies with the judgment of the surgeon and is limited by the degree of resulting microstomia, lip distortion, and wound tension.[10]

Advancement Flaps

Advancement flaps with perialar crescentic excision can be used for cutaneous defects involving the upper lip. Bilateral flaps are primarily used for central cutaneous defects. For defects just off the midline, a unilateral flap may suffice. This flap is designed with placement of incisions along the

boundaries of subunits of the lip; however, the flaps can be of differing lengths. In the upper lip, incisions are placed just inferior to the nasal sill and at the vermilion-cutaneous border. Crescentic skin excision along the alar-facial sulcus allows room for the advancement of skin to occur (**Fig. 6**). In the lower lip, the incisions are placed along the vermilion-cutaneous border and the mental crease. The plane of dissection is superficial to the orbicularis oris muscle. The distribution of tension between the 2 flaps (instead of one) is advantageous for central defects in order to lessen tissue distortion and improve flap perfusion.

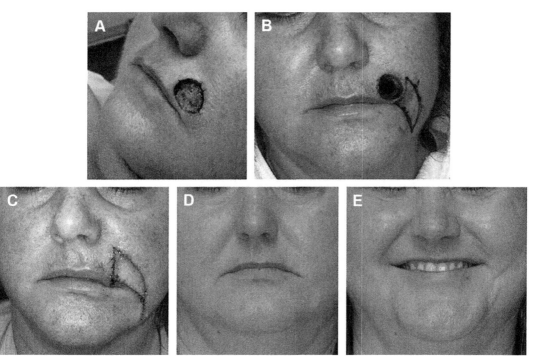

Fig. 8. V-to-Y advancement flap. (*A*) Mohs defect involving lateral segment of upper lip, sparing the adjacent vermilion. Note, less than 50% of the lateral lip segment. (*B*) Flap marked, preserving the vertical height of the medial side of the defect, and following the contour of the melolabial fold and the oral commissure. (*C*) Immediate result. Note slight overcorrection of height. (*D*) Reconstructive result at 6 months, repose. (*E*) Reconstructive result at 6 months, smiling.

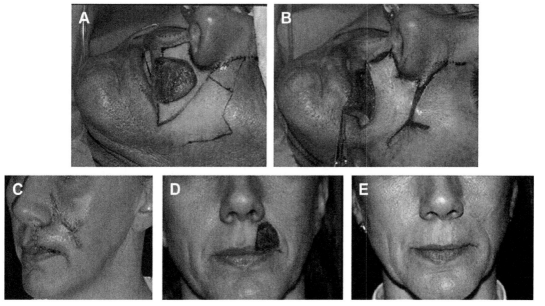

Fig. 9. Melolabial transposition flap and mucosal advancement flap with primary fat graft. (*A*) Mohs defect involving lateral segment of upper lip and adjacent vermilion. Proposed melolabial transposition flap for replacement of the entire lateral subunit. (*B*) Flap partially sutured into position, highlighting the extent of the vermilion defect. (*C*) Result at 1 week following reconstruction. Mucosal advancement flap with primary fat graft used to reconstruct vermilion defect. Note the skin fold left oral commissure. (*D*) Mohs defect involving the left upper lip. (*E*) Reconstructive result at 1 year, which included revision of deformity seen in panel (*C*).

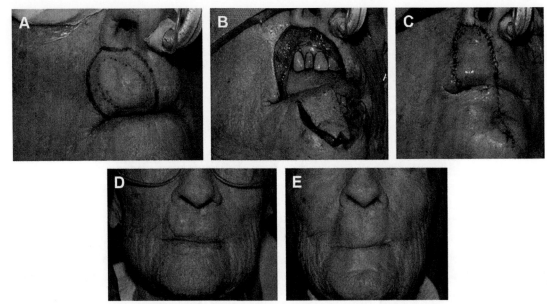

Fig. 10. Abbe flap. (*A*) Low-grade sarcoma right upper lip. (*B*) Defect following resection with Abbe flap incised. (*C*) Abbe flap sutured into position with pedicle from lower lip intact. (*D*) Preoperative photographs demonstrating mass right upper lip. (*E*) Postoperative result at 9 months.

Rotation advancement flaps can also be used effectively for small to moderate lip defects[17,18] (**Fig. 7**).

O-to-T Plasty

The O-to-T plasty can also be a useful technique for small cutaneous lip defects. Wide undermining can assist in the soft tissue advancement and help to decrease the tension and risk of distortion of surrounding structures. The "T" design closure leaves 3 standing cutaneous deformities. The vertical limb of the T is created from excision of a standing cutaneous deformity and should be placed along a natural skin crease or a subunit boundary. This technique results in a trifurcation that requires careful approximation. The O-to-T is a versatile closure technique for lateral upper lip defects, central and lateral lower lip defects with incisions placed along the vermilion-cutaneous border.[17,18]

V-to-Y Island Advancement Flaps

Defects in the lateral cutaneous lip larger than 1 cm^2 are amenable to closure with a V-to-Y flap.[19] This flap is a subcutaneous pedicle advancement flap with incisions placed adjacent to the alar-facial sulcus and along the vermilion border, designed in the shape of a V with the defect present at the base of the flap (**Fig. 8**). This flap provides advancement of the mobile skin and soft tissue of the inferior medial cheek.[17] With the pedicle

anchored to the soft tissue and fascia adjacent to the modiolus, the soft tissue can be mobilized to the philtrum.[19] In planning the flap, the width is equal to the height of the defect and the length of the incisions is 2 times the width of the defect, equal in distance and tapered to a point.[19] The pedicle can be narrowed, leaving at least the central one-third of the total flap surface attached to the underlying subcutaneous tissue for adequate blood supply. Closure of the donor site is completed with care to ensure no deformity of the vermilion border or surrounding structures. Defects as large as 3 cm^2 have been reconstructed with this technique with a 47% revision rate. Defects with alar or vermilion involvement were most likely to require revision.[19] For larger defects, the flap design is modified to include skin lateral to the melolabial crease and includes a superior peninsula of skin to re-create the alar-facial sulcus.[19]

Melolabial Flaps

Cutaneous lip defects can be restored with transposition or advancement of skin from the medial cheek or melolabial fold.[8] These flaps can be designed as transposition flaps or as V-to-Y subcutaneous tissue pedicled melolabial advancement island flaps.

The transposition flap can have a superior or inferior pedicle depending on the location of the defect.[8] An inferior pedicled flap can be considered for lateral upper or lower lip defects, whereas

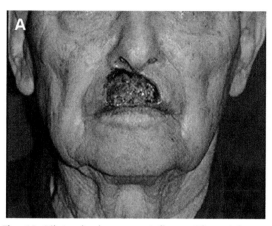
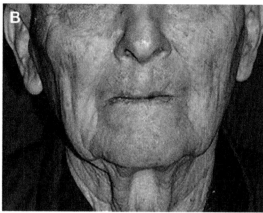

Fig. 11. Bilateral advancement flaps with perialar crescentic excision and Abbe flap. Demonstrates bilateral advancement flaps and Abbe flap reconstruction of central lip defect. (*A*) Defect involving right, left, and central upper lip. (*B*) Postoperative result at 6 months, following perialar crescentic excision, bilateral advancement flaps and Abbe flap.

a superiorly based pedicle is often considered in the reconstruction of the central upper lip.[8] As in any reconstruction, use of the contralateral normal anatomy can provide the template for incision planning. The flap is designed with the medial incision along the melolabial crease (**Fig. 9**). The transposed tissue is only slightly wider than the defect to allow for wound contracture.[8] The distal portion of the transposition flap can be thinned to match the thickness of the surrounding tissue. Revision of the pedicle in a second stage may be completed

to align the scars parallel to the melolabial crease.[8] Burget and Hsiao[20] have described their experience with a similar flap for reconstruction of large cutaneous defects of the upper lip but refer to it as a nasolabial rotation flap. This flap is rotated from a vertical orientation to a transverse orientation with the medial border of the flap becoming adjacent to the vermilion and the lateral border the nasolabial sulcus. The secondary defect can be closed with undermining and advancement or a Burow's triangle. Considerations when using

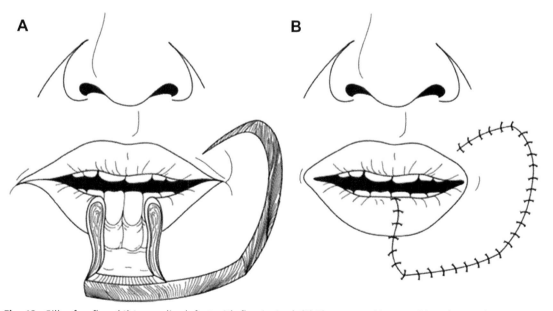

Fig. 12. Gilles fan flap. (*A*) Lower lip defect with flap incised. (*B*) Flap sutured into position. (*From* Ishii LE, Byrne PJ. Lip reconstruction. Facial Plastic Clin North Am 2009;17:451; with permission.)

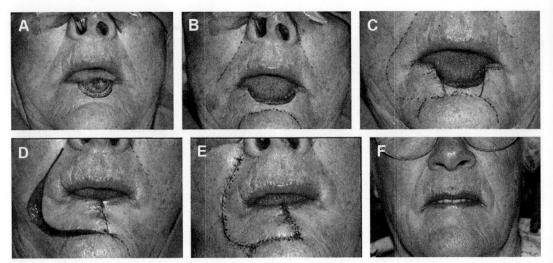

Fig. 13. Unilateral Karapandzic flap. (*A*) Squamous cell carcinoma lower lip with marked proposed excision. (*B*) Defect mid lower lip after resection with negative margins. (*C*) Proposed Karapandzic flap with marked boundaries of chin. (*D*) Dissection with rotation-advancement flap in position. (*E*) Immediate result following closure. (*F*) Result at 4 months.

these flaps include the risk of trapdoor deformity, flattening of the melolabial fold, and transposition of hair-bearing skin in an altered orientation.[8] Transposition of hair-bearing skin into non-hair-bearing regions should be avoided.

Another option for large (≥2 cm) lateral upper lip cutaneous defects is the V-to-Y subcutaneous tissue pedicled melolabial advancement island flap (Baker book). The principles of this flap are those as described previously in the V-to-Y Island Advancement Flaps.[19]

FULL-THICKNESS DEFECTS
Abbe and Estlander Flaps

The Abbe and Estlander flaps are ideal choices for reconstruction of full-thickness defects involving 30% to 60% of the lip.[8] They both allow transfer of the skin, muscle, and mucosa, thus restoring all layers with the goal of maintaining lip competence and function.

The Abbe flap is used for defects medial to the commissure, and the Estlander flap is used for defects involving the oral commissure. These cross

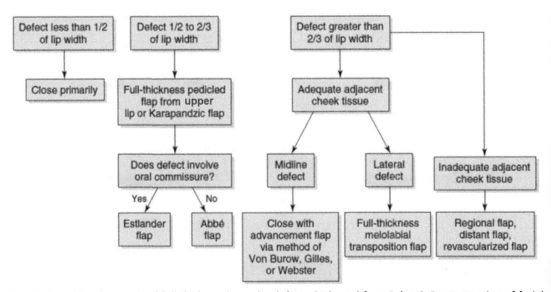

Fig. 14. Algorithm for repair of full-thickness lower lip defects. (*Adapted from* Baker S. Reconstruction of facial defects. [Chapter 24]. In: Flint PW, Haughey BH, Lund V, et al, editors. Cummings otolaryngology—head and neck surgery. 6th edition. Philadelphia: Elsevier Saunders; 2015. p. 363; with permission.)

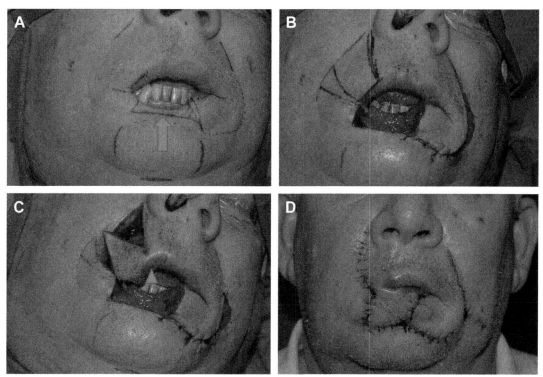

Fig. 15. Secondary reconstruction technique: Estlander and Karapandzic flaps. (*A*) Lower lip defect following failed prior Karapandzic flap performed elsewhere after resection and extensive squamous cell carcinoma of the lower lip. Proposed hinge flap (*arrow*) marked to re-create the gingivolabial sulcus. Markings for revision left Karapandzic flap. (*B*) Hinge flap elevated into position and attached to adjacent mucosa. Left Karapandzic flap in position. (*C*) Right Estlander flap has been designed, incised, and partially rotated. Triangle denotes site of new oral commissure. (*D*) Result at 1 week following hinge flap, Karapandzic flap, and Estlander flap.

lip flaps are designed of equal height of the defect; however, the width is approximately one-half to two-thirds of the defect (**Fig. 10**). Both flaps are designed with a lateral labial artery pedicle.[17] A vertical labiomental branch off the inferior labial artery supplies the lower lip and chin all the way into the submental region.[21] Thus, an extended Abbe flap can be designed for patients with large composite defects involving the upper lip. The extended Abbe flap is useful for lip defects involving the central face, such as the columella, perialar, or premaxillary regions, especially for those who lack adequate adjacent cheek tissue for defect closure.[21]

With the Estlander flap, the height and width dimensions are planned as in the Abbe flap. However, the lateral incisions are designed to include the oral commissure and to lie in the melolabial sulcus.[8] The flap is rotated 180° with the new oral commissure now residing at the pivot point of the flap.

The Abbe flap is a 2-stage flap with the pedicle remaining in place for approximately 14 to 21 days before division and inset. For upper lip defects, it is typically designed so that the flap donor site is centered on the midpoint of the lower lip (**Fig. 11**). With both flaps, the transferred tissue is temporarily denervated with a return of innervation, motor, and sensory, in about 1 year.[22] In an Abbe flap, the motor supply is replaced through the same facial nerve branches that supplied the original upper lip, and the lip function returns normally without the need for special training.[22] In an Estlander flap, the modiolus is displaced, and although the facial nerve innervation has not been transected, the muscles of the lower lip have been replaced into the upper lip, so retraining is a part of recovery.[22]

Gilles Flap

The Gilles flap is a rotation advancement flap that ultimately restores the continuity of the orbicularis oris (**Fig. 12**). It can be used to reconstruct defects involving 70% to 80% of the lower lip.[17] It is a composite flap based on the superior labial artery and is created parallel to the orbicularis oris. Incisions are full thickness from the inferior edge of

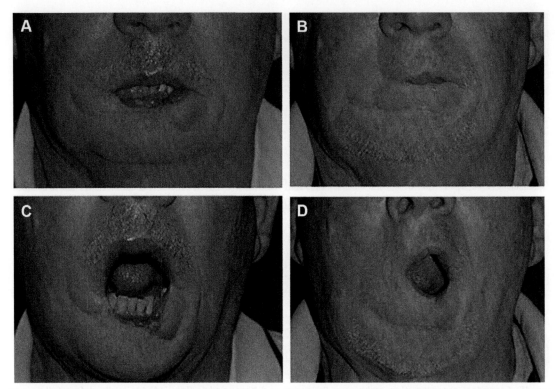

Fig. 16. Secondary reconstruction results: Karapandzic and Estlander flaps. (*A, C*) Preoperative photograph after failed Karapandzic flap reconstruction of extensive lower lip defect, performed elsewhere. Exposure of teeth with significant oral incompetence. (*B, D*) Postoperative result at 18 months, following reconstruction with right Estlander flap and left Karapandzic flap.

the defect lateral then, superior lateral around the commissure into the melolabial crease with an incision toward the upper lip vermilion border. Once the flap is rotated into position, it is closed in a multilayer fashion. The Gilles flap can be unilateral or bilateral. Disadvantages of this repair include potential microstomia, vermilion deficiency, and blunted oral commissure.[2,10] Oral incompetence may result from denervation of the orbicularis oris.[3] However, this denervation is often temporary with a gain partial reinnervation at 12 to 18 m postoperatively.[3,10]

Karapandzic Flap

The Karapandzic flap is a bilateral rotation-advancement flap that maintains the continuity of the orbicularis oris. It works best in reconstruction of major lower lip defects but can be inverted for upper lip defects.[2] Incisions are planned in a curvilinear fashion from the inferior edge of the defect superolaterally into the melolabial crease and nasolabial crease. The width of the flap corresponds to the height of the lip. Meticulous dissection is needed to ensure uniform thickness of the flap and preserve the neurovascular supply to

the flap, which includes the superior and inferior labial artery branches and branches of the buccal nerve.[9] The neurovascular bundle is found near the oral commissure between the orbicularis oris and the underlying facial musculature and soft tissue.[1] Preservation of the neurovascular bundle maintains lip mobility and sensation.[1] Maintaining symmetric vertical height of both flaps is an important principle that affects both function and cosmesis. Once the flap is fully incised and dissected, it is rotated into position and closed in a layered fashion. The disadvantages are microstomia and blunted commissures.[8] The senior author has applied the concept of the "sequential Karapandzic flap" for moderate lower lip defects. In this situation, a unilateral Karapandzic flap is created on the side with the most intact native tissue and advanced into position. If the closure is on too much tension or creates a short lower lip, the contralateral Karapandzic flap is dissected (**Fig. 13**).

Bernard-von Burow Flap

The Bernard-von Burow flap can be considered in near-total lower lip and total lip defects sparing the

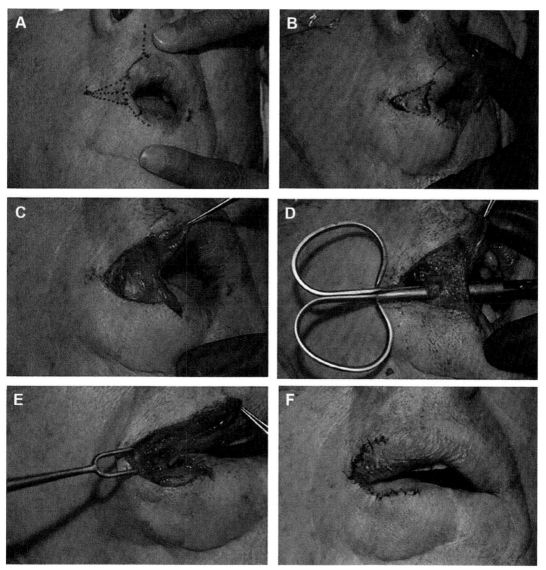

Fig. 17. Commissuroplasty technique. (*A*) Proposed excision of skin with site of new oral commissure at apex of triangle. (*B*) Triangle of skin excised. (*C*) Superiorly based vermilion flap onto lower lip. Point of flap goes to new oral commissure. (*D*) Exposure of orbicularis oris muscle, before transection. (*E*) Two ends of orbicularis muscle sutured to new oral commissure. (*F*) Immediate result following closure, demonstrating vermilion flap as well as mucosal advancement flap.

oral commissure. A brief description is included here, but other texts and articles can be sought for detailed explanation and illustration. Conceptually, this is a bilateral advancement flap of medial cheek soft tissue (which lacks orbicularis oris) and mucosa into a central defect. The horizontal length of each opposing cheek limb is half of the desired horizontal length of the reconstructed lip.[8] The height of each opposing cheek limb is the height of the desired reconstructed lip. In upper lip reconstruction, the soft tissue is advanced from the tissue adjacent to the melolabial sulcus, and in the lower lip, the soft tissue is

advanced from the tissue adjacent to the labiomental sulcus. To accomplish the amount of soft tissue advancement needed, a configuration of triangles, both superior and inferiorly based, is excised to minimize the secondary deformities. There have been many modifications described for this technique. One must consider the perfusion from the facial artery in patients with a history of neck dissection or radiation therapy.[9] These flaps are associated with significant neuromuscular dysfunction and facial deformity so they are typically a "last resort" in the reconstructive algorithm.

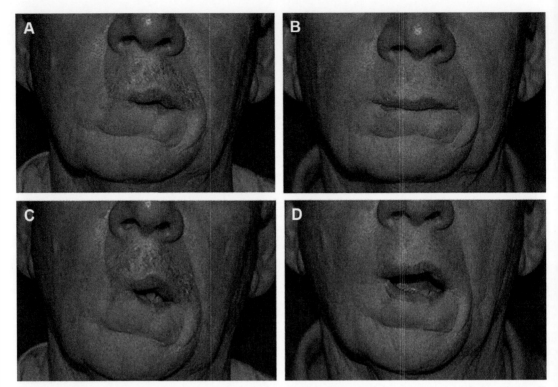

Fig. 18. Commissuroplasty results. (*A, C*) Relative microstomia, blunted oral commissure, and short lower lip following extensive reconstruction of lower lip defect. (*B, D*) Postoperative result at 3 months demonstrating improved symmetry of oral commissure, better lip contour, and longer lower lip.

Full-thickness defects of the lip offer a significant reconstructive challenge. **Fig. 14** represents the algorithm proposed by Baker for full-thickness defects of the lower lip.[23] In general, the authors prefer to avoid the use of an Abbe flap when the upper lip serves as the donor site. Instead, they would perform a Karapandzic flap for reconstruction of an extensive defect.

SECONDARY RECONSTRUCTION
Full-Thickness Defects

There are many circumstances in which secondary reconstruction of lip defects may be necessary. Whether the defect arises from cancer, trauma, burns, radiation, or failed reconstruction, the reconstructive techniques remain the same. The authors emphasize one technical point that applies to this set of patients. In lower lip defects, it is supremely important to try to maintain an intact labiogingival sulcus, thus minimizing the risk of postoperative salivary leakage. For this reason, hinge flaps are often used so that a new suture line does not exist at the inferior aspect of the sulcus. Instead, adjacent mucosa or skin is elevated as a hinge flap, and thus, there is a much lower likelihood there will be leakage because the sulcus

is intact. A case example is presented in **Figs. 15** and **16**.

Commissuroplasty

One may consider a commissuroplasty in patients with a blunted, round commissure after Estlander flap reconstruction. One method involves a full-thickness incision laterally from the blunted commissure ending at the point of the new apex of the commissure with advancement of the labial mucosa to restore the vermilion. A triangle of skin and subcutaneous tissue may be excised laterally to accommodate the new apex of the commissure.[8]

Another method is described as a vermilion and orbicularis muscle flap.[8] To create this, a triangle of skin and subcutaneous tissue is excised lateral to the blunted commissure. Here, the apex of the triangle is the new apex of the commissure, and the inferior and superior incisions should align with the level of the contralateral commissure. Then, a vermilion flap is elevated from the orbicularis muscle, and the length of this flap is that of the distance to the apex of the new commissure. A transverse incision is then completed through the orbicularis muscle at the level of the new commissure. The superior and inferior muscle ends are

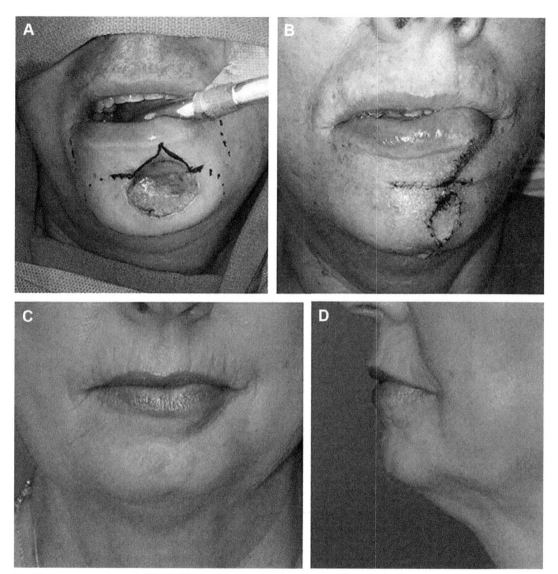

Fig. 19. Reconstruction of chin defect with bilateral advancement flaps and submental island flap. (*A*) Mohs defect involving 50% of chin skin and soft tissue as well as a segment of lower lip beyond the mentolabial sulcus; lip advancement flaps (A-to-T closure) marked dividing the defect into 2 defects involving 2 facial units. (*B*) Lower lip flaps advanced using the mentolabial crease. Island flap transposed from below the submental crease. (*C*) Reconstructive result at 18 months: frontal view. (*D*) Reconstructive result at 18 months: lateral view. Note preservation of chin projection.

then advanced into the point of the new commissure. The vermilion flap is the placed over the muscle, and a mucosal flap is elevated and advanced to restore the inferior vermilion.[8] This latter technique is favored by the authors (**Figs. 17** and **18**).

CHIN RECONSTRUCTION
H-Plasty, O-to-T, and V-to-Y Flaps

H-plasty is an ideal method to reconstruct defects of the central chin.[17] Incisions are placed parallel to the vermilion border to avoid distortion, and if possible, in the mental crease to retain this facial landmark. Burow triangles maybe excised laterally. The tissue is then advanced into the central defect.

The O-to-T flap is particularly useful for defects of the central or lateral chin. The flaps are designed with a vertical limb to excise a standing cutaneous deformity. The lateral limbs can be placed along the mandibular margin or along the boundary of the chin. Larrabee and Moyer[17] describe an asymmetric O-to-T used for defects of the lateral chin to allow for more lateral advancement of tissue.

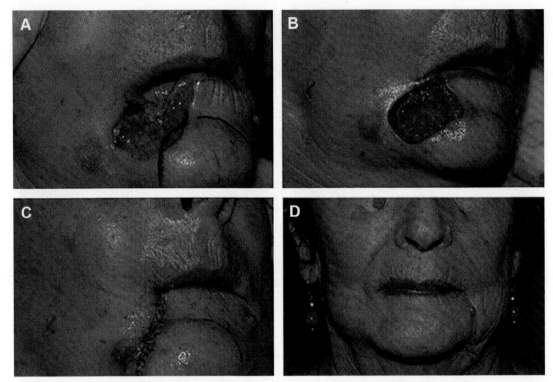

Fig. 20. Reconstruction of lip and chin defect with cheek advancement flap. (*A*) Mohs defect involving full-thickness lower lip and partial thickness of chin. Aesthetic boundaries of chin delineated. (*B*) Closure of muscle, vermilion, and mucosa. (*C*) Immediate result following closure of lip and chin defect, using cheek advancement flap. (*D*) Postoperative result at 5 months.

Lateral chin defects can also be reconstructed with a V-to-Y flap. When possible, the incisions are placed in the melolabial crease using the subunit principle.

Submental Island Flap

The submental island flap is a reliable flap for soft tissue reconstruction of the face and can be considered for the reconstruction of chin defects. It can be a cutaneous, musculocutaneous, musculofascial, or composite flap.[24,25] The blood supply for this flap is the submental artery, a branch of the facial artery, and the submental vein, which drains into the facial vein.[24] A Doppler can be used in planning, and the flap is designed with the arch of the mandible in the submentum, and the inferior extent (width of the flap) is largely based on the ease of closure after the flap has been elevated.[24] The subcutaneous adipose tissue, platysma, and mylohyoid can be harvested as well to provide a convexity for the chin.[25] In general, the laxity of the skin in this area and the cervical rhytids camouflage the incisions well. Also, the skin and soft tissue can be approximated to the hyoid to create a sharp cervicomental angle after the flap elevation and inset. **Fig. 19** demonstrates the use of

bilateral advancement flaps in combination with a submental island flap for reconstruction of a subtotal chin defect.

Fig. 20 demonstrates the use of a unilateral cheek advancement flap for an extensive defect of the lip and chin.

REFERENCES

1. Coppit GL, Lin DT, Burkey BB. Current concepts in lip reconstruction. Curr Opin Otolaryngol Head Neck Surg 2004;12:281–7.
2. Nabili V, Knott PD. Advanced lip reconstruction: functional and aesthetic considerations. Facial Plast Surg 2008;24:92–104.
3. Neligan PC. In: Neligan PC, editor. Lip reconstruction: plastic surgery. 4th edition. New York: Elsevier Saunders; 2018. p. 306–28.
4. Mulliken JB, Pensler JM, Kozakewich HPW. The anatomy of Cupid's bow in normal and cleft lip. Plast Reconstr Surg 1993;92(3):395–403.
5. Rogers CR, Meara JG, Mulliken JB. The philtrum in cleft lip: review of anatomy and techniques for construction. J Craniofac Surg 2014;25(1):9–13.
6. Ishii LE, Byrne PJ. Lip reconstruction. Facial Plast Surg Clin North Am 2009;17:445–53.

7. Saladin K. Anatomy and physiology: the unity of form and function. 5th edition. New York: McGraw Hill; 2009. p. 330.

8. Renner G. In: Baker SR, editor. Reconstruction of the lips: local flaps in facial reconstruction. 3rd edition. Philadelphia: Elsevier Saunders; 2014. p. 481–529.

9. Baumann D, Robb G. Lip reconstruction. Semin Plast Surg 2008;22:269–80.

10. McCarn KE, Park SS. Lip reconstruction. Facial Plast Surg Clin North Am 2005;13:301–14.

11. Becker GD, Adams LA, Levin BC. Outcome analysis of Mohs surgery of the lip and chin: comparing secondary intention healing and surgery. Laryngoscope 1995;105(11):1176–83.

12. Gloster HM Jr. The use of second-intention healing for partial-thickness Mohs defects involving the vermilion and/or mucosal surfaces of the lip. J Am Acad Dermatol 2002;47(6):893–7.

13. Leonard AL, Hanke CW. Second intention healing for intermediate and large postsurgical defects of the lip. J Am Acad Dermatol 2007;57(5):832–5.

14. Zitelli JA. Wound healing by secondary intention: a cosmetic appraisal. J Am Acad Dermatol 1983; 9(3):407–15.

15. Harris L, Higgins K, Enepekides D. Local flap reconstruction of acquired lip defects. Curr Opin Otolaryngol Head Neck Surg 2012;20:254–61.

16. Pepper JP, Baker SR. Local flaps: cheek and lip reconstruction. JAMA Facial Plast Surg 2013;15(5): 374–82.

17. Larrabee YC, Moyer JS. Reconstruction of Mohs defects of the lips and chin. Facial Plast Surg Clin North Am 2017;25:427–42.

18. Shew M. Flap basics II: advancement flaps. Facial Plast Surg Clin North Am 2017;25(3):323–35.

19. Griffin GR, Weber S, Baker SR. Outcomes following V to Y advancement flap reconstruction of large upper lip defects. Arch Facial Plast Surg 2012;14(3): 193–7.

20. Burget GC, Hsiao YC. Nasolabial rotation flaps based on the upper lateral lip subunit for superficial and large defects of the upper lateral lip. Plast Reconstr Surg 2012;130(3):556–60.

21. Kriet JD, Cupp CL, Sherris DA, et al. The extended Abbe flap. Laryngoscope 1995;105(9):988–92.

22. Burget GC, Menick FJ. Aesthetic restoration of one-half the upper lip. Plast Reconstr Surg 1986;78(5): 583–93.

23. Baker S. In: Flint PW, Haughey BH, Lund V, et al, editors. Cummings otolaryngology-head and neck surgery. 6th edition. Philadelphia: Elsevier Saunders; 2015. p. 351–70.

24. Martin D, Pascal JF, Baudet J, et al. The submental island flap: a new donor site. Anatomy and clinical applications as a free or pedicled flap. Plast Reconstr Surg 1993;92(5):867–73.

25. Howard BE, Nagel TH, Barrs DM, et al. Reconstruction of lateral skull base defects: a comparison of the submental flap to free and regional flaps. Otolaryngol Head Neck Surg 2016;154(6):1014–8.

Reconstruction of the Forehead and Scalp

Benjamin D. Bradford, MD, Judy W. Lee, MD*

KEYWORDS

- Scalp reconstruction • Forehead reconstruction • Scalp anatomy • Forehead anatomy • Skin graft
- Microsurgery • Tissue expansion

KEY POINTS

- Tissue inelasticity and the hair-bearing nature of the scalp and forehead pose unique challenges during reconstruction.
- Thorough understanding of the surgical anatomy of the scalp and forehead is paramount for optimal reconstructive outcomes.
- Primary wound closure is usually preferred to secondary intention healing and skin grafting when feasible.
- Use of dermal alternatives and tissue expansion are adjunctive therapies to facilitate scalp wound closure.
- Local skin and soft tissue flaps are most commonly used for small to medium sized defects; however, microsurgical free tissue transfer can be considered for large full-thickness skin defects of the forehead and scalp.

INTRODUCTION

Management of patients with scalp and forehead defects continues to be a challenge for the head and neck reconstructive surgeon. These defects are often encountered in the context of oncologic treatment but can be a result of trauma, burn injury, or the excision of a congenital lesion.[1] Although aesthetic and functional principles of scalp and forehead reconstruction have been well-described, the best results require a thoughtful, individualized approach.

The factors common to most scalp and forehead reconstructions are an inherent resistance to tissue distension, potential involvement of neurovascular structures, and cosmetically conspicuous areas such as the hairline and brows that frame the upper third of the face. Defects may range in complexity from a small skin defect to a full-thickness wound involving the skull or dura.

Defects of the scalp often tend to be larger, which can be challenging to reconstruct due to relative scalp immobility. Tissue quality and coverage goals may vary in patients with a history of previous surgery, radiation, or significant comorbidities.

Simply providing coverage of a defect is not enough. Surgical planning that optimizes both the preservation of function and aesthetic relationships to surrounding structures cannot be overlooked. An advanced understanding of the anatomy of the scalp and forehead, as well as an awareness of the full complement of reconstructive options, is essential to providing the patient the best result.

ANATOMY

An excellent understanding of the surgical anatomy of the scalp and forehead is paramount for optimal reconstructive outcomes. For the purposes

Disclosure Statement: None.
Department of Otolaryngology–Head and Neck Surgery, New York University School of Medicine, 240 East 38th Street, 14th Floor, New York, NY 10016, USA
* Corresponding author. NYU Otolaryngology Associates, 240 East 38th Street, 14th Floor, New York, NY 10016.
E-mail address: judy.lee@nyulangone.org

Facial Plast Surg Clin N Am 27 (2019) 85–94
https://doi.org/10.1016/j.fsc.2018.08.009
1064-7406/19/© 2018 Elsevier Inc. All rights reserved.

of reconstruction, it is convenient to conceptualize the forehead and the temporal region as a subunit separate from the rest of the scalp.

Forehead and Temples

The forehead comprises the area between the supraorbital rim inferiorly to the temporal-frontal hairline superiorly, and is bound laterally by the temporal hairline and zygoma. The paired frontalis muscles arise superiorly as a continuation of the galea aponeuroses and interdigitate with the paired corrugator supercilii muscles, midline procerus, and the orbicularis oculi muscles before inserting inferiorly into the dermis at the level of the brow. The temporal region continues posteriorly to the mastoid and is bound superiorly by the temporal line and inferiorly by the zygomatic arch.[2]

The forehead and temples are supplied by an extensive vascular network (**Fig. 1**). The supratrochlear artery takes off from the ophthalmic branch of the internal carotid system and pierces the orbital septum superior to the trochlea to emerge medially through its notch or foramen between the corrugator and frontalis muscles. As the vessel travels vertically toward the frontal scalp, it lies just beneath the frontalis muscle. At the midforehead level, it passes through the muscle to ascend into the subdermal plane as it approaches the hairline. The supratrochlear artery and its corresponding nerve are reliably located 1.7 to 2.2 cm from the midline, corresponding to the medial border of the eyebrow.[3]

Additionally, the supraorbital artery, which is typically the smaller of the terminal branches of the ophthalmic artery, passes through the supraorbital notch 2.4 to 2.7 cm lateral to midline and penetrates the corrugator as it divides into superficial and deep branches. The superficial branch courses in the galea frontalis layer and the deep branch supplies the pericranium. The artery then forms anastomoses with the supratrochlear and anterior superficial temporal artery (STA) branches, which are highly variable.[2]

Laterally, the forehead and temple derive their blood supplies from the anastomoses of the supratrochlear and supraorbital arteries with the anterior branches of the STA, a terminal branch of the external carotid system. The STA ascends into the face and scalp from deep within the parotid gland and emerges between the mandibular condyle and external auditory meatus.[2,4–6] As it courses toward the zygomatic arch, it lies within the temporoparietal fascia. Before crossing the zygomatic arch, the STA takes off the horizontally oriented transverse facial artery, which supplies the area of the lateral canthus. A second branch, the middle temporal artery, traverses the superficial layer of the deep temporal fascia to supply the temporal fat pad and deep temporalis fascia with minor contributions to the temporalis muscle. Finally, the STA divides into 2 or 3 terminal branches within 2 cm of crossing the zygomatic arch. The anterior branch supplies the lateral forehead. The posterior branch supplies a large area over the parietal scalp and forms rich anastomoses with adjacent arteries.[2,7] As the longest and largest of scalp vessels, the STA supplies the greatest area of temporal-parietal scalp.

The motor and sensory input to the forehead and temple may be compromised by the original pathologic condition; however, every effort should be made to preserve these structures during reconstruction. The motor innervation to the frontalis and corrugator muscle is the temporal branch of the facial nerve (cranial nerve [CN] VII). The procerus, on the other hand, receives its innervation from the contributions of the zygomatic and deep buccal branches of CN VII.[2]

It is critical to understand the course of the extratemporal facial nerve, especially as it courses over the zygomatic arch into the temporal scalp and forehead. The temporal branch can be found along a line starting from a point 0.5 cm below the tragus and passing 1.5 cm above the lateral brow, known as the Pitanguy line, within the temporoparietal fascia (**Fig. 2**).[8] Dissection in the immediate subcutaneous plane or deep to the superficial layer of the deep temporal fascia when dissecting around the zygomatic arch will avoid trauma to this important structure.

The supratrochlear and supraorbital nerves, which course with their vascular counterparts, emerge from the ophthalmic division of the trigeminal nerve (CN V) to provide sensation to the forehead. Laterally, the zygomaticotemporal and auriculotemporal nerves from the maxillary and mandibular divisions of CN V provide the temple with sensation (see **Fig. 1**).[2,9]

Scalp

The scalp, made up of the 5 main tissue layers of skin, connective tissue, aponeurosis, loose areolar tissue, and periosteum or pericranium (SCALP is the acronym commonly used as a mnemonic), is the thick, robust covering of the calvarium (**Fig. 3**). The scalp is hair-bearing in the occipital, parietal, and (to varying extents) in the temporal and frontal regions. The scalp is thickest in areas of dense hair growth and thins with alopecia. The epidermis, dermis, and subcutaneous layer make up the outermost layer of the scalp, which contains

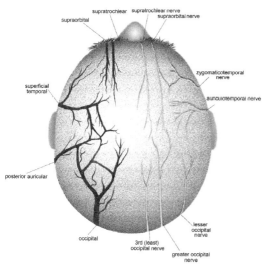

Fig. 1. Neurovascular supply of the forehead and scalp. (*Courtesy of* Graham Hadley, MD, New York, NY.)

the hair follicles, adnexal appendages, and fat. Underlying the skin and subcutaneous layers is the occipitofrontalis with its connecting galea aponeurosis, which overlies the pericranium. Laterally, the galea continues as the temporoparietal fascia and inferiorly as the superficial musculoaponeurotic system. The galea is most dense and inelastic in the central scalp and vertex, and more loose laterally in areas with underlying muscle and fascia. This is an important consideration when designing flaps within the scalp. The subgaleal plane, which contains loosely organized areolar tissue, is an avascular potential space conducive to blunt

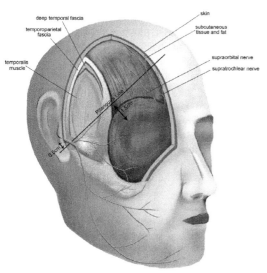

Fig. 2. Facial nerve anatomy. (*Courtesy of* Graham Hadley, MD, New York, NY.)

dissection, making it an excellent plane for wide undermining and flap development.[5,10]

Neurovascular supply to the central scalp and vertex overlaps somewhat with that of the forehead and temporal regions. The extensive blood supply that integrates anastomoses from the internal and external carotid systems is arranged in a centripetal fashion as vessels enter the scalp from the periphery. This allows for considerable latitude in reconstructive design because most areas of the scalp can survive on collateral circulation, even when axial blood supply is sacrificed. As previously discussed, the supraorbital and supratrochlear vessels supply the forehead and anterior scalp. Parietal branches of the STA, along with postauricular and occipital arteries from the external carotid circulation, supply the remainder of the scalp.[2,7,10]

The sensory innervation of the anterior scalp is derived from the supratrochlear and supraorbital nerves. The supratrochlear nerve exits its foramen and travels superiorly on its way to the scalp, coursing beneath the corrugator supercilii muscle to supply sensation to the medial upper eyelid, central forehead, and scalp. The supraorbital nerve leaves the supraorbital foramen more laterally at the midpupillary line and courses over the frontalis muscle to supply the central upper eyelid, ipsilateral forehead, and scalp. A deep branch of the supraorbital nerve travels between the frontalis and pericranium and galea to innervate the remaining anterior scalp and vertex. The posterior scalp territory is innervated by the greater and lesser occipital nerves from cervical spinal nerve (C)2 or C3. The temporal region is innervated by the auriculotemporal nerve, which travels with the STA above the zygomatic arch, as well as by contributions from the zygomaticotemporal nerve.[2]

RECONSTRUCTIVE OPTIONS
Secondary Intention Healing

Secondary intention healing is a nonsurgical option that can be a satisfactory option for select patients. In the absence of an intrinsic wound-healing challenge, such as heavy smoking or history of local radiation, allowing a wound to granulate and heal secondarily is best reserved for defects in non–hair-bearing areas of the scalp (eg, temple or vertex) in the setting of a partial-thickness wound. Patients who would not tolerate a surgical procedure or who are medically unfit to undergo anesthesia may also be considered.

The wound will close over weeks to months, depending on its size and depth, through a process of granulation, contraction, and reepithelialization.

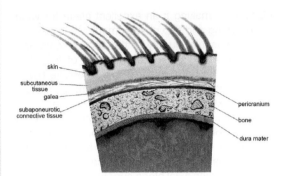

Fig. 3. Scalp layers. (*Courtesy of* Graham Hadley, MD, New York, NY.)

This treatment strategy requires a commitment on the part of the surgeon and the patient to prolonged, meticulous wound care to ensure the wound stays clean, moist, and covered. Smaller wounds (<2 cm) with a vascularized bed may heal over the course of a few weeks, whereas larger wounds may take several months to completely close.

If a vascularized bed is not present, such as in a full-thickness scalp defect with exposed skull bone, a burr may be used to drill down the outer calvarial table to expose the diploic vessels beneath and allow for formation of granulation tissue. If this option is chosen, the surgeon may elect to place a temporary skin substitute to protect the wound and provide a substrate for tissue growth.[11] Another option to expedite wound closure is judicious use of a purse-string suture to decrease the initial wound area.[12] A negative pressure wound vacuum-assisted closure device has also been used to decrease time to wound closure while keeping the site clean.

It should be noted that, although secondary intention can be effective and cosmetically acceptable, the wound will contract as much as 60% as it heals, potentially distorting adjacent tissue.[5,6,11] This is functionally and cosmetically important to consider in areas around the eyes and brow where asymmetry would be visually distracting. The scars from secondary healing tend to be atrophic and contain telangiectasias.[10] These factors should be discussed at length with patients and their caretakers when deciding to pursue this healing strategy.

Primary Wound Closure

Primary wound closure is usually preferred over secondary intention healing and skin grafting when feasible. The limiting factors for acceptable primary closure of scalp defects are its size and anatomic location. Scalp defects of 3 cm or less can usually be closed primarily, especially in the more distensible temporal and occipital scalp. Over the central scalp and vertex, even small defects may require significant tension to close. Wide, blunt subgaleal undermining can facilitate recruitment of 1 to 2 cm of adjacent tissue to reduce the tension on the closure.[11] In patients without vascular compromise, subcutaneous undermining around the periphery of the defect may further decrease wound tension.

Adjuncts to closure include rapid intraoperative tissue expansion[13] and the use of galea relaxing incisions called galeotomies. Rapid intraoperative tissue expansion, described by Sasaki,[14] involves cyclic expansion and deflation of a balloon device such as a Foley catheter beneath the closure site. The process, which can recruit an additional 1 to 2 cm, is most effective when the wound is held closed with clamps or sutures during expansion. Following rapid tissue expansion, the wound is immediately approximated in a multilayered closure. This process is believed to increase skin length through mechanical creep through disruption and realignment of elastic and collagen fibers, displacement of adjacent tissues, and reduction in interstitial fluids.[10,15] This technique should not be confused with prolonged tissue expansion (see later discussion). Galeotomies are full-thickness relaxing incisions made in the galea aponeurotica that may be performed parallel to the wound closure and serve to further reduce wound tension. It is critical to limit these incisions to the galea to avoid damage to the subcutaneous blood supply (**Fig. 4**).[16]

Primary closure of defects in the forehead and temple of lesions of 3 cm or less is made more favorable by the more distensible tissue.[17] However, this area challenges the surgeon to preserve the cosmetically conspicuous relationships of the forehead with the hairline and brow. Excision of cutaneous malignancies often leaves a circular defect amenable to conversion to fusiform, followed by primary closure. Ideally, this closure is hidden within a natural horizontal or less often, vertical rhytid. Care is taken to avoid changing the contour of the patient's hairline or distorting the ipsilateral brow by excessive tension on the wound.

Skin Grafting

As with secondary intention healing, skin grafting in the scalp has a limited role due to suboptimal cosmesis and lack of durability. However, this technique may be appealing in cases in which rapid, efficient defect closure is prioritized or close tumor surveillance is desired. Skin grafts can also

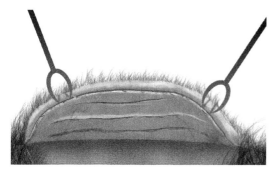

Fig. 4. Relaxing galeotomy incisions. (*Courtesy of* Graham Hadley, MD, New York, NY.)

be used as temporary coverage while awaiting definitive reconstruction with a vascularized flap or tissue expansion. The surgeon has the option of selecting a split-thickness skin graft (STSG) or a full-thickness skin graft (FTSG) for reconstruction. A commercial dermatome is commonly used for harvesting an STSG, often from the lateral thigh. Less commonly, an FTSG may be used in scalp and forehead reconstruction. Typical FTSG donor sites include supraclavicular or periauricular skin.

Both STSGs and FTSGs rely initially on nourishment by plasmatic imbibition, in which the graft passively absorbs the nutrients in the wound bed by diffusion. By 36 to 72 hours, a fine vascular network between the wound bed and the graft is established through inosculation and capillary ingrowth.[18,19] Survivability of skin grafts depends on a healthy wound bed, absence of infection, absence of shear forces, and hemostasis at the time of grafting. Patient-specific factors, such as peripheral vascular disease and history of local radiation, will also affect survivability. When healing is complete, skin grafts take on an atrophic, shiny appearance and tend to blend poorly with surrounding tissues. When used in areas of hair-bearing scalp, this can be especially distracting and is a major disadvantage of skin grafting.

Dermal Alternatives and Tissue Expansion

A variety of dermal alternatives have been described for coverage of scalp wounds in the acute setting following oncologic surgery, trauma, or burns. Products such as Integra (LifeScience Corp, Plainsboro, NJ, USA) and MatriDerm (Dr Suwelack Skin and Health Care AG, Billerbeck, Germany) were developed for use in burn patients but their use was later expanded to reconstructive surgery and management of chronic wounds.[20] Although microvascular free flap reconstruction is often most appropriate for reconstruction of large scalp defects, dermal substitutes may be selected as an alternative in some patients.

Integra is a bilaminate synthetic construct consisting of an outer silicone layer and a porous inner collagen-glycosaminoglycan (chondroitin-6-sulfate) matrix. Glycosaminoglycans lend elasticity to the matrix, control the rate of biodegradation, and maintain a porous structure, which promotes cellular migration and integration into the matrix.[21] Integra may be placed onto vascularized soft tissue, such as muscle, fat, or pericranium, or directly onto calvarium that has been drilled to the diploic space. The matrix is then sutured into place and secured with a bolster dressing. Granulation tissue formation over the subsequent 3 to 4 weeks will prepare the wound bed to receive a staged skin graft or, in some cases, the wound may be left to close secondarily.

MatriDerm is a thin (1 mm or 2 mm) porous membrane composed of coupled bovine collagen (types I, II, and V) and elastin, which provides a scaffold for connective tissue regeneration without the formation of a granulation tissue bed. There are several reports of successful single-stage procedures using 1 mm thick MatriDerm and STSG on full-thickness wounds.[22–24] Although this 1-stage option for scalp reconstruction is promising, current clinical data for use in full-thickness scalp defects is lacking. Disadvantages of dermal alternatives include the potential need for a second-stage procedure with prolonged local wound care before and after skin grafting.

Since Neumann first described the expansion of skin by progressive distension of a subcutaneous balloon in the 1950s,[25] tissue expansion techniques have undergone significant advances and are now used widely in reconstructive surgery. This technology is especially useful in the scalp and forehead where tissue inelasticity results in inability to mobilize tissue adjacent tissue for defect closure, and expansion facilitates closure of defects that would have otherwise required reconstruction with distant tissue. Additionally, the use of expanders allows for recruitment of hair-bearing scalp and provides an ideal match to the thickness, texture, and color of nearby scalp skin. Due to the thickness of the overlying skin and subcutaneous tissue, and the stability of the bony calvarium, the scalp is an ideal location for use of tissue expansion.[5,7,10,26]

Some surgeons advocate expansion of scalp before resection of the primary lesion; however, concern for tumor seeding in cases of malignancy may preclude this. More often, tissue expanders are placed after confirmation of negative pathologic margins. If a large defect is present and skin grafting is performed, tissue expanders should be planned as a second stage after the grafts are fully healed. Tissue expander placement under irradiated skin should be avoided due to the increased risk for vascular compromise and soft tissue necrosis.

This technique of gradual tissue expansion relies on the phenomenon of biologic creep, which refers to permanent elongation of tissues subjected to an external force. At a cellular level, biologic creep causes an increase in collagen production, angiogenesis, and epidermal proliferation. This process takes weeks to months for larger defects. It should be noted that when expanding areas of hair-bearing scalp, the number of follicular units does not increase. This translates to a decrease in hair density; however, this is usually well-tolerated with minimal aesthetic penalty. Approximately 50% of the scalp can be reconstructed with tissue expansion without causing significant hair thinning.[27]

Tissue expansion involves placement of a silicone elastomer expander into a subgaleal plane, which will ultimately be inflated by percutaneous injection of sterile saline solution through a remote port.[10,15] Two to 3 weeks of healing is allowed after placement, at which time the implant may start to be expanded. This may be performed 1 to 2 times per week at the surgeon's discretion and depending on the comfort of the patient. Overaggressive inflation may result in blanching of the skin, patient discomfort, and vascular compromise of the overlying tissue.

When choosing implant size, a general guideline is that the base diameter of the expander should be 2 to 2.5 times the defect diameter.[10] The shape of the expander depends on the location; crescent shapes are frequently used in the scalp. Ducic[11] maintains that the amount of tissue gained in the expansion process correlates to expander geometry with an increase in biologic creep when going from a round to crescent-shaped to rectangular expanders (with percentage of expansion 25%, 32%, and 38%, respectively). The amount of tissue available from each expander can be estimated by measuring the convex (dome) length and subtracting the base diameter.[10] To further increase scalp distensibility during expansion, galeotomies may be considered at the time of expander placement.

Potential complications of tissue expansion include infection, exposure of implant or port, implant leak, hematoma, seroma, skin necrosis, and neuropraxia overlying the implant. Most of these complications can be minimized by correct placement of implant, postoperative drains, and antibiotic prophylaxis for 2 to 3 weeks. In the case of implant exposure, further inflation of the device is not advised due to the risk of further extrusion without the benefit of additional tissue expansion.[10]

Local Flaps

In cases in which primary closure is not feasible or aesthetically favorable, the workhorse of forehead and scalp reconstruction is the local soft tissue flap or adjacent tissue transfer. These are best suited for small or medium sized defects but may also be considered for reconstruction of select large defects.[28–30] In general, local flaps can be categorized as an advancement, rotation, or transposition flaps, although many reconstructions are hybrids of these techniques.

There are key differences between the forehead and scalp that must be kept in mind during surgical planning. First, the scalp is largely immobile (see previous discussion), whereas the forehead and temporal areas are less adherent and feature relaxed skin tension lines. This may allow camouflage of scars within horizontal and, occasionally, vertical rhytides. The forehead region is cosmetically conspicuous and unintended alteration of the adjacent anterior hairline or brow position may create aesthetic disharmony and patient dissatisfaction. Finally, important neurovascular structures traverse the forehead and temporal regions and should not be sacrificed to make reconstruction more convenient. Disruption of motor and sensory nerves has significant long-term consequences for the patient, including paresis of the ipsilateral forehead and uncomfortable paresthesia that may extend well into the scalp.

As extensions of primary closure, unilateral or bilateral advancement flaps can be useful for reconstructing small (<3 cm) forehead defects.[29,30] These flaps are raised and widely undermined in the middle subcutaneous plane superficial to the frontalis muscle and allow for horizontal closures that can be hidden within forehead wrinkles. A vertical closure can also be aesthetically favorable for defects in the midline and paramedian forehead.

Advancement flaps rely on random blood supply from the dermal and subdermal plexus, and the viable length of a random pattern flap is determined by perfusion pressure in the distal flap. Classically, these flaps should be planned with a length-to-width ratio of at least 4:1.[29–32] Recruitment of the adjacent tissue provides an excellent skin thickness, texture, and color match. The temple offers some laxity and can be mobilized to facilitate closure of paramedian or lateral forehead defects, provided the frontotemporal hairline and brows are not distorted. In patients with sufficient skin laxity, neck and cheek skin can be mobilized superiorly as a cervicofacial advancement flap to reconstruct the non–hair-bearing temple and lateral forehead.

In the scalp, pure advancement flaps are seldom used because adequate tissue recruitment cannot be achieved for defects greater than 3 to 4 cm, despite using wide subgaleal undermining, rapid intraoperative tissue expansion, and parallel galeotomies.[28,30–32] Advancement flaps have the disadvantage of producing standing cutaneous cones, which can be excised in a delayed fashion or with removal of Burrows triangles at the time of reconstruction.[31] Hwang and colleagues[32] recently described the visor flap, a bipedicled advancement flap that uses wide undermining with a V-to-V advancement to allow redistribution of scalp tissue from a remote donor site. In a 7-subject series, all subjects were able to achieve complete, durable defect coverage without need for skin grafting to either the defect or donor sites. Defect size in this study ranged from 3 to 50 cm^2 (mean 17.9 cm^2). A variety of other flap designs have been described in scalp reconstruction, including the commonly used A-T, O-T, and V-Y advancement flaps (**Fig. 5**).[11,28,29,31]

Rotational flaps or rotation-advancement flaps are used in the reconstruction of most medium and large scalp defects. These flaps are ideally planned as wide-based flaps with an axial blood supply and may be based laterally (STA), posteriorly (occipital artery), or (less commonly) anteriorly (supratrochlear artery).[2,7,10] Flaps are generally raised in the subgaleal plane, and galeotomies should be considered when additional tissue recruitment is needed. When extending onto the convexity of the skull, these flaps are typically 4 to 6 times longer than they are wide.[7,11,31] If a back cut is used to extend the reach of the flap and to decrease tension at the recipient site, care is taken to maintain an adequate vascular pedicle to optimize flap viability. This may create a need for skin grafting or healing by secondary intention at the donor site, which is ideally remote and less cosmetically conspicuous than the original defect.

When anterior scalp defects are being reconstructed, preservation or recreation of the hairline deserves careful consideration. Trichophytic closure in hair-bearing skin, avoiding transection of follicles, and judicious use of electrocautery may help avoid postoperative alopecia, which distracts from an otherwise excellent reconstruction.[30] The ideal approach to defects involving the boundary between aesthetic subunits, especially from hair-bearing scalp into the forehead, is to reconstruct each subunit separately. When

possible, incisions should be placed at the interface of a subunit where a natural crease, shadow, or hairline will help camouflage the scar.

A large body of literature is available describing variations of rotational flaps used in the reconstruction of the scalp and forehead, and a detailed description of each is beyond the scope of this article. Often, multiple separate rotational advancement flaps can be used to distribute the tension of the closure over a wider area of the scalp.[29,30,32] Common examples include bilateral opposing rotational flaps (eg, O-Z) and 3-armed or 4-armed pinwheel flaps (**Fig. 6**).[31,33] As the rotational flap is placed into its recipient site, a proximal standing cutaneous cone is often present. Most will resolve within 1 to 2 months and may be easily excised if they continue to be a concern.[30]

Transposition flaps, defined by rotation over an intervening area of normal skin to reach the recipient site, are rarely used in scalp reconstruction. In 1975, Jose Juri[34] described a temporoparietal occipital flap for aesthetic hair restoration of the frontal hairline. This axial pattern flap, based on the superficial temporal vessels, is no longer used by most contemporary hair restoration surgeons but still may have limited application as a reconstructive flap. Fincher and Gladstone[35] described a case report of dual transposition flap for delayed closure of a 78.5 cm^2 defect following Mohs micrographic surgery. This flap was designed to borrow tissue from the occipitoparietal regions with coronally oriented axial blood supply. The orticochea banana peel flap is well described and may be used for very large defects in debilitated patients unable to undergo microsurgical reconstruction.[33] In cases in which a forehead defect does not involve the hairline, especially in the temple, a single (rhombic) or double (bilobed) flap may be considered.

Microsurgical Reconstruction

The use of muscular microvascular free flaps has become the gold standard for immediate or delayed vascularized reconstruction of large (larger than 6–8 cm diameter) scalp and forehead defects where a local flap cannot provide reliable coverage.[36] Microvascular tissue transfer is often planned to cover defects left by ablation of malignant or benign tumors and traumatic avulsions. As opposed to local flaps, free flaps can be used to safely cover large full-thickness wounds and cranial defects. Furthermore, vascularized free flaps can tolerate postoperative radiation therapy with reduced risk of wound healing complications. Flap selection is highly variable and depends on defect location, as well as surgeon preference.

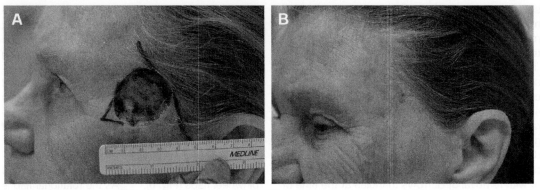

Fig. 5. O-T advancement flap repair of a temple defect. (*A*) Left temple defect with O-T advancement flap markings. (*B*) Left temple following O-T advancement flap reconstruction.

The latissimus dorsi and anterolateral thigh flaps have become the workhorse free flaps for reconstruction of large scalp defects. However, use of many other flaps for this purpose have been well-described, including radial forearm, serratus anterior, scapula, rectus abdominis, and free omentum flaps.[28–30,32,33] Muscular flaps without an attached skin paddle are typically surfaced with a meshed STSG at the time of reconstruction. Though muscle-based flaps are often initially bulky, flap atrophy over time yields an acceptable cosmetic result with tissue thickness comparable to adjacent scalp tissue.[10,11,30,31] Though alopecia is among the disadvantages of microvascular free

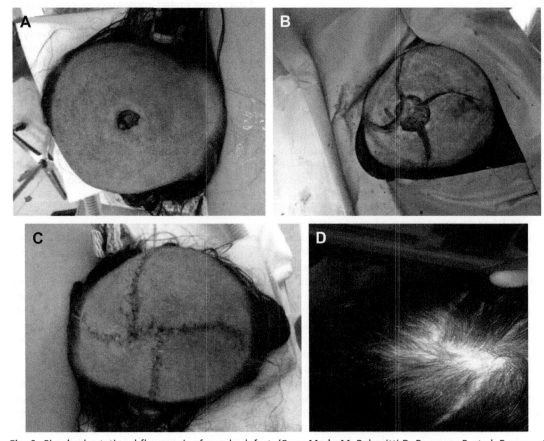

Fig. 6. Pinwheel rotational flap repair of a scalp defect. (*From* Marks M, Polecritti D, Bergman P, et al. Emergent soft tissue repair in facial trauma. Facial Plast Surg Clin North Am 2017;25(4):597; with permission.)

flap reconstruction in the scalp, case studies have described delayed hair transplantation into a latissimus dorsi microvascular flap with fair aesthetic outcome.[37] Microvascular reconstruction is an invaluable part of a reconstructive surgeons' armamentarium given its durability, flexibility, and versatility.

SUMMARY

Successful reconstruction of the scalp and forehead requires a thoughtful, individualized approach with attention to both functional and aesthetic goals. The best outcomes are achieved through detailed knowledge of anatomy and understanding of the full complement of reconstructive options. Primary wound closure is usually preferred to secondary intention healing and skin grafting when feasible. Use of dermal alternatives and tissue expansion are adjunctive therapies to facilitate scalp wound closure. Local skin and soft tissue flaps are most commonly used for most small to medium sized defects; however, microsurgical free tissue transfer can be considered for large full-thickness skin defects of the forehead and scalp.

ACKNOWLEDGMENTS

Special thanks to Graham Hadley, MD, for his outstanding artistic talent in creating the illustrations.

REFERENCES

1. Jurkiewicz MJ, Hill HL. Open wounds of the scalp: an account of methods of repair. J Trauma 1981; 21(9):769–78.
2. Larrabee WF, Makielski KH, Henderson JL. Surgical anatomy of the face. Philadelphia: Lippincott Williams & Wilkins; 2004.
3. Menick FJ. A modern approach to nasal reconstruction with a forehead flap. Nasal Reconstruction: art and practice; 2009. p. 109–54.
4. Stuzin JM, Wagstrom L, Kawamoto HK, et al. Anatomy of the frontal branch of the facial nerve. Plast Reconstr Surg 1989;83(2):265–71.
5. Seline PC, Siegle RJ. Scalp reconstruction. Dermatol Clin 2005;23(1):13–21.
6. Temple CL, Ross DC. Scalp and forehead reconstruction. Clin Plast Surg 2005;32(3):377–90.
7. Earnest LM, Byrne PJ. Scalp reconstruction. Facial Plast Surg Clin North Am 2005;13(2):345–53.
8. Pitanguy I, Ramos AS. The frontal branch of the facial nerve. Plast Reconstr Surg 1966;38(4):352–6.
9. Moore KL, Dalley AF, Agur AMR. Clinically oriented anatomy. Philadelphia: Wolters Kluwer; 2018.
10. Cheney ML, Hadlock TA. Facial surgery: plastic and reconstructive. Boca Raton (FL): CRC Press, Taylor & Francis Group; 2015.
11. Ducic Y. Reconstruction of the scalp. Facial Plast Surg Clin North Am 2009;17(2):177–87.
12. Bentz ML. Circular excision of hemangioma and purse-string closure: the smallest possible scar. Arch Facial Plast Surg 2003;5(1):117.
13. Baker SR, Swanson NA. Rapid intraoperative tissue expansion in reconstruction of the head and neck. Arch Otolaryngol Head Neck Surg 1990;116(12): 1431–4.
14. Sasaki G. Intraoperative expansion as an immediate reconstructive technique. Facial Plast Surg 1988; 5(04):362–78.
15. Baker SR, Swanson NA. Tissue expansion of the head and neck: indications, technique, and complications. Arch Otolaryngol Head Neck Surg 1990; 116(10):1147–53.
16. Barry R, Lawrence C, Langtry J. The use of galeotomies to aid the closure of surgical defects on the forehead and scalp. Br J Dermatol 2009;160(4): 875–7.
17. Olson MD, Hamilton GS. Scalp and forehead defects in the post-Mohs surgery patient. Facial Plast Surg Clin North Am 2017;25(3):365–75.
18. Ratner DCACA. Skin grafting. From here to there. Dermatol Clin 1998;16(1):75–90.
19. Robson MC, Krizek TJ. Predicting skin graft survival. Plast Reconstr Surg 1973;52(3):330.
20. Campagnari M, Jafelicci AS, Carneiro HA, et al. Dermal substitutes use in reconstructive surgery for skin tumors: a single-center experience. Int J Surg Oncol 2017;2017:1–8.
21. Moiemen NS, Vlachou E, Staiano JJ, et al. Reconstructive surgery with Integra dermal regeneration template: histologic study, clinical evaluation, and current practice. Plast Reconstr Surg 2006;117(7 Suppl):160S–74S.
22. Min JH, Yun IS, Lew DH, et al. The use of Matriderm and autologous skin graft in the treatment of full thickness skin defects. Arch Plast Surg 2014;41(4): 330.
23. Santi GD, Greca CL, Bruno A, et al. The use of dermal regeneration template (Matriderm 1 mm) for reconstruction of a large full-thickness scalp and calvaria exposure. J Burn Care Res 2016;37(5): e497–8.
24. Bertolli E, Campagnari M, Molina AS, et al. Artificial dermis (Matriderm®) followed by skin graft as an option in dermatofibrosarcoma protuberans with complete circumferential and peripheral deep margin assessment. Int Wound J 2013;12(5): 545–7.
25. Neumann CG. The expansion of an area of skin by progressive distention of a subcutaneous balloon. Plast Reconstr Surg 1957;19(2):124–30.

26. Angelos PC, Downs BW. Options for the management of forehead and scalp defects. Facial Plast Surg Clin North Am 2009;17(3): 379–93.

27. Argenta LC. Tissue expansion. Ann Plast Surg 1993; 31(6):574.

28. Dedhia R, Luu Q. Scalp reconstruction. Curr Opin Otolaryngol Head Neck Surg 2015;23(5): 407–14.

29. Fowler NM, Futran ND. Achievements in scalp reconstruction. Curr Opin Otolaryngol Head Neck Surg 2014;22(2):127–30.

30. Hoffmann JF. Management of scalp defects. Otolaryngol Clin North Am 2001;34(3):571–82.

31. Lee S, Rafii AA, Sykes J. Advances in scalp reconstruction. Curr Opin Otolaryngol Head Neck Surg 2006;14(4):249–53.

32. Hwang L, Ford N-K, Spitz J, et al. The visor flap: a novel design for scalp wound closure. J Craniofac Surg 2017;28(2):e146–8.

33. Frodel JL, Ahlstrom K. Reconstruction of complex scalp defects. Arch Facial Plast Surg 2004;6(1):54.

34. Juri J, Valotta MF. The use of the Juri Temporo-Parieto-Occipital Flap. Semin Plast Surg 2005; 19(02):128–36.

35. Fincher EF, Gladstone HB. Dual transposition flaps for the reconstruction of large scalp defects. J Am Acad Dermatol 2009;60(6):985–9.

36. Kim YH, Kim GH, Kim SW. Reconstruction of a complex scalp defect after the failure of free flaps: changing plans and strategy. Arch Craniofac Surg 2017;18(2):112.

37. Veir Z, Kisić H, Mijatović D. Hair transplantation on a free microvascular latissimus dorsi flap. case report. Ann Plast Surg 2017;78(6):770.

Reconstruction of the Ear

Ryan M. Smith, MD*, Patrick J. Byrne, MBA, MD

KEYWORDS

• Ear reconstruction • Skin cancer • Auricular reconstruction • Mohs reconstruction of the ear

KEY POINTS

- Although the aesthetic and practical functions of the ear are often taken for granted, patients with auricular deformities are known to suffer both physically and psychologically.
- Auricular skin cancer accounts for 6% of all cutaneous malignancies found in the head and neck.
- Repair of skin cancer defects is the most common indication for reconstructive surgery of the ear.
- The unique anatomy of the external ear makes ear reconstruction challenging.
- The goal of ear reconstruction is to restore both form and function; a careful and detailed assessment of the defect will inform the best reconstructive strategy.

INTRODUCTION

The external ear is a complex anatomic structure with an intricate architecture and detailed topography. The ear is unique among facial features in that it projects away from the side of the head as a free-standing structure with high visibility from many angles. Its relationship to other facial landmarks helps to create the aesthetic balance of the face. The cosmetic importance of the ear is illustrated by the practice of ear piercing, one of the oldest known forms of body modification dating back through ancient history. Functionally, the external ear directs sound waves into the acoustic meatus. It also provides a platform for eyeglasses, allows the use of headphones, and accommodates hearing-assistance devices that are crucial for social interaction, quality of life and work place productivity.[1]

Although the aesthetic and practical functions of the ear are often taken for granted, patients with auricular deformities are known to suffer both physically and psychologically. In patients with facial defects in general, recent evidence using health utility and valuation metrics has demonstrated a significant quality of life penalty associated with facial deformity. Furthermore, reconstructive surgery was seen to eliminate this effect for most defects and was seen to have high societal value as an intervention.[2] Quality of life improvements in some domains have been measured in the use of prostheses for auricular reconstruction, although with less significance and a high rate of noncompliance.[3] The impact of auricular deformity, therefore, creates a challenging yet rewarding arena for the reconstructive surgeon and patient.

The past experience of treating traumatic and congenital deformities has allowed for the refinement of techniques that today are useful for a wider range of indications. Skin cancer-related defects represent one of the most common reasons for reconstructive surgery of the ear. As the population ages, the incidence of skin cancer is expected to continue to increase. The development of Mohs micrographic surgery as an effective treatment for nonmelanoma skin cancers requires the involvement of experienced reconstructive surgeons familiar with options for a variety of defect sizes and locations. Auricular skin cancer accounts for around 6% of all cutaneous malignancies found in the head and neck.[4] The

Disclosure Statement: The authors have nothing to disclose.
Division of Facial Plastic and Reconstructive Surgery, Department of Otolaryngology–Head and Neck Surgery, Johns Hopkins School of Medicine, 601 North Caroline Street, 6th Floor, Baltimore, MD 21287, USA
* Corresponding author. 1611 West Harrison Street, Suite 550, Chicago, IL 60612.
E-mail address: ryansmithrmc@gmail.com

Facial Plast Surg Clin N Am 27 (2019) 95–104
https://doi.org/10.1016/j.fsc.2018.08.010
1064-7406/19/© 2018 Elsevier Inc. All rights reserved.

exposure of the ear to chronic sun damage, a large skin surface area-to-size ratio, and contour irregularities that may harbor occult lesions all contribute to the risk of malignancy in this area.

This article discusses the relevant anatomy of the auricle, presents a categorization scheme based on defect location, and details a variety of reconstructive options and considerations. Last, surgical timing, postoperative care, and an algorithm for surgical decision making are presented.

ANATOMY

The shape of the auricle is defined by the convoluted structure of the underlying elastic cartilage, which is folded into a series of ridges that produce both concave and convex surfaces. The very thin and tightly adherent skin of the ear shows this framework in sharp relief, because the absence of subcutaneous fat allows direct adherence to the perichondrium. The auricle is subdivided into discretely named anatomic regions based on this surface structure (**Fig. 1**, **Table 1**).

The ear projects from its base of attachment to make a 30° angle with the skull, and is anchored by the superior, anterior, and posterior auricular muscles and corresponding ligaments. The conchal cartilage is contiguous with the cartilaginous portion of the external auditory canal, which provides fixation of the auricle around the auditory meatus.

Sensation of the ear is largely provided by the great auricular nerve, which branches from the third cervical nerve to innervate the anterior and posterior surfaces. The auriculotemporal nerve, a

Table 1 Anatomy of the auricle	
Helix	Outer rim that curves from the helical root to the helical tail above the lobule
Antihelix	Parallels the helix separated by the scapha
Crua	Anterior and posterior crua join to form the Y-shaped antihelix
Tragus	Raised point of cartilage located anterior to the auditory meatus
Antitragus	Raised point of cartilage at the base of the antihelix
Concha	Made up of the cymba and cavum conchae and divided by the helical crus
Scapha	Groove between the helix and the antihelix
Triangular fossa	Bounded by the helix and superior and inferior crura of the antihelix
Lobule	Inferior-most structure, mostly fibrofatty tissue instead of cartilage

branch of the third division of the trigeminal nerve, provides some sensation superiorly, as does the lesser occipital nerve. The conchal bowl is innervated by the auricular branch of the vagus nerve.

The external carotid system provides the blood supply to the ear mainly through the posterior auricular and superficial temporal arteries. The occipital artery supplies the postauricular scalp and mastoid area. The superficial temporal and posterior auricular veins provide venous drainage. Importantly, the elastic cartilage of the ear lacks its own vascularization and is reliant on the perichondrial blood supply.

RECONSTRUCTIVE GOALS

Auricular defects can vary greatly in terms of their size, depth, and location. Regardless of the defect, the goals of ear reconstruction remain the same and attempt to restore as many features of the normal ear as possible. This process includes restoration of the various subunits discussed elsewhere in this article with strict attention to the inherent concavity, convexity, and projection of the areas involved. The overall size and shape of the ear should not be altered dramatically. Although slight asymmetries with the contralateral ear are usually not noticed because both ears are rarely viewed at the same time, techniques that preserve the size of the auricle should be preferred. Just as

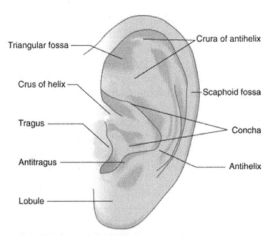

Fig. 1. Anatomy of the external ear. (*From* Wenig BM. Embryology, anatomy, and histology of the ear. In: Wenig BM, editors. Atlas of head and neck pathology. 1st edition. Philadelphia: Elsevier; 2016. p. 1076; with permission.)

repair of the vermillion border is essential for lip reconstruction, perfect alignment of the gentle curves found in the helix and antihelix are crucial to avoid easily discernible notching, height mismatch, or excessive bulk. In these areas, if the defect includes cartilage, then the repair must restore rigid support to avoid contour irregularity or scar contracture. In more central defects, this factor is less important and soft tissue coverage alone can often suffice. Reconstructive options that maintain the postauricular and superior sulci will avoid flattening of the ear or interference with the ability to wear glasses, although in many staged procedures the sulcus may be lost temporarily. Skin defects must be addressed using appropriately thin skin with good color and texture match with the surrounding tissue. Last, the reconstructive plan should address the specific concerns, perceptions, and expectations of the patient.

DEFECT ASSESSMENT

The chance for successful reconstruction is in large part determined well before the first cut is made. A thoughtful inspection of the defect with respect to its location, size, depth, subunits involved, and tissues affected is imperative during the preoperative assessment. As the first principle of plastic surgery dictates, "observation is the basis of surgical diagnosis."[5]

It is, therefore, useful to divide the ear into distinct zones to characterize the nature of the defect and plan the appropriate reconstruction. A simple and intuitive categorization scheme divides the ear into central and peripheral zones, with the central zone further divided into anterior and posterior defect locations. The peripheral zone includes the lobule and the helix. The helix can be divided into upper, middle, and lower thirds. The anterior central zone contains the concha, helical root, and antihelix.

The depth of the defect can be superficial, with skin loss but intact underlying cartilage, or may be deep if perichondrium and cartilage are missing as well. In some cases, a through-and-through defect may include both anterior and posterior skin layers as well as intervening cartilage. Partial auricular defects involve multiple subunits and at least 2 zones of the ear and can be categorized as upper-third, middle-third, or lower-third defects. A total auricular defect may result from total auriculectomy or in cases of multiply recurrent cancer.

RECONSTRUCTIVE OPTIONS

The reconstructive ladder provides a useful guide during any reconstructive procedure. It is always helpful to consider all options, including the simplest to the most complex. Simpler procedures may involve less operative time and patient morbidity, but also compromise the aesthetic result to a degree. They can also involve longer healing time and more involved wound care. Complex procedures may achieve excellent cosmesis but incur higher risk. Last, the use of auricular prostheses for extensive defects should always be considered as an alternative to surgery. An understanding of the goals, expectations, and motivations of the patient is crucial for decision making and patient satisfaction.

Primary Closure

Primary closure of auricular defects is possible for very small lesions, but limited by the adherent and nondistensible skin of the ear. This procedure can create tension at the closure, which can lead to scarring, contracture, and distortion. Closure can be considered for some posterior defects where the skin is less adherent and in the lobule, which lacks cartilage.

Secondary Intention

Healing by secondary intention can be quite effective for defect closure, but is thought to be less cosmetic than other methods. It requires patient compliance with wound care and tolerance of longer healing times, which may take up to 10 weeks. Difficulty visualizing the wound or poor manual dexterity may make this impossible for some patients. Healing by secondary intention will occur even in the absence of the perichondrium and can be facilitated by creating fenestrations in the cartilage to expose the opposing skin layer.[6] Because secondary intention will result in a depressed scar, this method is best suited for flat or concave surfaces. Defects of the anterior central zone, particularly the conchal bowl, are amenable to healing by secondary intention.

Skin Grafting

Skin grafting is a versatile and effective technique, especially in the case of superficial skin defects with intact underlying cartilage. Both full-thickness and split-thickness grafts can be used, and the choice is usually governed by the native skin thickness and the presence of perichondrium. Full-thickness skin grafts require the perichondrial layer for blood supply. They offer the advantages of less painful harvest without the need for a dermatome, direct closure of the donor site, options for facial harvest sites with closer color and texture match, and less contracture than split grafts.[7] The forehead, preauricular, postauricular, and supraclavicular skin can be used. Split-thickness skin grafts can be used for cartilage coverage in the absence of perichondrium. Split grafts can provide very thin coverage useful in the conchal bowl, meatus, and ear canal and may help to prevent stenosis. They may also be better compressed to the wound bed by bolstering, which can increase survival.

Local Flaps

Local flaps are versatile and offer tissue that can closely match native structures. They are useful for larger defects and rely on a random pattern blood supply. The geometry and design of local tissue flaps is important for successful healing because necrosis related to folding, narrowing of the pedicle, or constriction during inset may compromise the result. Specific local flap techniques are discussed in greater detail elsewhere in this article.

Regional Flaps and Free Tissue

Regional flap reconstruction and free tissue transfer can be used for the most severe defects or in the case of total auriculectomy. These techniques are useful when most of the ear framework is lost and extensive costal cartilage grafting is required to rebuild form. This vascularized tissue can cover cartilage constructs and decrease warping, absorption, and infection. Both fascia and skin can be incorporated into the flap design to provide thin covering and external lining. The radial forearm free flap and regional temporoparietal fascia flap have been used for this purpose. These techniques require a multistage approach and represent the most extensive means of auricular reconstruction.

STRATEGIES BASED ON LOCATION
Peripheral

Helix

The most important consideration in the reconstruction of helical defects is perfect approximation of the wound edges to avoid notching and contour irregularities that are highly visible in this area. Meticulous closure in multiple layers to achieve a tension-free repair will avoid these issues. The use of vertical mattress sutures to create eversion of skin edges is also helpful.

Small skin defects in the upper third of the helix may heal well by secondary intention or full-thickness skin grafting if no cartilage needs to be replaced. A composite graft including cartilage and skin can be harvested from the posterior ear and conchal bowl if cartilage must be replaced (**Figs. 2–6**). Another option is the helical cutaneous

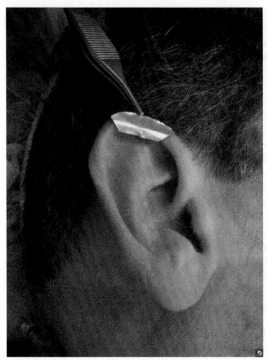

Fig. 2. Measurement of the defect and creation of a template.

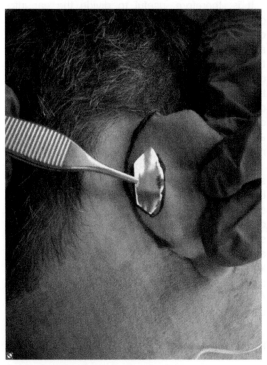

Fig. 3. Transposition of the template onto the posterior ear for composite graft harvest.

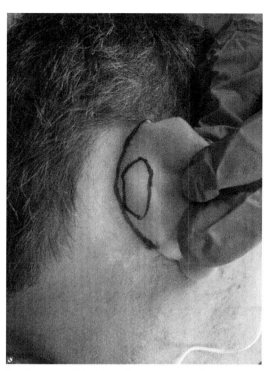

Fig. 4. Planned incisions for graft harvest.

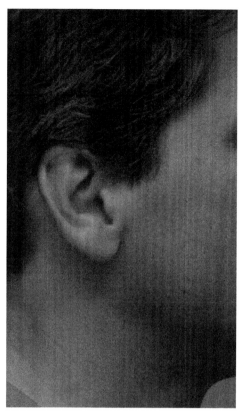

Fig. 6. Postoperative result.

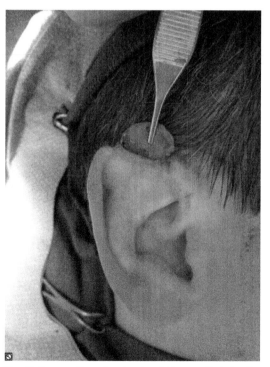

Fig. 5. Preparation for inset of the graft into the defect.

advancement flap, which is an anterior based skin flap created with incisions made parallel to the helix that is, advanced posteriorly. Preauricular cutaneous advancement or rotation flaps can provide skin coverage for upper third defects as well. Larger defects of the upper third that involve cartilage can be closed using helical chondrocutaneous flaps.[8] In this technique, a crescent-shaped incision is made in the scapha through the anterior skin and cartilage. The helix is mobilized on its posterior auricular skin and advanced for closure (**Fig. 7**). A modification of this technique converts the wound into 2 wedge-shaped defects and closure is performed with siding chondrocutaneous flaps (**Figs. 8–12**).

Full-thickness defects of the upper third require adequate tissue to restore the contour of the helical rim. A 3-staged postauricular tube flap can provide sufficient height to the helix. In the first stage, the mastoid skin is tubed and remains pedicled superiorly and inferiorly. During the second stage, the tube is lifted and remains pedicled inferiorly to be inset along the superior defect margin. The last stage completes the transfer.

Middle third defects may be closed using a wedge excision if small. Extension of the defect

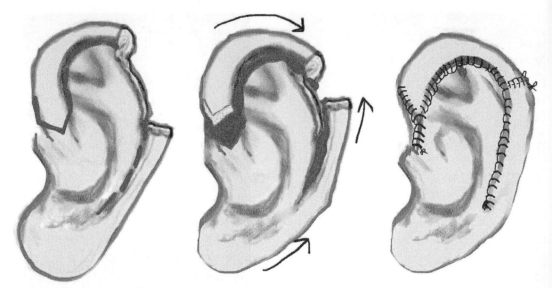

Fig. 7. The sliding chondrocutaneous flap for helical reconstruction. (*From* Sivam SK, Taylor CB, Stallworth CL. Reconstruction of upper third auricular defects. Op Tech Oto 2017;28(2):108; with permission.)

into a wedge shape allows closure without standing cutaneous deformities if the apex angle is 30° or less. In larger excisions, this angle is more obtuse and excision of Burow's triangles may be needed to convert the wedge into a stellate pattern. Wedge excision will make the ear smaller and can result in a cup ear deformity. It should be

reserved for small lesions. Modification of the chondrocutaneous advancement flap used for upper third defects into a bidirectional advancement flap can be used for the middle third of the helix.

A composite graft obtained from the helix of the contralateral ear has been used for wedge-shaped

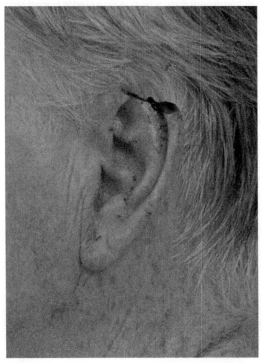

Fig. 8. Large defect of the upper third of the helix.

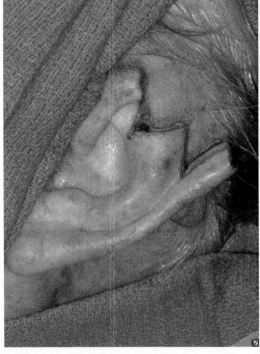

Fig. 9. Conversion of the wound into 2 wedge-shaped defects.

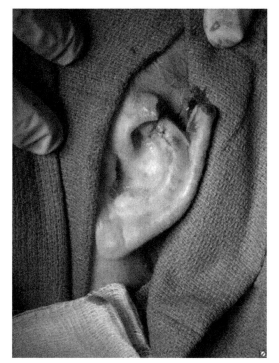

Fig. 10. Primary closure of the first wedge.

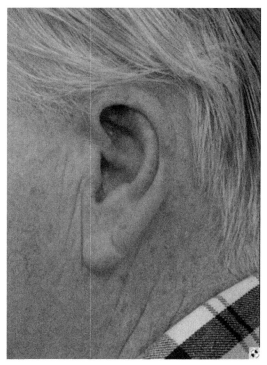

Fig. 12. Postoperative result.

defects of the middle third. A full-thickness composite graft is harvested that is one-half the size of the defect. This graft is turned 180° for inset into the ipsilateral ear and both defects are closed in layers. Use of this technique risks deforming the contralateral ear in the case of poor healing or if loss of the graft occurs.

Staged repair of middle third defects using posteriorly based advancement or rotation flaps are common. Retroauricular flaps are lifted from the posterior ear whereas postauricular flaps are lifted from the scalp and cross the sulcus (**Figs. 13–15**).

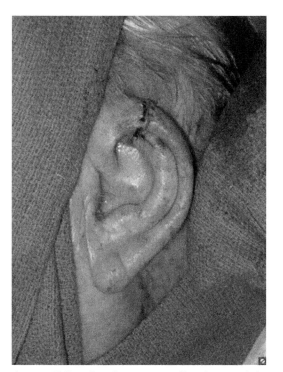

Fig. 11. Sliding chondrocutaneous flap closure of the second wedge.

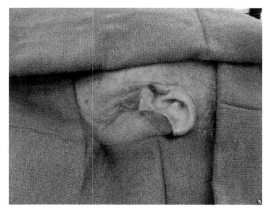

Fig. 13. Middle third defect involving skin only.

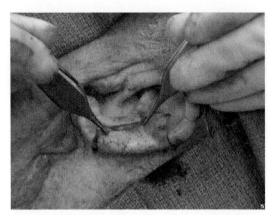

Fig. 14. Postauricular cutaneous advancement flap is lifted and prepared for inset.

The lower third of the helix is where the cartilage terminates at the helical tail just above the lobule. This area has greater skin mobility than the superior helix. Two-stage superior or inferior based transposition flaps can achieve coverage of larger lower third defects. Either conchal or rib cartilage can be included to prevent significant contracture of the flap if needed. Small defects are best treated with secondary intention or full-thickness skin grafting.

Lobule

The mobility of the lobular skin owing to the absence of cartilage in this region allows direct linear closure and wedge excision to be effective with less risk of notching seen in other areas. Vertical mattress sutures can further decrease this risk. Total lobular defects can be reconstructed with the Gavello technique, in which a bilobed flap with an anterior base is folded on itself.

Central Defects

Anterior

Concha Full-thickness skin grafting can be used for conchal defects with harvest from the

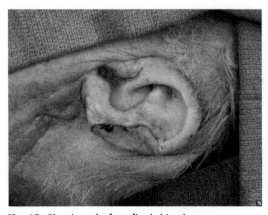

Fig. 15. Flap inset before final skin closure.

postauricular sulcus or mastoid skin. These areas provide adequate thickness and can be closed primarily. A well-placed bolster is crucial for graft survival given the concave nature of the conchal bowl. Quilting stitches can also be used to seat the graft in the wound bed.

Transposition flaps using a pull-through technique can be useful for defects of the concha that extend superiorly into the antihelix or into the auditory canal. Based superiorly or inferiorly, the flap is lifted from the retroauricular skin and tunneled through the defect for inset anteriorly. The tunneled portion of the pedicle can be deepithelialized. The retroauricular defect is closed primarily and a second stage allows division of the pedicle.

Island flaps are also used and are supplied by the posterior auricular artery. Both myocutaneous and cutaneous designs have been described. The flap is brought out through the defect anteriorly and inset. One advantage of this technique is that a large skin paddle can be used allowing a 2-layered closure of both the anterior primary and posterior secondary defects. This procedure can result in a significant reduction of the sulcus. The method described by Park in 1998 identifies the middle branch of the posterior auricular artery using Doppler ultrasound examination to base an island flap for anterior conchal defects.

Helical root Defects of the helical root can be repaired using the chondrocutaneous advancement flap method also used for the helical rim. Mobilization of the ascending helix and advancement inferiorly and posteriorly can reestablish the horizontal orientation of helical root.

Antihelix Posterior transposition flaps and island flaps based on the posterior auricular artery can be used for defects of the antihelix as previously described.

Posterior

The posterior auricular skin is slightly less adherent to the underlying perichondrium than the anterior skin. This property allows the use of bilobed transposition flaps to reconstruct defects 2 cm or less in size. The primary lobe of the flap is designed with equal size to the defect, whereas the secondary lobe is smaller than the defect. However, owing to the relative obscurity of the posterior ear, less involved methods of reconstruction, such as direct closure, skin grafting, and secondary intention, may be selected with little aesthetic cost. In defects that span the postauricular sulcus, direct closure can be used as it is when postauricular skin grafts are harvested. This strategy may narrow the sulcus and pin the ear back in an angle

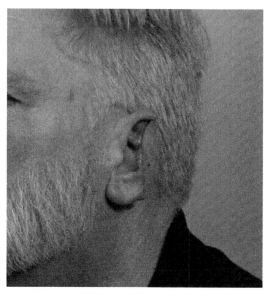

Fig. 16. Large defect involving the helix, antihelix, and crura.

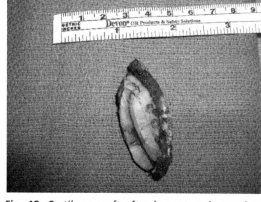

Fig. 18. Cartilage graft after harvest and carved to create specifically shaped construct.

less than the 30° of normal divergence from the skull. If this feature is noticed postoperatively at the time of suture removal, it can be corrected by pulling the wound edges apart and allowing healing by secondary intention.

If the donor skin is insufficient for use of a bilobed flap, an O-to-T flap may be used. This flap is especially effective for posterior defects that approximate the helical rim. This technique avoids a decrease in the size of the ear, unlike the wedge excision that is used for helical rim repairs. A longitudinal incision is created along the posterior auricle and the posterior skin is elevated, which is then advanced superiorly and incorporated into the T-shaped closure.

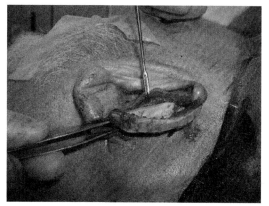

Fig. 19. Creation of subcutaneous pocket and placement of graft.

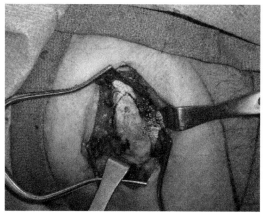

Fig. 17. Incision and exposure of costal cartilage for graft harvest.

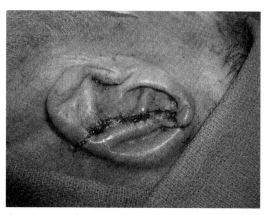

Fig. 20. Immediate postoperative result.

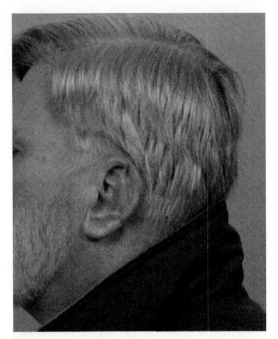

Fig. 21. Final postoperative result.

Partial Reconstruction

Reductive closures such as wedge excision, helical chondrocutaneous sliding flaps, or composite grafting from the contralateral ear can all be used for partial auriculectomy defects and have already been described. These procedures, however, will produce a smaller ear and incur a cosmetic cost in doing so. They should be reserved for patients with poor overall health, advanced age, or for those patients already bothered by large ears.

In 1920, Gillies was the first to use a carved autologous costal cartilage framework for partial ear reconstruction. This method has been refined over the last century and now represents a powerful tool for partial and total auricular reconstruction. Cartilage grafting supplies the framework needed to recreate multiple missing subunits, can be combined with soft tissue techniques for coverage, and is able to resist scar contracture that leads to distortion.

The synchondrosis of the sixth and seventh ribs is commonly harvested to have sufficient material.

The eighth rib provides 8 to 10 cm of cartilage that is well-suited for the helix. The contralateral concha can be harvested if very thin cartilage is needed. A variety of carving instruments and fixation materials have been used to tailor the graft and fit the specific need of the defect (**Figs. 16–21**).

Total Reconstruction

Total auricular reconstruction is beyond the focus of this article. Reconstruction of the entire auricle requires an extensively carved cartilage construct and full soft tissue coverage. A temporoparietal fascial flap or radial forearm free flap can be used. Alternatively, in some patients, use of a prosthesis may be the best option. Prosthetics that include osteointegrated implants can be more durable and reliable than traditional adhesive-based prostheses.

REFERENCES

1. Kozlowski L, Ribas A, Almeida G, et al. Satisfaction of elderly hearing aid users. Int Arch Otorhinolaryngol 2017;21(01):92–6.
2. Dey JK, Ishii LE, Joseph AW, et al. The cost of facial deformitya health utility and valuation study. JAMA Facial Plast Surg 2016;18(4):241–9.
3. Tam CK, McGrath CP, Ho SMY, et al. Psychosocial and quality of life outcomes of prosthetic auricular rehabilitation with CAD/CAM technology. Int J Dent 2014;2014:393571.
4. Arons MS, Savin RC. Auricular cancer: some surgical and pathologic considerations. Am J Surg 1971; 122(6):770–6.
5. Gillies H, Millard DR. The principles and art of plastic surgery. Boston: Little, Brown and Company; 1957. p. 48–54.
6. Levin BC, Adams LA, Becker GD. Healing by secondary intention of auricular defects after Mohs surgery. Arch Otolaryngol Head Neck Surg 1996;122(1): 59–66.
7. Brenner MJ, Moyer JS. Skin and composite grafting techniques in facial reconstruction for skin cancer. Facial Plast Surg Clin North Am 2017;25(1):347–63.
8. Shonka DC Jr, Park SS. Ear defects. Facial Plast Surg Clin North Am 2009;17(3):429–43.

Periocular Reconstruction

Kira L. Segal, MD*, Christine C. Nelson, MD

KEYWORDS

- Eyelid • Skin cancer • Eyelid reconstruction • Mohs • Flaps • Lacrimal system

KEY POINTS

- Periorbital reconstruction aims include restoring function and cosmesis.
- When operating near the eyelid, flaps and grafts should be designed to avoid retraction of the lower eyelid postoperatively.
- Flaps/grafts should approximate facial aesthetic units of the face.
- When defects include both the anterior and posterior lamellae of the eyelid, both elements must be replaced during reconstruction.

INTRODUCTION

The goals of periocular reconstruction include restoring function and cosmesis of the anatomic region. In the periocular area, particular care must be taken ensure that the reconstruction provides protection of the ocular surface and optimizes visual functioning. An understanding of the eyelid, orbital, and lacrimal anatomy is essential for surgical planning and preventing complications.

GENERAL PRINCIPLES

Periocular cutaneous malignancy accounts for 5% to 10% of all skin cancers. Basal cell carcinoma (BCC) is by far the most common followed by squamous cell carcinoma, sebaceous gland carcinoma, and cutaneous melanoma.[1] BCC typically occurs in older, fair-skin individuals, but when lesions present in younger patients, the growth pattern can be more aggressive.[2] Squamous cell carcinoma and BCC most commonly present in the lower eyelid followed by medial canthus, upper eyelid, and lateral canthus.[3] An evidence level rating of I (strong supporting evidence) is assigned for the treatment of BCC and squamous cell carcinoma with Mohs' micrographic surgery as well as excision with frozen or permanent section

control owing to a high cure rate. An evidence level rating of I is also applied for the treatment of sebaceous cell carcinoma with either Mohs' micrographic surgery or frozen or permanent section control with the addition of conjunctival map biopsies.[1] Less consensus exists regarding the optimal treatment of malignant pigmented lesions.

When performing periorbital reconstruction, a baseline ophthalmologic examination can aid in surgical planning. Measuring preoperative visual acuity is important, particularly if reconstruction might occlude vision in the better seeing eye, for example, when performing a Hughes flap or Frost tarsorrhaphy. Ectropion, entropion, eyelid retraction, trichiasis, and superficial punctate keratopathy should all be noted preoperatively and repaired during the reconstruction. Eyelid laxity must be addressed with a lid-tightening procedure when a defect may predispose to lateral eyelid retraction. A careful slit lamp examination of the eyelid should include eversion to expose the palpebral conjunctiva. The lesion of interest should be examined and described in detail with particular attention paid to the size, depth of invasion, involvement of the nasolacrimal system (or anticipated involvement with excision), and precise notation of the location. A thorough inspection of the lesion can aide in managing patient and operating

Disclosure Statement: The authors have no financial interests to disclose.
Kellogg Eye Center, Michigan Medicine, 1000 Wall Street, Ann Arbor, MI 48105, USA
* Corresponding author.
E-mail address: kira.segal@gmail.com

Facial Plast Surg Clin N Am 27 (2019) 105–118
https://doi.org/10.1016/j.fsc.2018.08.011

room team expectations, because the case may require special equipment, prolonged operating room time, or specific anesthesia.

As with any reconstruction, restoring function alone is not sufficient; the appearance of the final scar can have significant implications for a patient's social and professional functioning. Optimizing the aesthetic result is aided by good surgical technique and abiding by principles of the facial aesthetic unit. First reported by Gonzalez-Ulloa,[4] the regional aesthetic units of the face were described as a guide for skin grafting. The article premised that lost skin should be replaced with another region of similar skin quality with regard to histology, texture, and thickness. Cadaveric work ultimately led to the development of 14 aesthetic regions of the face, including the forehead, right and left cheeks, nose, right and left upper lids, right and left lower lids, right and left ears, upper lip, lower lip, mental region, and neck.[5] Further exploration by Burget and Menick[6] exposed the concept of regional or topographic subunits. These investigators posited that each aesthetic unit can be further described in terms of slightly convex or concave surfaces made up of valleys and ridges that reflect light and shadow. When scars, flaps, or graft borders are strategically placed between these regional subunits, they are more likely to be perceived as normal.

Most relevant to periorbital reconstruction are the forehead, upper and lower eyelid, cheek, and nasal aesthetic units. The boarders of the forehead unit include the hairline superiorly and laterally, the nasion inferomedially, and an imaginary line connecting the lateral orbital rims to the sideburns inferolaterally. The subunits of the forehead include the eyebrows and 2 imagined vertical lines separating a more convex medial from concave lateral forehead subunit. The upper and lower eyelid unit consists of 4 distinct subunits, the upper and lower eyelid and medial and lateral canthal subunits. The eyelid subunits extend from the gray line to the inferior aspect of the brow and the inferior orbital rim for upper and lower eyelids, respectively, as well as the to the lateral and medial orbital rims. The lateral canthal subunit forms a triangle that extends from the lateral commissure to the lateral orbital rim. The limbs of the triangle are formed by imaginary lines extending from the lateral eyelid margins. The medial canthal subunit forms a similarly shaped triangle that extends from the upper and lower eyelid puncta to the medial orbital wall.[7]

Relaxed skin tension lines (RSTLs) result from the orientation of collagen fibers of the skin and are reflected in the aging face as lines and wrinkles. In the periorbital region, the RSTLs are directed horizontally. When possible, incisions and skin closures should be performed parallel to RSTLs to minimize the appearance of scars and wound tension. In the periorbital area, closing wounds parallel to RSTLs creates vertical tension that can result in cicatricial retraction, and is typically avoided (**Box 1**).

PERIOCULAR ANATOMY

A thorough understanding of the normal eyelid anatomy and physiology aids I the selection of the reconstructive approach that optimizes function and cosmesis. The eyelid forms an elliptical palpebral fissure that measures 8 to 11 mm and 30 to 33 mm in vertical and horizontal dimensions, respectively. The palpebral fissure culminates in V-shaped medial and lateral commissures, with the lateral located 2 mm higher than the medial.

Box 1
Preoperative and perioperative surgical tips

- Topical proparacaine 0.5% or tetracaine 1% is used before preparation to anesthetize the ocular surface.

- Surgical preparation needs to be safe if the solution comes in contact with the eye (we suggest 5% betadine mixed 50:50 with tissue-sol).

- Local anesthesia varies somewhat by surgeon preference, but is typically 1% or 2% lidocaine with 1:100,000 epinephrine mixed 1:1 with bupivacaine 0.5% (adding hyaluronidase adds expense but enhances rapid spread of anesthetic and epinephrine).

- A 25-gauge needle or smaller is used in the eyelid.

- Subconjunctival injection is less painful than subcutaneous injection and is used for repairs involving the margin.

- Corneal shields with lubricating ointment or frequent rewetting with ophthalmic petrolatum ointment can prevent corneal drying, photophobia, and corneal abrasion.

- Tapered needles are preferred for partial thickness tarsal passes to prevent corneal perforation or an exposed suture rubbing against the cornea. Evert the eyelid after passing tarsal bites.

- When suturing the eyelid margin, use braided sutures.

- Aberrant lashes in contact with the globe should be epilated at the time of surgery.

- External photos are obtained preoperatively, after the lesion is excised, and postoperatively.

The bulbar conjunctiva wraps around the globe and is continuous as the posterior-most lining of the eyelids. The fornix in the upper and lower eyelid is formed by the redundant conjunctival continuity between the bulbar and palpebral conjunctiva. A smooth and continuous conjunctival surface is essential for a smooth blink that distributes tears over the corneal surface.

The layers of the upper eyelid at the margin include eyelid skin, orbicularis oculi, levator aponeurosis, tarsus, and conjunctiva. The eyelid skin consists of epidermis without a subcutaneous layer. At the eyelid crease (approximately 10 mm superior to the margin), the layers include skin, orbicularis oculi, septum, preaponeurotic fat, levator aponeurosis, Müller's muscle, and conjunctiva. The lower eyelid has a similar anatomy with capsulopalpebral fascia corresponding with the levator aponeurosis and the inferior tarsal muscle corresponding with Müller's muscle. The orbicularis oculi muscle serves as the protractor of the eyelid and contraction of the pretarsal component pumps tears into the lacrimal sac with active blinking. Laterally, the orbicularis muscle and fibers from the lateral tarsal plate form the lateral canthal ligament, which attaches to Whitnall's tubercle just inside the lateral orbital rim. The medial canthal ligament splits into anterior, superior, and posterior limbs. The anterior limb inserts on the maxillary bone and the thinner posterior limb inserts on the posterior lacrimal crest where it acts as a horizontal supporting band of the eyelid.[8,9] Recreating the deep attachments of the medial and lateral canthal ligaments is essential to avoiding eyelid malposition postoperatively.

The upper and lower eyelids can be divided into anterior and posterior lamellae. The anterior lamella consists of skin and the orbicularis oculi muscle and the posterior lamella consists of the conjunctiva, tarsus, and eyelid retractors (levator aponeurosis and capsulopalpebral fascia). The orbicularis oculi inserts into the eyelid margin forming the gray line. The tarsal plates in the upper and lower eyelid house the meibomian glands, which produce the oil component of the tear film. In the upper eyelid, the tarsal plate stretches for 10 to 12 mm superiorly from the margin, whereas the lower eyelid tarsus extends only 4 to 5 mm. The orbital septum is considered a middle lamella and although it is not reconstructed, it is used as an anatomic landmark.

LOCAL FLAPS FOR SUPERFICIAL AND ANTERIOR LAMELLAR DEFECTS

When defects involve the anterior lamella (skin and orbicularis muscle), local flaps are used for reconstruction. Flaps should be oriented parallel to RSTLs when possible, although minimizing unwanted vertical tension on the eyelids is essential to avoid postoperative eyelid retraction. Local flaps offer superior aesthetic results as compared with full-thickness skin grafts owing to better skin color and texture match, as well as less scar depression. Flaps undergo less contraction than skin grafts because they provide their own blood supply, optimizing the chance for success.[10] Flaps are particularly preferred in smokers owing to a high risk of skin graft failure. When reconstructing a hair-bearing area, such as the eyebrow or temple, flaps avoid unsightly gaps in facial hair.

The ellipse is the simplest and most commonly used flap in facial reconstruction. As compared with other regions of the face, in the periorbital area the ellipse should be oriented perpendicular to RSTLs to avoid vertical tension on the eyelid. Ellipses oriented in parallel to RSTLs can be used with caution in the lateral canthus, brow, glabella, and upper eyelid only when significant dermatochalasis is present. Modifications of the ellipse, such as the O-to-Z plasty, can be used to conserve tissue (**Fig. 1**). The double-S ellipse sacrifices less tissue by excising alternate halves of an ellipse. The wound is closed into an S-shaped configuration. An M-plasty, which is designed by drawing an M with 30° angles on either side of the defect, decreases the amount of tissue excised and also produces a shorter scar than a typical ellipse.

Advancement flaps are commonly used to repair anterior lamellar defects in the eyelid. "Advancement flap" refers the sliding movement of the flap toward the defect and is typically used in areas with skin elasticity. In the eyelid, advancement flaps are useful when designed such that the incisions can be hidden in the eyelid crease or eyebrow. Examples of commonly used advancement flaps include the unipedicle (**Figs. 2** and **3**), bipedicle, and V-Y (island pedicle) flaps.

In younger patients, when skin tension or laxity prevents the use of unipedicle advancement

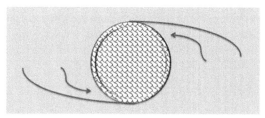

Fig. 1. O-to-Z plasty. Curved, tangential incisions on either end of the defect close tissue with a Z-shaped configuration.

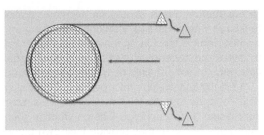

Fig. 2. Unipedicle advancement flap. Parallel incisions are designed beginning at 1 edge of the defect (the leading edge of the flap is made up of 1 edge of the defect). Standing cutaneous deformities are removed at the base of the advancement flap.

flap, bilateral unipedicle advancement can be designed such that the flaps are advanced from both sides of the defect. Closure results in an H- or T-shaped scar. The standing cutaneous deformity is excised perpendicular to the linear axis, inferior to the flap meeting point, or along the linear axis of the flaps. The flaps on either side of the defect need not be identical in length, with design determined by the potential for advancement from each side (**Fig. 4**).

The V-Y subcutaneous island pedicle advancement flap is commonly used to reconstruct defects located along the nasal sidewall extending into the medial canthus. It is easily combined with other flaps and/or a full-thickness skin graft to accommodate defects that extend across aesthetic units. The island pedicle flap is designed as a triangular island with the base of the flap formed by the inferior margin of the defect. The width of the flap is equivalent to the widest portion of the defect with the vector of the flap positioned parallel to or within the melolabial fold. Positioning of the trailing portion of the donor closure site within the melolabial fold or along the nasal sidewall optimally conceals the scar (**Box 2**, **Figs. 5** and **6**).

The depth of the flap can be modified to match the recipient site. In the cheek, where subcutaneous tissue is prevalent, the flap thickness is left intact, whereas in the medial canthus or eyelid the flap is thinned. A standing cutaneous deformity is not induced with the island pedicle advancement flap; therefore, no tissue is wasted.

Transposition flaps are linear flaps that move around a pivotal point and develop a standing cutaneous deformity at the base of the flap. Because of the location of the standing cutaneous deformity, the effective length of the flap is decreased and this property must be considered during flap design. Transposition flaps are extremely versatile. The flap can be designed contiguous to the defect or at some distance away, in areas of greater skin laxity, such that only the base of the defect is contiguous with the flap. Commonly used transposition flaps include rhomboid, switch, and bilobe flaps.

Rhomboid flaps are versatile in the periorbital region, particularly in the temple and medial and lateral canthal areas.[11,12] The flap can be easily combined with other flaps or full-thickness skin grafts. First reported by Limberg in 1966,[13] a rhombus shaped flap is designed with internal angles of 60° and 120°. Care must be taken when undermining the flap to ensure the vascular supply from dermal and subdermal plexuses remain uninjured (**Fig. 7**). Scars can be hidden in glabellar folds, the eyelid crease, and the medial and lateral canthal angles. When performing rhombic flaps near the lateral canthus, the vector of maximal wound closure tension can be directed vertically as long as the lateral canthal angle contour remains unchanged.

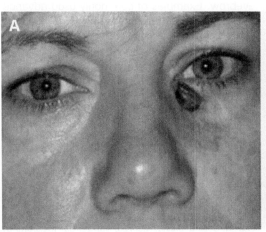
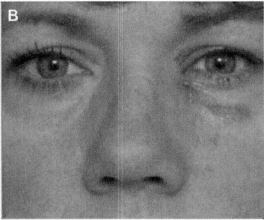

Fig. 3. (*A*) A 14 × 13-mm defect resulting from Mohs' micrographic surgery for basal cell carcinoma. (*B*) Postoperative week 1 after reconstruction with a unipedicle advancement flap.

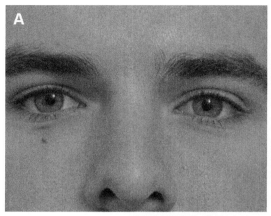
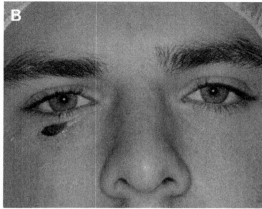
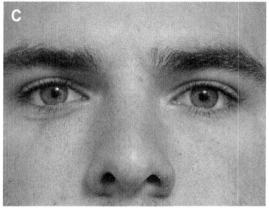

Fig. 4. (*A*) Basal cell carcinoma of the right lower eyelid. (*B*) Right lower eyelid anterior lamellar defect measuring 14 × 10 mm. (*C*) The 6 week postoperative view status post reconstruction with O-to-T plasty. Note that the scars hide in lower eyelid crease along the relaxed skin tension lines.

Box 2
Steps of island pedicle flap

- Skin is incised in the shape of a V.

- Blunt and sharp dissection is performed to the level of fascia along the length of the incision (dissection is performed with a slight bevel directed away from the center of the flap to avoid compromise of the vascular supply).

- The flap is divided into thirds such that the superior and inferior third of the flap are dissected free of subcutaneous attachments.

- The central one-third of the flap remains attached to the underlying subcutaneous tissue as the vascular pedicle.

- The flap is advanced superiorly with a skin hook and sutured to the periosteum.

- Wound surrounding the remaining flap is closed with subcutaneous sutures (these can be anchored to the periosteum to recreate the nasal sidewall contour).

- The trailing edge of the resulting defect transitions the wound from a V to a Y.

Modifications of the rhomboid flap can be used to close square or circular defects. When repairing circular defects with rhomboid flaps, the surface area of the defect is greater than the surface are

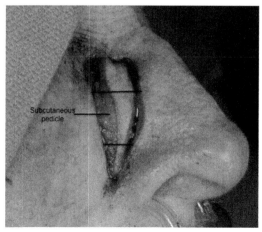

Fig. 5. V-Y subcutaneous tissue pedicle advancement flap with the central one-third of the flap attached to its subcutaneous pedicle.

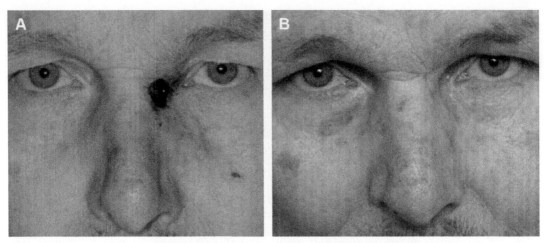

Fig. 6. (*A*) Nasal sidewall and medial canthal defect after Mohs' micrographic surgery for basal cell carcinoma. (*B*) Postoperative month 4 view after reconstruction with inferior V-Y island pedicle advancement flap and small rhomboid flap.

of the flap.[14] Additionally, the diagonal is about two-thirds the length of the diameter of the circular defect with the other side of the flap drawn at 60° and approximately equal to the extension (**Figs. 8** and **9**).

A switch flap is a transposition flap used to repair lower eyelid anterior lamellar defects. The flap is designed such that the upper eyelid skin acts as the distant flap site and is transposed into the lower eyelid defect. The pivot point and

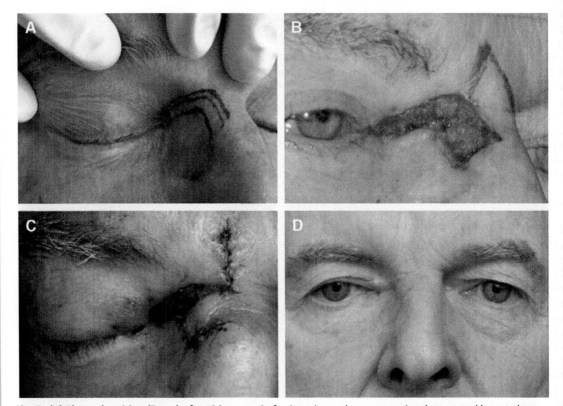

Fig. 7. (*A*) Planned excision (7 mm) of positive margin for invasive melanoma previously removed by another surgeon. (*B*) Plan for repair of a 37 × 10-mm defect with a rhombic flap measuring 12 × 12 mm. (*C*) Rhombic flap completed with wound closure. (*D*) Postoperative month 4 view status post rhombic flap plus a full-thickness skin graft.

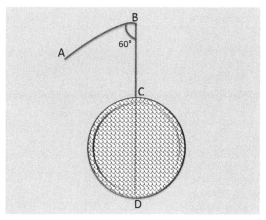

Fig. 8. Modified rhomboid flap. AB = BC = 2/3*CD. A standing cutaneous deformity is excised at the base of the flap.

vascular pedicle are located at the lateral canthus. Dermatochalasis is used for the flap, with the scar strategically hidden in the eyelid crease. The flap can be transposed as a cutaneous or musculocutaneous flap.

If there is concern for postoperative lower eyelid retraction a suborbicularis oculi fat lift and lateral canthal tightening procedure is performed prophylactically for additional flap support. The suborbicularis oculi fat lift is performed in combination with the myofascial flap when the defect borders the cheek. At the inferior border of the defect, dissection is performed in a preperiosteal plane to isolate and free the suborbicularis oculi fat from its attachments. Care is taken in the area of the infraorbital and seventh nerves to avoid injury. The suborbicularis oculi fat is then affixed to periosteum at the lateral orbital rim (**Fig. 10**).

FULL-THICKNESS DEFECTS OF THE EYELID

Classically, the percentage of the eyelid margin excised is used to determine the type of reconstruction used. By this teaching, if less than 30% of the margin is missing, the defect is primarily closed. If between 30% and 50% of the margin is excised, a Tenzel flap is used, and if more than 50% of the margin is missing, a tarsoconjunctival flap is required. These rules generally hold true; however, the laxity of the eyelid should be considered and reconstruction customized to the patient.

For small defects involving a full-thickness eyelid margin, reconstruction is achieved via direct closure with or without an anterior lamellar flap. Direct closure recreates a smooth margin contour and reconstitutes the lashes and tarsal plate. To

get a rough estimate of whether the wound can be closed primarily, 2 forceps are used to grasp the edges of the defect to bring them in contact (**Fig. 11**). Often, elderly patients or those with sleep apnea have so much laxity preoperatively that after wedge excision patients experience an improvement in ocular surface comfort. If forceps can bring the wound edges together but there is tension or hammocking of the eyelid underneath of the globe, canthotomy can be performed with or without a Frost suture. A small canthotomy is performed using a sharp scissor without a cantholysis and is usually left open to heal by secondary intention. A temporary Frost suture secured to the brow with Steri-Strips or sutures is left in place during the first postoperative week to aide in preventing eyelid retraction.

A pentagonal wedge excision is performed if the defect involves only partial thickness tarsus. Excision of the pentagonal wedge helps to create a sharp tarsal border, which ultimately results in a smoother margin postoperatively. One limb of the wedge is incised with a scissor and then the edges are overlapped to determine the appropriate size of the pentagonal wedge to be removed. Once the pentagon is excised and the tarsal borders are sharply demarcated, the margin repair is performed (**Box 3, Fig. 12**).

For defects encompassing 30% to 50% of the eyelid margin, a Tenzel semicircle flap is typically selected for reconstruction.[15] The Tenzel semicircular flap is performed with a skin muscle incision beginning at the lateral canthal angle and extending laterally and superiorly in a semicircle. The flap is undermined and rotated medially until it meets the tarsal edge of the defect. The skin muscle flap is then sutured to the lateral edge of tarsus and secured to periosteum at the lateral orbital rim. A Frost suture can be added for vertical support.

When full-thickness defects encompass more than 50% of the lower eyelid margin, a staged Hughes flap is performed. During the first stage, a tarsoconjunctival flap (**Fig. 13**) is left in place for 4 to 6 weeks to promote vascularization. During this period, vision is completely occluded in the postoperative eye. The flap provides replacement of the posterior lamella in the form of autogenous vascularized tarsus. The anterior lamella is replaced by a full-thickness skin graft, local advancement flap, or switch flap. Takedown of the flap is performed during the second stage (**Fig. 14**) between postoperative weeks 4 and 6. During the procedure, a groove director or narrow malleable is inserted posterior to the flap and the flap is separated at the desired lower eyelid margin height using an angled cut

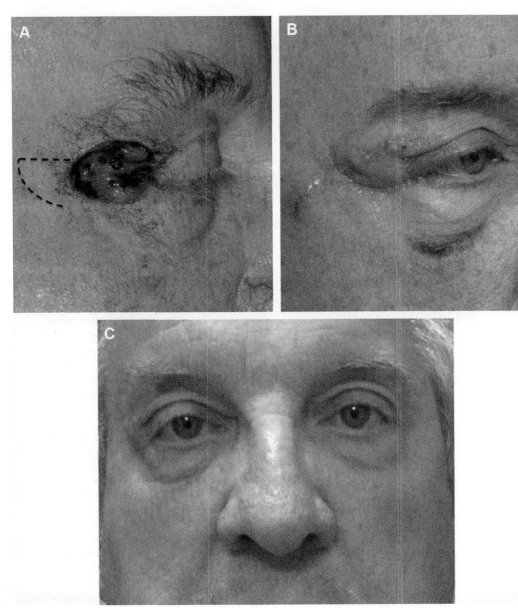

Fig. 9. Reconstruction of a temple defect with modified rhomboid flap. (*A*) The defect measuring 25 × 25 mm after Mohs' micrographic surgery for basal cell carcinoma (planned flap represented by *dashed line*). (*B*) Postoperative week 1 view after reconstruction with modified rhomboid flap. (*C*) Postoperative view at 3 months.

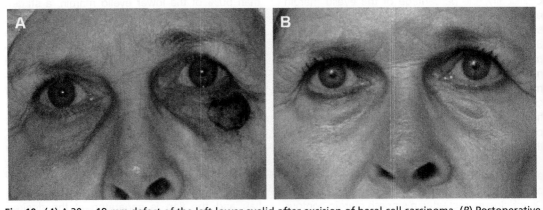

Fig. 10. (*A*) A 30 × 19-mm defect of the left lower eyelid after excision of basal cell carcinoma. (*B*) Postoperative month 2 after reconstruction with O-to-T plasty, suborbicularis oculi fat lift, lateral canthal tightening via canthal-sparing canthoplasty, and Frost tarsorrhaphy.

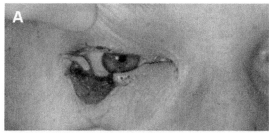
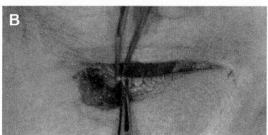
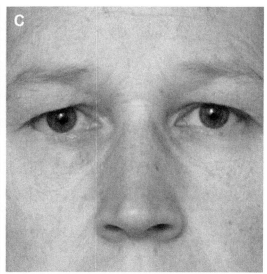

Fig. 11. (A) A 30% full thickness eyelid margin and a 12 × 14-mm anterior lamella defect status post excision of pigmented lesion. (B) Two forceps bring the edges of the defect together to demonstrate result of direct closure. (C) Four month postoperative view status post direct margin repair plus canthotomy, O-to-T plasty, and Frost suture.

to preserve a beveled edge of conjunctiva. The conjunctiva is sutured anteriorly to the superior edge of skin using a running chromic suture. Recession of the levator is performed during the takedown to avoid upper eyelid retraction postoperatively.

Regardless of the procedure selected for reconstruction, it is essential to replace the anterior and posterior lamellae of the eyelid with appropriate substitutes and to provide adequate vascular supply. Either the posterior or anterior lamella component in the reconstruction must bring along a vascular pedicle. In the Hughes flap, the vascular pedicle is composed of a tarsoconjunctival flap from the upper eyelid. Other options for vascular supply include a musculocutaneous switch flap from the upper eyelid or a "bucket handle" musculocutaneous flap from the lower eyelid.[16,17] When

the anterior lamella provides the vascular supply, the posterior lamella can be selected from a number of sources, including the hard palate, ear cartilage, or other autologous substitute.

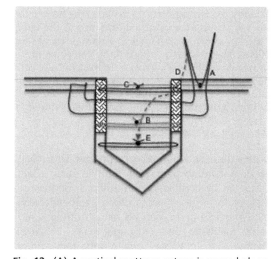

Fig. 12. (A) A vertical mattress suture is passed along the gray line and through the tarsal plate. Once the suture is placed, the wound should evert into a pouting configuration. The tails are left long. (B) Partial thickness tarsal bites are passed and tied deep to the skin. In the upper eyelid, the longer tarsal plates allows for 2 to 4 of these sutures to be placed. (C) A suture is placed through the lash line, including the tarsus. (D) The tails from the vertical mattress (A) are tied into the skin and lash line sutures (C, E) to avoid contact with the cornea. (E) The skin is sutured with or without buried orbicularis closure.

Box 3
Tips for direct margin repair

- Dissolving (6-0 Vicryl) or permanent (6-0 silk) sutures are suggested for repair.

- A monofilament suture is not recommended owing to a propensity for corneal irritation or abrasion.

- Margin sutures are left in place at least 2 weeks.

- A spatulated needle is recommended for partial thickness tarsal bites.

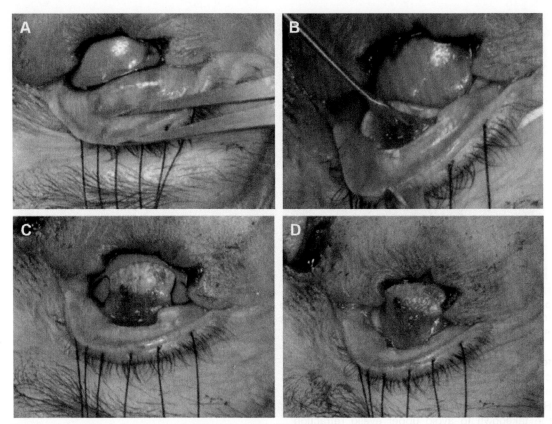

Fig. 13. Steps of Hughes stage 1 tarsoconjunctival flap. (*A*) The upper eyelid is everted and a caliper set on 4 mm measures the tarsus to remain in place. The horizontal length of the tarsus needed is also marked and measured and is typically just smaller than the size of the defect. (*B*) An incision through tarsus is performed with a #15 blade. A 2-pronged skin hook is used to lift and reflect the tarsus while the conjunctival flap is dissected. The Müeller muscle is left as a part of the flap when procedure performed in smokers. (*C*) With adequate dissection, the flap should lie easily across the defect without vertical retraction. The corneal protector should be removed at this stage. (*D*) The tarsoconjunctival flap is sutured to the free ends of the remaining tarsal tissue and superior border of conjunctiva/inferior retractors with 6-0 Vicryl. Suture tails should be tied so as to limit the risk of corneal abrasion. A full-thickness skin graft is then sutured in place.

PERIOCULAR SKIN GRAFTS

When a defect cannot be reconstructed with a flap alone, a full-thickness skin graft is used. Skin grafts can be combined with a flap or performed in isolation. When defects cross aesthetic facial units, multiple grafts can be placed strategically within aesthetic units to hide scars in facial shadows and transition zones. In the thin skin of the eyelid, full-thickness skin grafts are preferred to split or composite grafts. Full-thickness grafts tend to heal with better color and texture match, are easily harvested, and do not require special equipment. Disadvantages include longer healing time and decreased graft survival compared with other methods. Ideal locations to harvest skin grafts for periocular defects include the upper eyelid, preauricular, postauricular, and supraclavicular areas. Before selecting the harvest site, the skin should be examined for lesions, solar

damage, hair growth, and tissue laxity to anticipate ease of reconstruction of the defect site.

Harvest of the skin graft is performed by creating a template of the defect site and then marking the harvest site using the template as a guide. When performing skin grafts in the lower eyelid, a traction suture is helpful to place the lower eyelid on stretch for more accurate gauge of skin graft size. Otherwise, the graft can be slightly oversized to accommodate the stretch created by downward pull of the face with the patient in an upright position. In other periocular sites, the graft is designed true to fit and not oversized (**Box 4**, see **Fig. 16**).

RECONSTRUCTION INVOLVING THE NASOLACRIMAL SYSTEM

When defects involve the medial upper or lower eyelid, the canalicular system is examined to

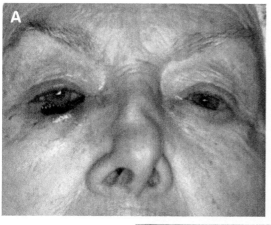
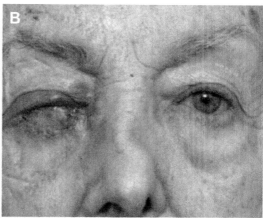
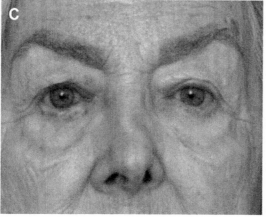

Fig. 14. (*A*) A 70% full-thickness eyelid defect after Mohs' micrographic surgery. (*B*) View postoperative week 1 after stage 1 Hughes tarsoconjunctival flap and full-thickness skin graft from left preauricular area. (*C*) View postoperative week 5 after flap takedown (stage 2).

Box 4
Steps of full-thickness skin graft

- The borders of the graft site are incised with a #15 blade

- The graft is harvested using a no-touch technique (typically a 2-pronged skin hook provides tension while dissection is performed with either a #15 blade or a scissor).

- The graft defect site can be reconfigured into an ellipse to optimize closure.

- The graft is thinned to the layer of the rete pegs (these look like small cobblestones; **Fig. 15**).

- The graft is laid over the defect and trimmed to a perfect fit.

- The graft is sutured to the defect site using multiple 6-0 Vicryl cardinal sutures followed by a 360° running suture (6-0 chromic or fast gut absorbing suture).

- A bolster providing pressure on the graft is secured (**Fig. 16**).

determine if punctum or canaliculus has been violated (**Fig. 17**). A Bowman probe is inserted into the punctum and ampulla perpendicular to the eyelid margin for a distance of 2 mm. The probe is then rotated 90° such that the probe is

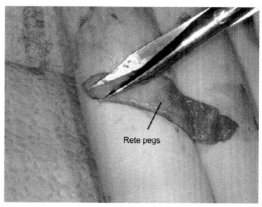

Rete pegs

Fig. 15. The skin graft is thinned, using a Westcott scissor, down to the layer of the rete pegs.

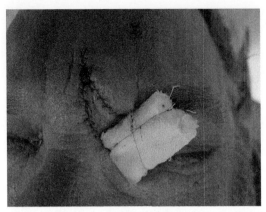

Fig. 16. A bolster is constructed by wrapping a dental roll in xeroform sterile petrolatum gauze. Sutures are affixed to sites around the wound and are tied into position around the bolster. Sutures are not secured to the upper eyelid. The bolster is removed at postoperative week 1.

parallel with the eyelid margin. Lateral tension is then applied to the eyelid as the probe is smoothly directed through the canaliculus to a bony stop at the nasal sidewall. The probe should slide easily without tension or force. If the probe is not visible and is in contact with the nasal sidewall, then the canalicular system is intact.

Defects that involve the canalicular system are repaired with a nasolacrimal stent at the time of primary reconstruction. Defects involving the upper or lower eyelid canalicular system are repaired with a monocanalicular stent, such as the Mini-Monoka or Mono-Crawford (FCI Ophthalmics, Pembroke, MA). If the upper and lower systems have been violated, a Crawford (FCI Ophthalmics) or Jackson tube (Bausch & Lomb, Rochester, NY) are preferred (**Fig. 18**). These stents are retrieved

under the inferior turbinate with a Crawford hook, forceps, or clamp. If retrieval in the nose is anticipated, hemostasis and anesthesia are optimized by packing the nose with oxymetazoline, lidocaine, or topical cocaine-soaked cottonoids during the surgical preparation. The tubes can be tied to each other in a simple knot, sutured together with a dissolving suture, sutured to the nasal sidewall, or left hanging loose. In-office removal of the tubes is performed between 3 and 6 months postoperatively. Affixing the tubes with too great a tension can cause punctal erosion. Tubes should be handled with smooth forceps, because sharp instruments can puncture, stretch or fracture the stent. Once the stents are positioned, the pericanalicular tissue is carefully sutured around the stent on 3 sides using 7-0 Vicryl such that the tube is completely covered by canalicular tissue. If the entire canaliculus and punctum are excised, then a conjunctivodacryocystorhinostomy with a Jones tube is required. This procedure can be performed secondarily if a specialist is needed.

COMPLICATIONS OF EYELID RECONSTRUCTION

Eyelid retraction is a common complication of facial and periorbital reconstruction. Etiologies for eyelid retraction include anterior lamellar shortening, vertical tension from a flap, and medial/punctal ectropion. Common errors leading to these outcomes include poor fixation of the lateral canthal ligament to the lateral orbital wall, improper or lack of fixation of the posterior portion of the medial canthal ligament, undersizing a skin graft or flap, and/or improper deep fixation of a flap.

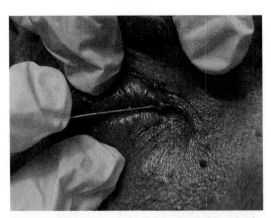

Fig. 17. A Bowman probe is inserted through the punctum and visualized emerging through the cut end of the canaliculus.

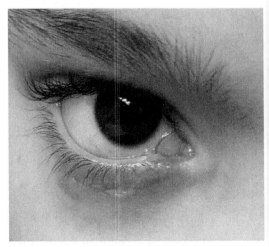

Fig. 18. A Crawford tube in good position at the medial commissure.

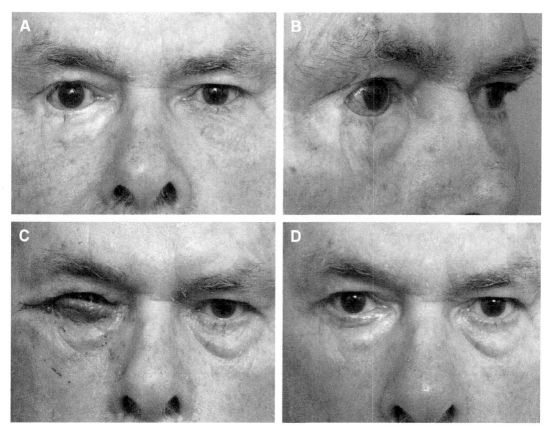

Fig. 19. (A) Eyelid retraction 10 years status post reconstruction of Mohs defect with a V-to-Y flap. (B) Preoperative side view demonstrates inferior eyelid retraction and corneal exposure. (C) Postoperative week 1 status post scar lysis via subciliary incision, suborbicularis oculi fat lift, lateral canthal tightening, full-thickness preauricular skin graft, and Frost suture tarsorrhaphy. (D) Postoperative month 2 view demonstrating improved lower eyelid position.

When eyelid retraction is caused by shortening of the anterior lamella, a full-thickness skin graft is required. An incision is made at the junction between the flap or graft and the native skin. This step is followed by complete scar lysis. As scar lysis is performed, the lower eyelid position should improve and the anterior lamellar defect will manifest. Once all scar bands are dissected free, a

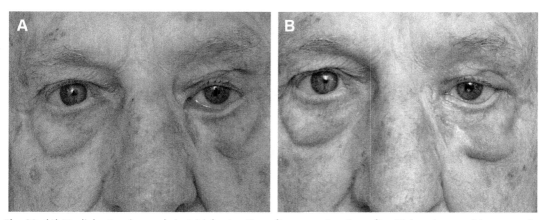

Fig. 20. (A) Medial ectropion and cicatricial retraction after reconstruction after Mohs micrographic surgery for basal cell carcinoma. (B) Postoperative month 2 view status post scar lysis, full-thickness preauricular skin graft, suborbicularis oculi fat lift, lateral canthal tightening, medial canthal tightening, and probing of the lower lid canaliculus.

Frost suture is placed through the lower eyelid margin to provide vertical support through the lower eyelid and to ensure sufficient graft size. Often, a midface lift and lateral canthal tightening are required in addition to a skin graft (**Fig. 19**). If cicatricial retraction is greatest medially, fixation of the medial canthal ligament[18] in addition to a full-thickness skin graft and scar lysis is essential for complete correction of malposition (**Fig. 20**).

Other common complications to be avoided when operating in the periorbital area include corneal abrasion, lid malposition such as entropion or ectropion, and trichiasis. When using upper eyelid dermatochalasis as a graft donor site, at least 20 mm of skin should be left in place to avoid postoperative lagophthalmos.

REFERENCES

1. Cook BE, Bartley GB. Treatment options and future prospects for the management of eyelid malignancies: an evidence-based update. Ophthalmology 2001;108(11):2088–98.

2. Leffell DJ, Headington JT, Wong DS, et al. Aggressive-growth basal cell carcinoma in young adults. Arch Dermatol 1991;127(11):1663–7.

3. Cook BE, Bartley GB. Epidemiologic characteristics and clinical course of patients with malignant eyelid tumors in an incidence cohort in Olmsted County, Minnesota. Ophthalmology 1999;106(4):746–50.

4. Gonzalez-ulloa M. Restoration of the face covering by means of selected skin in regional aesthetic units. Br J Plast Surg 1956;9(3):212–21.

5. Gonzalez-ulloa M. Regional aesthetic units of the face. Plast Reconstr Surg 1987;79(3):489–90.

6. Burget GC, Menick FJ. The subunit principle in nasal reconstruction. Plast Reconstr Surg 1985;76(2):239–47.

7. Fattahi TT. An overview of facial aesthetic units. J Oral Maxillofac Surg 2003;61(10):1207–11.

8. Anderson RL. Medial canthal tendon branches out. Arch Ophthalmol 1977;95(11):2051–2.

9. Baker SR. Local flaps in facial reconstruction. Elsevier Health Sciences; 2007.

10. Patrinely JR, Marines HM, Anderson RL. Skin flaps in periorbital reconstruction. Surv Ophthalmol 1987;31(4):249–61.

11. Ng SG, Inkster CF, Leatherbarrow B. The rhomboid flap in medial canthal reconstruction. Br J Ophthalmol 2001;85(5):556–9.

12. Bullock JD, Koss N, Flagg SV. Rhomboid flap in ophthalmic plastic surgery. Arch Ophthalmol 1973;90(3):203–5.

13. Limberg AA. Design of local flaps. Mod Trends Plast Surg 1966;2:38–61.

14. Quaba AA, Sommerlad BC. "A square peg into a round hole": a modified rhomboid flap and its clinical application. Br J Plast Surg 1987;40(2):163–70.

15. Tenzel RR, Stewart WB. Eyelid reconstruction by the semicircle flap technique. Ophthalmology 1978;85(11):1164–9.

16. Rajabi MT, Bazvand F, Hosseini SS, et al. Total lower lid reconstruction: clinical outcomes of utilizing three-layer flap and graft in one session. Int J Ophthalmol 2014;7(3):507–11.

17. Czyz CN, Cahill KV, Foster JA, et al. Reconstructive options for the medial canthus and eyelids following tumor excision. Saudi J Ophthalmol 2011;25(1):67–74.

18. Fante RG, Elner VM. Transcaruncular approach to medial canthal tendon plication for lower eyelid laxity. Ophthal Plast Reconstr Surg 2001;17(1):16–27.

The Role of Sentinel Lymph Node Biopsy in the Management of Cutaneous Malignancies

Faisal I. Ahmad, MD, Shirley Y. Su, MBBS, FRACS,
Neil D. Gross, MD, FACS*

KEYWORDS

- Sentinel lymph node biopsy • Microscopic nodal disease • Prognostic information
- Cutaneous malignancies • Nonmelanoma skin cancer

KEY POINTS

- Cutaneous malignancies are the most common type of cancer diagnosed in the United States.
- Regional nodal basins have been traditionally evaluated with physical examination and imaging, which allows for the detection of macroscopic metastatic disease but can miss microscopic disease.
- Sentinel lymph node biopsy, with the ability to detect microscopic nodal disease and prognostic information that may inform treatment selection, has become an increasingly important diagnostic procedure for the evaluation of lymph node status over the last 3 decades.

INTRODUCTION

Cutaneous malignancies are the most common type of cancer diagnosed in the United States. It is estimated that more than 2 million cases of non-melanoma skin cancer[1] and almost 200,000 cases of melanoma skin cancer are diagnosed every year.[2] Cutaneous malignancies may metastasize to regional lymph nodes through a rich network of dermal lymphatics, which is associated with a poorer prognosis.[3,4] Regional nodal basins have been traditionally evaluated with physical examination and imaging (including ultrasound examination, computed tomography [CT] scans, and PET), which allows for the detection of macroscopic metastatic disease but can miss microscopic disease. As such, routine elective neck treatment with either surgery or radiation was often advocated even for early tumor (T)-stage cutaneous malignancies with high risk features, resulting in potential overtreatment of patients without nodal disease. Sentinel lymph node biopsy (SLNB), with the ability to detect microscopic nodal disease and prognostic information that may inform treatment selection, has become an increasingly important diagnostic procedure for evaluation of lymph node status over the last 3 decades.

The term "sentinel node" was first used in 1960 by Gould and colleagues[5,6] to describe a lymph node found at the junction of the anterior and posterior facial vein, which was often the first involved node with the spread of parotid cancers. Later, several other authors used this term to describe lymph node metastases from penile and testicular cancers.[7,8] Although these descriptions were largely based on anatomic location, it was not until

Disclosure: Dr. Gross: Research Support (Regeneron).
Department of Head and Neck Surgery, The University of Texas MD Anderson Cancer Center, 1515 Holcombe Boulevard, Unit 1445, Houston, TX 77030-4009, USA
* Corresponding author.
E-mail address: NGross@mdanderson.org

Facial Plast Surg Clin N Am 27 (2019) 119–129
https://doi.org/10.1016/j.fsc.2018.08.004

1992 when Morton and colleagues[9] defined the "sentinel node" on the basis of the physiology of lymphatic drainage and the idea of selective lymphatic drainage. In this seminal article, the authors demonstrated that metastatic melanoma would spread in a predictable manner to a sentinel node and then to secondary and tertiary lymph nodes. Furthermore, they applied the principle of intraoperative lymphatic mapping to detection of nodal metastases in patients with early stage melanoma. As predicted by the scientific rationale behind their study, the application of SLNB has spread to other cutaneous malignancies.

SKIN LYMPHATICS AND THE HEAD AND NODAL BASINS

Lymphatic vessels, in the skin and elsewhere, are relatively permeable and are closely associated with adjacent interstitial spaces, which allows for free passage of fluid and proteins.[10] Like the blood microvasculature, the lymphatic microvasculature of the skin is organized into 2 horizontal plexuses. The superficial plexus originates from vertical projections in the dermal papillae and is located in the subpapillary region. The superficial plexus drains through larger vertical branches into the deep lymphatic plexus, which is situated in the lower dermis and the superficial zone of the subcutaneous tissue. The deep plexus leads into larger collecting ducts and then subsequently regional lymph nodes. Although there is some controversy regarding the role of lymphangiogenesis on lymphatic metastases, peritumoral lymphatics ultimately serve as the route of spread of cutaneous malignancies to regional lymph nodes.[11] Similarly, interstitial injection of dyes and radiolabeled molecules into the skin adjacent to a malignancy allow the tracer to be taken up by peritumoral lymphatics and subsequently drain into the deep plexus and regional lymph nodes and serves as the basis for the SLNB technique.[9,10]

In addition to the commonly known cervical levels I to VI, the postauricular, suboccipital, superficial temporal, parotid, and external jugular nodal groups also play an important role in cutaneous malignancies of the head and neck. Whereas the cutaneous drainage patterns elsewhere in the body are more predictable and often reliably drain to a single nodal basin, drainage patterns in the head and neck are more complex.[12] For example, a melanoma of the lower extremity would be expected to drain to the ipsilateral inguinal nodes. In the head and neck, a cutaneous malignancy may drain to multiple nodal basins. Lesions near the midline also have potential for spread to bilateral or even contralateral nodes.

Lymphatic drainage may also skip an adjacent nodal basin for a more distant basin. As emphasized by Uren and colleagues,[12] the complexity of lymphatic drainage in the head and neck "reinforce[s] the concept that the sentinel node is not simply the node closest to the primary" lesion. The complexity of drainage in this region is also likely the reason why SLNB was not widely adopted for head and neck melanoma when identification was based solely on the injection of dye.[13]

Even though lymphatic drainage for head and neck cutaneous malignancies can be complex, several commonly noted patterns occur.[14] For example, lesions of the forehead, upper face, and lower face tend to drain to the parotid nodes and levels I to III. Lesions of the coronal scalp and peri-auricular regions can metastasize to the parotid and levels II to V. In contrast, lesions of the posterior scalp are less likely to metastasize to the parotid, but can drain the suboccipital nodes and levels II to V. Furthermore, metastases to the external jugular chain are almost exclusively associated with cutaneous malignancy (vs tumors of upper aerodigestive origin).

SENTINEL LYMPH NODE BIOPSY TECHNIQUE

In their original description, Morton and colleagues[9] performed intradermal injections of blue dye (patent blue-V or isosulfan blue) into the melanoma or prior scar after the induction of anesthesia. The injection site would be massaged to promote passage of dye along the lymphatics, and an incision would be made over the expected draining nodal basin. The sentinel lymph node (SLN) could then be identified with the arrival of the blue dye through lymphatics and by findings the node(s) that stained blue. With this technique, they were able to detect the sentinel node in 194 of 237 nodal basins (82%) with a false-negative rate of less than 1%. Although this technique works well for melanomas with known drainage pathways, it was more challenging to apply to head and neck melanomas owing to variable drainage patterns and the frequent proximity of the SLN to the primary tumor site.

The use of blue dye is simple and intuitive, because it allows for the visual inspection of the nodal basin to identify the SLN. The use of blue dye in the head and neck can be challenging because of multiple possible drainage pathways. Blue dye can also stain and obscure the primary site surgical field, making the dissection of vessels and nerves difficult. Over exuberant injection of dye, particularly in the subdermal plane, can lead to staining of the epidermis that can last up to a

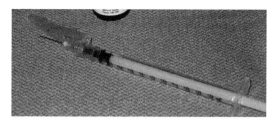

Fig. 1. A tuberculin syringe with the correct volume (0.1–0.2 mL) of dye required for sentinel lymph node mapping.

few weeks, which is unsightly in a prominent location like the head and neck.[15] The use of blue dye has been associated with rare anaphylactic reactions and interference with pulse oximetry measurements when used in high volumes.[15,16] For these reasons, some head and neck surgeons prefer to forgo the use of blue dye during SLNB. However, in experienced hands it can be administered safely and can serve in a complementary role to radionuclide tracers.

Owing to their nonspecific binding, these dyes pass quickly through the lymphatics and lymph nodes, further underscoring the importance of low-volume injection (0.1–0.2 mL) into the dermal plexus (**Fig. 1**).[9] Isosulfan blue has a slower transit time than methylene blue, and therefore is generally preferred. The use of blue dye can also influence the sequence of the procedure. For example, depending on the proximity of the SLN to the primary, it is often beneficial to start the procedure with the SLN dissection (rather than resection of the primary) to visualize the blue dye before it exits the SLN. When blue dye identification is coupled with the use of a radionuclide tracer, it is important to direct the collimator away from the primary site so as to avoid "shine through" from the primary.

RADIONUCLIDE TRACERS

The introduction of radionuclide tracers has been credited with improving the identification of SLN[17] and allowed for better applicability of SLNB to head and neck cutaneous malignancies.[13] Shortly after the description of the blue dye-based SLNB technique, Alex and Krag[18] described the use of a radionuclide tracer (technetium-99 sulfur colloid) and a gamma-probe to intraoperatively localize SLN. With this technique, a radionuclide tracer was injected into a lesion and allowed to spread through lymphatics, ultimately reaching the primary draining nodal basin. A gamma probe (ie, a radiation detector) could then be used intraoperatively to guide the dissection of SLN. This technique can help to localize where an SLN resides, and is particularly important when there are multiple possible draining basins (eg, midline lesion with possible bilateral drainage).

In addition to node localization, the gamma probe allows verification that the correct node has been removed by checking its activity count ex vivo. Furthermore, checking the activity count of the nodal basin after removal of the sentinel node can help to determine the presence of residual lymph nodes.[18,19] More specifically, if only the most radioactive node is removed from the nodal basin, it is estimated that about 13% of SLN will be missed. Consequently, it is recommended that all nodes that measure 10% or higher than the ex vivo count of the most radioactive node should be removed to ensure optimal detection of the true SLN.[20]

The most widely used radionuclide tracer for SLNB is technetium-99 sulfur colloid. This radionuclide had previously been used for nuclear mapping of the lymphatic system (lymphoscintigraphy) and was easily transitioned to intraoperative lymph node detection.[18] As SLNB became more popular in head and neck malignancies (particularly oral cavity cancer), several limitations of the radiolabeled colloid became apparent. In prospective clinical trials using SLNB for oral cavity and oropharynx cancer, sulfur colloid was noted to have a false-negative rate of 5% to 13%,[21,22] which was attributed to the particulate nature of the colloid and a lack of specific binding.[23] Radiolabeled colloids have differently sized particles (100–1000 nm) and nonstandardized preparations, which results in retention of particles at the injection site.[24] This radiotracer retention results in a shine-through phenomenon, particularly when the primary site is close to the draining nodal basin, making it more challenging to identify SLNs. The lack of specific binding of colloid to nodal tissue also allows free passage of the radiotracer from first echelon nodes to downstream nodes, thus potentially bypassing a true SLN and making the procedure more time dependent (usually performed within hours of surgery).

Improved SLN identification and a decreased false-negative rate has been demonstrated with technetium-99 tilmanocept.[23] This radiotracer is small (7 nm), nonparticulate, and targets CD206 mannose-binding receptors found on the reticuloendothelial cells within lymph nodes.[25] Tilmanocept can clear more rapidly from the injection site, and will bind avidly to first echelon lymph nodes, minimizing movement downstream to distal lymph nodes. Accordingly, this radiotracer has been demonstrated to identify SLN in 97.6% of patients with a false-negative rate of 2.6%. The specificity of technetium-99 tilmanocept binding to CD206 also decreases the time

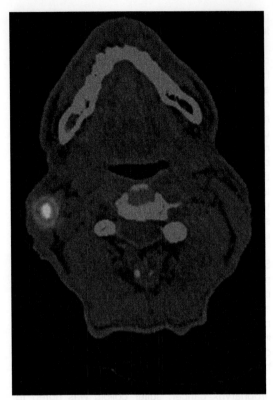

Fig. 2. A single photon emission computed tomography/computed tomography hybrid image demonstrating an external jugular chain sentinel lymph node from a temple primary. Without the anatomic detail provided by the computed tomography scan, it would be difficult to determine whether this lymph node was in level II or a part of the external jugular chain.

dependence of injections and allows for more flexibility with regard to injection time and subsequent procedures.[23] Specifically, patients can be injected the day before surgery for imaging studies without the need for reinjection before surgery. Despite some biologic advantages and compelling data from a single nonrandomized trial, tilmanocept has not been compared directly with sulfur colloid. A prospective, randomized trial is warranted for head and neck cutaneous malignancies.

PREOPERATIVE IMAGING OF SENTINEL LYMPH NODES

The use of preoperative lymph node imaging before SLNB is particularly valuable for head and neck cutaneous malignancies because it allows for a targeted approach to operative planning. The simplest mode of imaging SLNs is lymphoscintigraphy, which provides a planar 2-dimensional

image. This technique can provide the general location of an SLN, but is limited by its resolution and a lack of anatomic detail. For instance, a lymphoscintigram could provide laterality of drainage for a midline lesion, but would not be able to distinguish between a parotid or level II node.

Single photon emission CT with CT (SPECT/CT) has become increasing popular for SLN mapping. This hybrid imaging technique merges the radioactivity distribution provided by SPECT with anatomic detail provided by a CT scan (**Fig. 2**).[26] In particular, the image processing associated CT (vs a raw gamma camera signal) allows for better visualization of the sentinel node with less scatter, whereas the CT scan allows for the visualization of the sentinel node in relationship to anatomic structures. Because of the complex and multiple potential drainage patterns in the head and neck, this imaging technique has been particularly useful. For example, Vermeeren and colleagues,[27] in their comparison study found that SPECT/CT (vs lymphoscintigraphy), were able to detect additional SLNs in about a fifth of patients, and data from SPECT/CT altered the surgical plan more than 50% of the time. Accordingly, the use of radionuclide tracers and the introduction of hybrid imaging techniques has increased the applicability and success of SLNB in head and neck cutaneous malignancies.

OPERATIVE TECHNIQUE AND CONSIDERATIONS

At our institution, most patients with head and neck cutaneous malignancies undergo preoperative lymphatic mapping with SPECT/CT. This procedure provides information about drainage patterns and allows for surgical planning. If lymphatic mapping is done with technetium-99 tilmanocept and is performed within 24 hours of surgery, reinjection of the lesion is usually not required at the time of surgery. Excision of the primary tumor and SLNB is performed under the same general anesthetic. Before incision planning, a hand-held gamma probe is used to verify the location(s) of the SLN, and the overlying skin is then marked (**Fig. 3**). Whenever possible, incisions are then designed such that they could be used as a part of a larger incision if a completion lymphadenectomy is required at a later date and potentially to facilitate closure. This strategy allows for a small incision without compromising future surgical planning. Blue dye is used at the discretion of the surgeon. Proper technique is critical in cases where blue dye is used. A 1.0-mL tuberculin syringe should be used with a 27-guage needle. Blue dye should be injected very superficially into

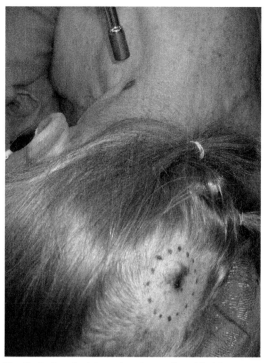

Fig. 3. Before incision planning, a hand-held gamma probe is used to verify the location(s) of the sentinel lymph node, and the overlying skin is then marked.

the epidermis at an angle near parallel to the skin and with the needle beveled away from the skin surface (**Fig. 4**). A maximum of 0.2 mL should be injected immediately before prepping the skin.

Surgeon preference can also influence the sequence of the surgery. If blue dye is used, then the SLN dissection is typically performed first. If not, or if the SLN maps very close to the primary

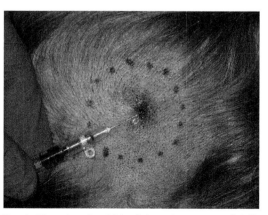

Fig. 4. Blue dye should be injected very superficially into the epidermis at an angle near parallel to the skin and with the needle beveled away from the skin surface.

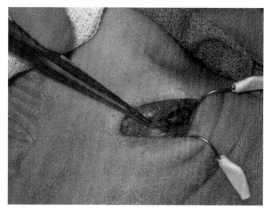

Fig. 5. When a sentinel lymph node is detected, it is carefully dissected free from the surrounding fat and fascia, and the associated lymphatic and blood vessels are cauterized and or ligated.

site, then the primary resection will be completed first to reduce shine-through. Some surgeons will change gloves and instruments between dissection of the primary site and the SLN. During the SLN dissection the hand-held gamma probe can placed in sterile sheath and used intraoperatively. The gamma probe is directional in nature, and can be used to guide the path of dissection by following the trajectory of highest counts. When a potential lymph node is detected, it is carefully dissected free from the surrounding fat and fascia, and the associated lymphatic and blood vessels are cauterized and or ligated (**Fig. 5**). Once the lymph node has been removed, the gamma probe is used to obtain an ex vivo radioactivity count. The gamma probe can then be used to obtain a count from the nodal bed. If the residual count in the nodal bed is greater than 10% of the SLN ex vivo count, additional lymph nodes are sought and dissected. The incision(s) can then be closed according to surgeon preference.

SURGEON EXPERIENCE

The reliability of SLNB is highly dependent on surgeon experience. This finding is particularly true in the head and neck, given the complex anatomy of the head and neck and proximity of pathology to critical structures. In a study from the early 1990s, Morton and colleagues[28] reported that approximately 30 cases was the threshold for a surgeon to become comfortable with intraoperative lymphatic mapping in the head and neck. They found that one surgeon's success in finding the SLN improved from 79% to 100% during the latter one-half his experience with 58 cases. Data from the Multicenter Selective Lymphadenectomy Trial (MSLT-I) demonstrated improved accuracy even after 30 cases, with an additional 25 cases required to identify the SLN with at least 95% accuracy.[29] Furthermore, in the final trial report of the MSLT-I, the authors demonstrated decreasing rates of false-negative results with increasing surgeon experience.[30]

COMPLICATIONS

SLNB is usually well-tolerated by patients with low morbidity. In a recent systematic review encompassing 21 studies and 9047 patients (all body sites), the overall rate of complications from SLNB was 11.3%.[31] The most common complication was seroma (5.1%). The incidence of hematoma was 0.5% and wound infection was 2.9%. Although a breakdown of specific complications for head and neck SLNB were not available for this analysis, the overall complication for the head and neck was 3.5%. The risk of nerve injury was exceedingly low at 0.3%. However, injury to the facial nerve is a concern when SLN localizes to the parotid gland, because the facial nerve is not routinely identified during the dissection. Fortunately, sentinel nodes in the parotid are often located superficial to the plane of the facial nerve and can be removed safely by experienced surgeons.[19] For SLNs localized to the parotid gland, the rate of temporary weakness of the facial nerve can be as high as 10%, underscoring the importance of preoperative patient counseling.[32] Allergic reactions ranging from urticaria to anaphylaxis have been observed in up to 2.7% of patients undergoing SLNB.[33,34]

Arguably, the most serious potential complication of SLNB is a false-negative result, whereby a patient develops nodal disease after a biopsy in which the removed "sentinel node" is reported negative. This outcome typically represents a failure of the SLNB to detect the true SLN, and is reasoned to occur when radiotracer and or dye passes from first-tier nodes to second-tier nodes, and the second-tier nodes are identified and removed as the "sentinel node." Initial reports for SLNB for head and neck melanoma demonstrated false-negative rates as high as 20%.[19,35] However, more recent studies of cutaneous melanomas of the head and neck have demonstrated false negative rates between 3.4% to 9%, which is comparable with non–head and neck sites.[36–38]

APPLICATIONS OF SENTINEL LYMPH NODE BIOPSY

SLNB was originally described in the management of cutaneous melanoma. This technique has demonstrated value in detecting occult metastases, allowing for accurate regional staging, and thus its applications have expanded to other cutaneous malignancies as well as mucosal malignancies of the upper aerodigestive tract. We briefly describe the application of SLNB in several head and neck cutaneous malignancies, including melanoma, Merkel cell carcinoma (MCC), and high-risk squamous cell carcinoma.

Melanoma

In 2017, more than 87,000 new cases of melanoma were diagnosed.[39] Although melanoma accounts for about 5% of all cutaneous malignancies in the United States, it is the leading cause of skin cancer mortality.[40] Local disease can be treated effectively with surgical excision with wide margins. However, the presence of regional nodal disease, which has a positive association with tumor thickness, is the most important prognostic factor associated with survival.[4,30] Before SLNB, patients with obvious nodal disease or at those at high risk of occult nodal disease underwent lymphadenectomy, and patients with a low risk of occult disease underwent nodal observation. SLNB has now become standard of care for melanoma at risk of occult nodal disease, because it provides a more precise evaluation of nodal status and allows for effective staging to guide therapeutic options.[41]

The MSLT-I study, which commenced in 1994 and enrolled 1347 patients, was designed to determine whether SLNB should be performed in patients with intermediate thickness melanomas (Breslow thickness of 1.2–3.5 mm) to identify occult nodal metastases and to determine whether immediate completion lymphadenectomy yielded better outcomes compared with observation followed by lymphadenectomy for nodal recurrences.[42] In this study, the rate of identification of a SLN was 99.4%, and 16% of patients who underwent SLNB had occult disease, establishing SLNB as a valid method for detection of occult disease. At 5 years, the disease-free survival rate was 53.4% (±4.9%) for patients with positive SLNB compared with 83.2% (±1.6%) for negative SLNB (P < .001), confirming that nodal disease was associated with a poor survival. Patients undergoing SLNB and subsequent completion lymphadenectomy had a 5-year disease-free survival rate of 72.3% (±4.6%) compared with 52.4% (±5.9%; P = .004) for patients who underwent observation and lymphadenectomy after recurrence. This study demonstrated the benefits of early lymphadenectomy for occult disease versus observation without SLNB and delayed lymphadenectomy.

In a subsequent international trial, the second Multicenter Selective Lymphadenectomy Trial (MSLT-II) compared immediate lymphadenectomy after a positive SLNB with observation.[43] The authors found that immediate completion lymphadenectomy was associated with improved 3-year regional control (92% ± 1.0% vs 77% ± 1.5%; P < .001), but no difference in 3-year melanoma-specific survival rates. Similar results were found in a German Dermatologic Cooperative Oncology Group study examining complete lymph node dissection versus observation for SLN positive melanoma.[44] Consequently, the authors of the MSLT-II trial and other studies have suggested that, in addition to being a diagnostic technique, SLNB may have some therapeutic usefulness/benefit in a certain subset of patients with micrometastatic nodal disease.[43–45] Furthermore, the benefits of adjuvant systemic therapies (including immunotherapy and targeted therapies) for this subset of patients with node-positive disease is currently an area of active research interest.[46–48] Taken together, the decision regarding completion lymphadenectomy after a positive SLNB for head and neck melanoma has become more complex. At MD Anderson Cancer Center, this decision is currently made on a case-by-case basis after a comprehensive discussion with the multidisciplinary team.

Because of the significance of clinically occult nodes and SLNB in melanoma, the eighth edition of the American Joint Committee on Cancer Cancer Staging manual includes SLN status as part of the staging system for melanoma.[49] The presence of a single, 2 to 3, or more than 4 clinically occult nodes as found by SLNB are staged as N1a, N2a, and N3a, respectively. The presence of micrometastases was included in the staging system because of the improved survival with occult disease versus clinically evident nodal disease.[50] Based on the new staging system, the American Society of Clinical Oncology and the Society of Surgical Oncology recommend the routine use of SLNB in patients with thin melanomas with high-risk features such as ulceration (T1b, 0.8–1.0 mm), intermediate thickness melanomas (T2 or T3, >1.0–4.0 mm), and thick melanomas (T4, >4.0 mm).[39] These guidelines for SLNB apply to melanomas arising from the head and neck.

Merkel Cell Carcinoma

MCC is a rare and aggressive cutaneous malignancy that was first described in 1972.[51] This malignancy is thought to arise from Merkel cells in the basal layer of the epidermis that are associated with skin mechanoreceptors.[52] A viral pathogenesis with Merkel cell polyomavirus has been implicated as well.[53] About 1500 cases are diagnosed a year in the United States, with the malignancy affecting persons with light skin, immunosuppression, those with concurrent malignancies, and those who are older.[54,55] The most frequent anatomic location for MCC is the head and neck (43%).[56] Involvement of regional lymph nodes is the most important predictor of survival, with a 5-year overall survival of 51%, 35%, and 14% for local, nodal, and distant disease at first presentation, respectively.[57] For patients with local disease that is treated with wide local excision only, the rate of nodal recurrence is between 58% and 65%.[58,59] Furthermore, the 5-year overall survival rates are 40% and 27% for clinically occult and clinically apparent nodal disease, respectively.[57]

Owing to the importance of nodal disease and the high rates of nodal recurrence, the National Comprehensive Cancer Network guidelines for MCC recommend SLNB in cases where there is no clinical or radiographic evidence of nodal involvement.[60] SLNB for MCC has rates of SLN detection between 96% and 100%.[61,62] SLNB is positive for occult nodal metastases in 32% to 45% of patients with clinical node negative disease. A recent meta-analysis, however, demonstrated a false-negative rate of 17% for SLNB for MCC, which is higher than melanoma.[63]

The Surveillance, Epidemiology, and End Results database data reported an improved 5-year survival for patients with a negative SLNB compared with those with a positive biopsy (85% vs 65%).[64] Patients with a negative SLN also do not require a completion lymphadenectomy, but may undergo observation of the nodal basin or radiation therapy.[60] However, there are some data to suggest that adjuvant regional radiotherapy after a negative SLNB does not improve regional recurrence rates and observation is an appropriate option.[63] Patients with a positive SLNB may be treated with either completion lymphadenectomy and radiation or radiation alone. Both treatment approaches have been shown to improve regional control rates, although there is no consensus regarding the optimal treatment for patients with positive SLNB.[65–67] There are no data to suggest that the excision of SLN in MCC confers a therapeutic benefit, as there is with melanoma. As such, SLNB in MCC can provide important prognostic information and allow tailoring of treatment, but further prospective studies are required to determine the therapeutic benefits of SLNB.

High-Risk Cutaneous Squamous Cell Carcinoma

Cutaneous squamous cell carcinoma (CSCC) is the second most common nonmelanoma skin cancer and accounts for approximately 20% of nonmelanoma skin cancers.[68] The incidence of CSCC has increased in the United States over the last 20 years and it is estimated that more than 700,000 cases are diagnosed each year.[69] In additional to known risk factors such as age, fair skin, and UV exposure, the degree and duration of immunosuppression also increases the risk of developing CSCC.[70,71] The rate of metastases to regional lymph nodes of CSCC is between 2% and 5%.[72–74] High-risk features such as a tumor thickness of greater than 4 mm, a Clark level of 4 or greater, size greater than 20 mm, ear and lip primary sites, perineural invasion, and poorly differentiated histology are associated with rates of nodal metastases[75] of between 11% and 50%. Similar to head and neck melanoma, the presence of regional metastasis to cervical lymph nodes is an important prognostic factor and is associated with a decreased overall survival of 25% to 35% at 5 years compared with 98% for nonmetastatic CSCC.[76,77] Considering the disparity in survival for metastatic CSCC compared with nonmetastatic disease, there has been increasing interest in SLNB as a prognostic indicator.

In a systematic review examining SLNB for high-risk CSCC (including non–head and neck sites), the rate of SLN identification was 98.5%.[78] The authors found that the probability of SLN positivity was 14.1% and the false-negative rate was 2% in studies that had a follow-up of greater than 2 years. A systematic review of SLNB for head and neck CSCC had similar findings, with a 100% SLN identification rate, 13.5% SLN positivity rate, and 4.7% false-positive rate.[79] These studies demonstrate that SLNB is a valid technique for staging patients with high-risk CSCC cancer, with results similar to SLNB in melanoma.

Although SLNB can be used to detect occult metastases in high-risk CSCC, the present data are retrospective in nature. There are also limited data on the indications for SLNB and the prognostic significance of a positive SLN. Patients with positive SLN could likely benefit from completion lymphadenectomy and/or adjuvant treatment with radiation, but outcomes data are lacking. Future prospective studies are required to define the role of SLNB in high-risk CSCC and to determine whether this technique can be used to improve regional control and survival.

SUMMARY

SLNB has developed into an important technique in the management of head and neck cutaneous malignancies. Although SLNB was initially considered challenging in the head and neck owing to complex drainage patterns, the development of radionuclide dyes and advances in imaging (ie, SPECT/CT) have improved SLN localization and reliability. This technique is extremely valuable in cutaneous malignancies with a high risk of harboring occult metastases, where nodal status and prognostic information is vital in selecting the appropriate regional lymph node treatment and systemic therapy.

REFERENCES

1. Rogers HW, Weinstock MA, Feldman SR, et al. Incidence estimate of nonmelanoma skin cancer (Keratinocyte Carcinomas) in the U.S. Population, 2012. JAMA Dermatol 2015;151:1081–6.
2. Siegel RL, Miller KD, Jemal A. Cancer statistics, 2018. CA Cancer J Clin 2018;68:7–30.
3. Dinehart SM, Pollack SV. Metastases from squamous cell carcinoma of the skin and lip. An analysis of twenty-seven cases. J Am Acad Dermatol 1989;21:241–8.
4. Gershenwald JE, Thompson W, Mansfield PF, et al. Multi-institutional melanoma lymphatic mapping experience: the prognostic value of sentinel lymph node status in 612 stage I or II melanoma patients. J Clin Oncol 1999;17:976–83.
5. Gould EA, Winship T, Philbin PH, et al. Observations on a "sentinel node" in cancer of the parotid. Cancer 1960;13:77–8.
6. Nieweg OE, Uren RF, Thompson JF. The history of sentinel lymph node biopsy. Cancer J 2015;21:3–6.
7. Sayegh E, Brooks T, Sacher E, et al. Lymphangiography of the retroperitoneal lymph nodes through the inguinal route. J Urol 1966;95:102–7.
8. Cabanas RM. An approach for the treatment of penile carcinoma. Cancer 1977;39:456–66.
9. Morton DL, Wen DR, Wong JH, et al. Technical details of intraoperative lymphatic mapping for early stage melanoma. Arch Surg 1992;127:392–9.
10. Skobe M, Detmar M. Structure, function, and molecular control of the skin lymphatic system. J Investig Dermatol Symp Proc 2000;5:14–9.
11. Stacker SA, Achen MG, Jussila L, et al. Lymphangiogenesis and cancer metastasis. Nat Rev Cancer 2002;2:573–83.
12. Uren RF, Howman-Giles R, Thompson JF. Patterns of lymphatic drainage from the skin in patients with melanoma. J Nucl Med 2003;44:570–82.
13. Dwojak S, Emerick KS. Sentinel lymph node biopsy for cutaneous head and neck malignancies. Expert Rev Anticancer Ther 2015;15:305–15.

14. Pathak I, O'Brien CJ, Petersen-Schaeffer K, et al. Do nodal metastases from cutaneous melanoma of the head and neck follow a clinically predictable pattern? Head Neck 2001;23:785–90.

15. van der Ploeg IM, Madu MF, van der Hage JA, et al. Blue dye can be safely omitted in most sentinel node procedures for melanoma. Melanoma Res 2016;26: 464–8.

16. Howard JD, Moo V, Sivalingam P. Anaphylaxis and other adverse reactions to blue dyes: a case series. Anaesth Intensive Care 2011;39:287–92.

17. Albertini JJ, Cruse CW, Rapaport D, et al. Intraoperative radio-lympho-scintigraphy improves sentinel lymph node identification for patients with melanoma. Ann Surg 1996;223:217–24.

18. Alex JC, Krag DN. Gamma-probe guided localization of lymph nodes. Surg Oncol 1993;2:137–43.

19. Bagaria SP, Faries MB, Morton DL. Sentinel node biopsy in melanoma: technical considerations of the procedure as performed at the John Wayne Cancer Institute. J Surg Oncol 2010;101:669–76.

20. McMasters KM, Reintgen DS, Ross MI, et al. Sentinel lymph node biopsy for melanoma: how many radioactive nodes should be removed? Ann Surg Oncol 2001;8:192–7.

21. Alkureishi LW, Ross GL, Shoaib T, et al. Sentinel node biopsy in head and neck squamous cell cancer: 5-year follow-up of a European multicenter trial. Ann Surg Oncol 2010;17:2459–64.

22. Civantos FJ, Zitsch RP, Schuller DE, et al. Sentinel lymph node biopsy accurately stages the regional lymph nodes for T1-T2 oral squamous cell carcinomas: results of a prospective multi-institutional trial. J Clin Oncol 2010;28:1395–400.

23. Agrawal A, Civantos FJ, Brumund KT, et al. [(99m) Tc]Tilmanocept accurately detects sentinel lymph nodes and predicts node pathology status in patients with oral squamous cell carcinoma of the head and neck: results of a phase iii multi-institutional trial. Ann Surg Oncol 2015;22:3708–15.

24. Wallace AM, Hoh CK, Limmer KK, et al. Sentinel lymph node accumulation of Lymphoseek and Tc-99m-sulfur colloid using a "2-day" protocol. Nucl Med Biol 2009;36:687–92.

25. Azad AK, Rajaram MV, Metz WL, et al. gamma-tilmanocept, a new radiopharmaceutical tracer for cancer sentinel lymph nodes, binds to the mannose receptor (CD206). J Immunol 2015;195: 2019–29.

26. Veenstra HJ, Vermeeren L, Olmos RA, et al. The additional value of lymphatic mapping with routine SPECT/CT in unselected patients with clinically localized melanoma. Ann Surg Oncol 2012;19: 1018–23.

27. Vermeeren L, Valdes Olmos RA, Klop WM, et al. SPECT/CT for sentinel lymph node mapping in head and neck melanoma. Head Neck 2011;33:1–6.

28. Morton DL, Wen DR, Foshag LJ, et al. Intraoperative lymphatic mapping and selective cervical lymphadenectomy for early-stage melanomas of the head and neck. J Clin Oncol 1993;11:1751–6.

29. Morton DL, Cochran AJ, Thompson JF, et al. Sentinel node biopsy for early-stage melanoma: accuracy and morbidity in MSLT-I, an international multicenter trial. Ann Surg 2005;242:302–11 [discussion: 11–3].

30. Morton DL, Thompson JF, Cochran AJ, et al. Final trial report of sentinel-node biopsy versus nodal observation in melanoma. N Engl J Med 2014;370: 599–609.

31. Moody JA, Ali RF, Carbone AC, et al. Complications of sentinel lymph node biopsy for melanoma - a systematic review of the literature. Eur J Surg Oncol 2017;43:270–7.

32. Picon AI, Coit DG, Shaha AR, et al. Sentinel lymph node biopsy for cutaneous head and neck melanoma: mapping the parotid gland. Ann Surg Oncol 2016;23:9001–9.

33. Scherer K, Studer W, Figueiredo V, et al. Anaphylaxis to isosulfan blue and cross-reactivity to patent blue V: case report and review of the nomenclature of vital blue dyes. Ann Allergy Asthma Immunol 2006;96: 497–500.

34. Tripathy S, Nair PV. Adverse drug reaction, patent blue V dye and anaesthesia. Indian J Anaesth 2012;56:563–6.

35. de Rosa N, Lyman GH, Silbermins D, et al. Sentinel node biopsy for head and neck melanoma: a systematic review. Otolaryngol Head Neck Surg 2011; 145:375–82.

36. Davis-Malesevich MV, Goepfert R, Kubik M, et al. Recurrence of cutaneous melanoma of the head and neck after negative sentinel lymph node biopsy. Head Neck 2015;37:1116–21.

37. Erman AB, Collar RM, Griffith KA, et al. Sentinel lymph node biopsy is accurate and prognostic in head and neck melanoma. Cancer 2012;118: 1040–7.

38. Miller MW, Vetto JT, Monroe MM, et al. False-negative sentinel lymph node biopsy in head and neck melanoma. Otolaryngol Head Neck Surg 2011;145:606–11.

39. Wong SL, Faries MB, Kennedy EB, et al. Sentinel lymph node biopsy and management of regional lymph nodes in melanoma: American Society of Clinical Oncology and Society of Surgical Oncology clinical practice guideline update. J Clin Oncol 2018;36:399–413.

40. Miller AJ, Mihm MC Jr. Melanoma. N Engl J Med 2006;355:51–65.

41. Balch CM, Morton DL, Gershenwald JE, et al. Sentinel node biopsy and standard of care for melanoma. J Am Acad Dermatol 2009;60:872–5.

42. Morton DL, Thompson JF, Cochran AJ, et al. Sentinel-node biopsy or nodal observation in melanoma. N Engl J Med 2006;355:1307–17.

43. Faries MB, Thompson JF, Cochran AJ, et al. Completion dissection or observation for sentinel-node metastasis in melanoma. N Engl J Med 2017; 376:2211–22.

44. Leiter U, Stadler R, Mauch C, et al. Complete lymph node dissection versus no dissection in patients with sentinel lymph node biopsy positive melanoma (De-COG-SLT): a multicentre, randomised, phase 3 trial. Lancet Oncol 2016;17:757–67.

45. Geimer T, Sattler EC, Flaig MJ, et al. The impact of sentinel node dissection on disease-free and overall tumour-specific survival in melanoma patients: a single centre group-matched analysis of 1192 patients. J Eur Acad Dermatol Venereol 2017;31: 629–35.

46. Weber J, Mandala M, Del Vecchio M, et al. Adjuvant nivolumab versus ipilimumab in resected stage III or IV melanoma. N Engl J Med 2017;377:1824–35.

47. Eggermont AM, Chiarion-Sileni V, Grob JJ, et al. Prolonged survival in stage III melanoma with ipilimumab adjuvant therapy. N Engl J Med 2016;375: 1845–55.

48. Long GV, Hauschild A, Santinami M, et al. Adjuvant dabrafenib plus trametinib in stage III BRAF-mutated melanoma. N Engl J Med 2017;377: 1813–23.

49. Amin MB. AJCC cancer staging manual. 18th edition. New York: Springer; 2017. p. 563–88.

50. Gershenwald JE, Scolyer RA, Hess KR, et al. Melanoma staging: evidence-based changes in the American Joint Committee on Cancer eighth edition cancer staging manual. CA Cancer J Clin 2017;67: 472–92.

51. Toker C. Trabecular carcinoma of the skin. Arch Dermatol 1972;105:107–10.

52. Ratner D, Nelson BR, Brown MD, et al. Merkel cell carcinoma. J Am Acad Dermatol 1993;29: 143–56.

53. Leroux-Kozal V, Leveque N, Brodard V, et al. Merkel cell carcinoma: histopathologic and prognostic features according to the immunohistochemical expression of Merkel cell polyomavirus large T antigen correlated with viral load. Hum Pathol 2015;46: 443–53.

54. Lemos B, Nghiem P. Merkel cell carcinoma: more deaths but still no pathway to blame. J Invest Dermatol 2007;127:2100–3.

55. Howard RA, Dores GM, Curtis RE, et al. Merkel cell carcinoma and multiple primary cancers. Cancer Epidemiol Biomarkers Prev 2006;15:1545–9.

56. Smith VA, Camp ER, Lentsch EJ. Merkel cell carcinoma: identification of prognostic factors unique to tumors located in the head and neck based on analysis of SEER data. Laryngoscope 2012;122: 1283–90.

57. Harms KL, Healy MA, Nghiem P, et al. Analysis of prognostic factors from 9387 Merkel cell carcinoma cases forms the basis for the new 8th edition AJCC staging system. Ann Surg Oncol 2016;23:3564–71.

58. Smith DE, Bielamowicz S, Kagan AR, et al. Cutaneous neuroendocrine (Merkel cell) carcinoma. A report of 35 cases. Am J Clin Oncol 1995;18: 199–203.

59. Gillenwater AM, Hessel AC, Morrison WH, et al. Merkel cell carcinoma of the head and neck: effect of surgical excision and radiation on recurrence and survival. Arch Otolaryngol Head Neck Surg 2001; 127:149–54.

60. Schwartz JL, Wong SL, McLean SA, et al. NCCN guidelines implementation in the multidisciplinary Merkel cell carcinoma program at the University of Michigan. J Natl Compr Canc Netw 2014;12: 434–41.

61. Schwartz JL, Griffith KA, Lowe L, et al. Features predicting sentinel lymph node positivity in Merkel cell carcinoma. J Clin Oncol 2011;29:1036–41.

62. Gupta SG, Wang LC, Penas PF, et al. Sentinel lymph node biopsy for evaluation and treatment of patients with Merkel cell carcinoma: the Dana-Farber experience and meta-analysis of the literature. Arch Dermatol 2006;142:685–90.

63. Gunaratne DA, Howle JR, Veness MJ. Sentinel lymph node biopsy in Merkel cell carcinoma: a 15-year institutional experience and statistical analysis of 721 reported cases. Br J Dermatol 2016;174: 273–81.

64. Kachare SD, Wong JH, Vohra NA, et al. Sentinel lymph node biopsy is associated with improved survival in Merkel cell carcinoma. Ann Surg Oncol 2014; 21:1624–30.

65. Fang LC, Lemos B, Douglas J, et al. Radiation monotherapy as regional treatment for lymph node-positive Merkel cell carcinoma. Cancer 2010; 116:1783–90.

66. Cassler NM, Merrill D, Bichakjian CK, et al. Merkel cell carcinoma therapeutic update. Curr Treat Options Oncol 2016;17:36.

67. Servy A, Maubec E, Sugier PE, et al. Merkel cell carcinoma: value of sentinel lymph-node status and adjuvant radiation therapy. Ann Oncol 2016;27: 914–9.

68. Alam M, Ratner D. Cutaneous squamous-cell carcinoma. N Engl J Med 2001;344:975–83.

69. Rogers HW, Weinstock MA, Harris AR, et al. Incidence estimate of nonmelanoma skin cancer in the United States, 2006. Arch Dermatol 2010;146: 283–7.

70. Ramsay HM, Reece SM, Fryer AA, et al. Seven-year prospective study of nonmelanoma skin cancer incidence in U.K. renal transplant recipients. Transplantation 2007;84:437–9.

71. Fortina AB, Piaserico S, Caforio AL, et al. Immunosuppressive level and other risk factors for basal cell carcinoma and squamous cell carcinoma in

heart transplant recipients. Arch Dermatol 2004;140: 1079–85.

72. Brougham ND, Dennett ER, Cameron R, et al. The incidence of metastasis from cutaneous squamous cell carcinoma and the impact of its risk factors. J Surg Oncol 2012;106:811–5.

73. Brantsch KD, Meisner C, Schonflsch B, et al. Analysis of risk factors determining prognosis of cutaneous squamous-cell carcinoma: a prospective study. Lancet Oncol 2008;9:713–20.

74. Joseph MG, Zulueta WP, Kennedy PJ. Squamous cell carcinoma of the skin of the trunk and limbs: the incidence of metastases and their outcome. Aust N Z J Surg 1992;62:697–701.

75. Schmults CD, Karia PS, Carter JB, et al. Factors predictive of recurrence and death from cutaneous squamous cell carcinoma: a 10-year, single-institution cohort study. JAMA Dermatol 2013;149: 541–7.

76. Kraus DH, Carew JF, Harrison LB. Regional lymph node metastasis from cutaneous squamous cell carcinoma. Arch Otolaryngol Head Neck Surg 1998; 124:582–7.

77. Rowe DE, Carroll RJ, Day CL Jr. Prognostic factors for local recurrence, metastasis, and survival rates in squamous cell carcinoma of the skin, ear, and lip. Implications for treatment modality selection. J Am Acad Dermatol 1992;26: 976–90.

78. Kwon S, Dong ZM, Wu PC. Sentinel lymph node biopsy for high-risk cutaneous squamous cell carcinoma: clinical experience and review of literature. World J Surg Oncol 2011;9:80.

79. Ahmed MM, Moore BA, Schmalbach CE. Utility of head and neck cutaneous squamous cell carcinoma sentinel node biopsy: a systematic review. Otolaryngol Head Neck Surg 2014;150: 180–7.

Radiotherapy for Skin Cancers of the Face, Head, and Neck

Michelle L. Mierzwa, MD

KEYWORDS

- Radiation • Electrons • Skin cancer • Melanoma • Merkel cell carcinoma • Orthovoltage
- Cutaneous squamous cell carcinoma • Basal cell carcinoma

KEY POINTS

- Definitive radiotherapy is a reasonable treatment option for early stage nonmelanoma skin cancers with favorable local control and toxicity results.
- Adjuvant radiotherapy improves locoregional control in high-risk nonmelanoma skin cancers.
- Radiotherapy plays a limited role in the management of melanoma, primarily as adjuvant therapy in patients at high risk for progressive regional disease.

INTRODUCTION

Radiotherapy (RT) plays a role in the definitive or adjuvant management of early and late stage skin cancers including nonmelanoma basal cell carcinoma (BCC) and cutaneous squamous cell carcinoma (cSCC), melanoma, and Merkel cell carcinoma (**Fig. 1**). This article reviews the background, indications, and technical aspects of RT in skin cancer.

NONMELANOMA SKIN CANCER

Nonmelanoma skin cancer of the head and neck is a largely curable condition that typically presents in early stages in geriatric populations with good overall prognosis. This is composed primarily of BCC and cSCC, which are the two most common malignancies in the United States with an estimated 3 million new cases annually. BCC and cSCC are increasing in incidence with an estimated occurrence in up to 26% of light-skinned patients older than the age of 65. These are typically associated with high cumulative UV sun exposure.

Basal Cell Carcinoma

BCC is the most common malignancy in the United States, occurring most frequently in light-skinned elderly men with increasing incidence over lifetime. The 5-year cause-specific survival is 99% with low rates (0.1%) of regional lymph node metastases or distant metastases and low 1% rate of perineural spread. BCCs typically present in early stages and are associated with UV exposure and immunosuppression. Initial treatment typically includes excision, curettage, or electrodissection.

However, left untreated, BCC can become locally invasive and destructive requiring multimodality therapy to achieve local control. Histologically more aggressive tumors include sclerosing, basosquamous, mixed infiltrative types, and morpheaform. Other risk factors for aggressive behavior include perineural invasion (PNI), diameter greater than 2 cm, long-standing presence or prior therapy (incomplete excision or prior RT), history of immunosuppression, or poorly defined borders.

Disclosure Statement: Nothing to disclose.
Department of Radiation Oncology, University of Michigan, 1500 East Medical Center Boulevard, Ann Arbor, MI 48109, USA
E-mail address: mmierzwa@med.umich.edu

Facial Plast Surg Clin N Am 27 (2019) 131–138
https://doi.org/10.1016/j.fsc.2018.08.005
1064-7406/19/© 2018 Elsevier Inc. All rights reserved.

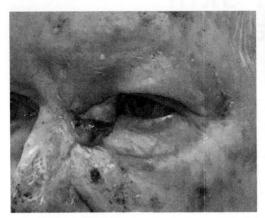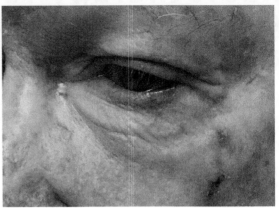

Fig. 1. (*Left*) Pre-RT photograph of CT1N0 cSCC of the medial canthus/nasal bridge. (*Right*) A 6-months post-RT photograph of the same lesion.

Because BCC typically presents at advanced age and frequently in patients with multiple medical comorbidities making them medically inoperable, RT is considered as definitive therapy for early lesions or as adjuvant therapy for more advanced lesions. RT is also considered for definitive management in cases where cosmetic or functional outcomes may be unacceptable with definitive surgical management, such as eyelids, nasal tip or ala, or lips. If RT is used in the adjuvant setting, it is typically given to the postoperative bed alone because of low risk of nodal or perineural spread.

Cutaneous Squamous Cell Carcinoma

cSCC is the second most common malignancy in the United States with similar features to BCCs with higher risk of regional and distant metastases. cSCC are also frequently associated with cumulative sun exposure and fair complexions. Other risk factors include advanced age, acquired immunosuppression (after solid organ transplantation, treatment of leukemia/lymphoma, or autoimmune disease), depth greater than 3 mm, poorly differentiated histology, and PNI. The 5-year metastases

rate of cSCC is low, but may be up to 30% in tumors greater than 2 cm.[1]

Management of Low-Risk Localized Nonmelanoma Skin Cancer

Local excision is the standard of care, but RT plays an important role with high local control rates especially in the geriatric population, which may not be able to undergo anesthesia for definitive oncologic surgery. Primary RT for medically inoperable patients or in areas of poor surgical cosmetic outcome is commonly done with good results. Areas of the face where primary RT is considered include eyelids, nasal tip/ala, and lips. Result of several contemporary institutional series are shown in **Table 1**. Using a variety of fractionation schemes from 1 to 30 fractions, local control rates are typically quoted to be 95% for BCCs, greater than or equal to 90% for cSCC, and with less than or equal to 6% rates of skin necrosis or ulceration.

With lateral or deep positive margin, the recurrence rate of BCC may be 33% to 50% and that of SCC is typically higher. Indications for adjuvant RT in nonmelanoma skin cancers include: positive

Table 1
Contemporary series of definitive radiotherapy treatment of early stage non-melanoma skin cancers and outcomes

	N	Histology	Dose Per Fraction/ Total Dose (Gy)	Outcome	Complications
Chan et al,[31] 2007	806	BCC + SCC	18–22 single dose	10 y LRR 4%	6% skin necrosis
Schulte et al,[32] 2005	1267	BCC + SCC	5/45–60	10 y LRR for T1 5%, T2 10%	6.3% skin ulceration
Locke et al,[33] 2001	531	BCC + SCC	2–4/40–60	5 y LRR 10% BCC, 18% SCC	5.8% skin necrosis
Cognetta et al,[34] 2012	1715	BCC + SCC	5–7/35	5 y LRR 4% BCC, 6% SCC	Not reported

margin that cannot be reresected, PNI, muscle/ cartilage or bony involvement, and nodal involvement. Nodal treatment with radiation should be considered for recurrences after surgery, poorly differentiated tumors, primary tumor greater than 3 cm, and large infiltrative ulcerative SCC.

High-Risk Aggressive Cutaneous Squamous Cell Carcinoma

The overall prognosis of cSCC is good, but poor prognosis has been associated with involvement of the parotid gland, advancing cervical nodal metastases (single lymph node >3 cm, multiple positive lymph nodes, or extracapsular extension), immunosuppression, and bony involvement. Local failure in the postoperative bed or along cranial nerves and regional nodal failure account for most definitive treatment.[2] Overall survival at 2 years in retrospective studies[3,4] has been 70% to 80% for N1 parotid and/or neck involvement, but 25% to 50% for N2-3 patients. It has also been reported that immunocompromised patients have a 7.2-fold increased risk of local recurrence and a 5.3-fold increased risk of any recurrence after treatment of cutaneous squamous cell carcinoma of the head and neck. Skin cancer cause-specific mortality is also increased in the setting of immunosuppression; skin cancer was the fourth most common cause of death in a reported renal transplant cohort.[5] Additionally, multiple patient series have reported that histopathology of cSCC in immunocompromised patients is more aggressive, with tumor size being less important.[6,7]

PNI has been identified as a poor prognostic factor in cSCC. PNI along cutaneous nerves may occur in up to 15% of cSCCs and has also been associated with poor prognosis.[8] Discontinuous skip lesions commonly recur despite aggressive surgical management and areas of the forehead and midface have a higher incidence of neurotropism. Involvement of both major nerve trunks and smaller nerve involvement have been associated with increased risk of regional failure and local failure in the postoperative bed or along cranial nerves. In 102 patients reviewed, PNI was defined as gross PNI (cranial nerve deficit or evidence on MRI), microscopic extensive PNI (>2 nerves involved in the resection specimen), or microscopic focal PNI (1–2 nerves involved in resection specimen). The 2-year recurrence-free survival in nerves was 94% versus 25% ($P = .01$) in those managed with and without adjuvant RT that including the course of dermatomal nerves. Disease-free survival was also significantly improved in those patients treated with adjuvant RT (73 vs 40%; $P = .05$).[9]

Management of Aggressive Cutaneous Squamous Cell Carcinoma

cSCC is most commonly managed with primary surgery, although very locally advanced lesions can be treated with primary RT. Including patients salvaged with surgery, larger skin cancers can have control rates of 80% with primary RT treatment.[10] After radical resection, indications for postoperative RT include positive surgical margins, PNI, positive lymph nodes, invasion of bone or cartilage, and extensive skeletal muscle infiltration. Despite surgery and postoperative RT, approximately 25% patients experience locoregional failure, 25% develop distant metastases, and the 2-year overall survival in several large series is reported to be 40% to 55%.[11–13]

Adjuvant radiotherapy

Postoperative RT alone is the current standard of care for patients with locally advanced cSCC of the head and neck. Radiation fields for adjuvant treatment typically include the postoperative bed and a generous radial and deep margin of approximately 1 to 2 cm treated to 60 to 66 Gy. Because many recurrences are the result of marginal miss, computed tomography (CT) and/or MRI are often helpful in the delineation of appropriate treatment lateral and deep margin. For patients with positive lymph nodes, the nodal basins at risk are included in treatment volume. Depending on indication, this frequently includes the ipsilateral parotid and ipsilateral neck (**Fig. 2**). For close margins, the primary tumor bed and margin may be included in a boost volume to 66 to 70 Gy. In patients with PNI, trigeminal and facial nerve pathways are frequently at risk. Clinical target volumes in patients with PNI should include pathways along cranial nerves that supply the primary tumor site.[14]

Adjuvant concurrent chemoradiation

Although many have extrapolated the use of adjuvant chemoradiation from mucosal head and neck squamous cell carcinomas, there is currently no prospective positive evidence for the addition of concurrent cytotoxic chemotherapy or cetuximab. A recent negative prospective trial reported by TROG randomized 321 patients with high-risk cSCC patients to adjuvant RT alone or RT plus concurrent weekly carboplatin (AUC 2), showing no observed benefit from the addition of weekly carboplatin.[15] The lack of significant benefit on this trial has been in part attributed to a high rate of freedom from locoregional recurrence (88%) observed for adjuvant RT alone.

Several studies have demonstrated high epidermal growth factor receptor (EGFR) expression in cSCC, thus leading scientists to believe

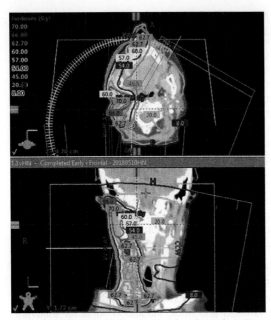

Fig. 2. Adjuvant radiotherapy field with isodose lines for a patient with nodal recurrence of cSCC on right cheek/nasal ala. Pathology demonstrated 2/50 positive lymph nodes in the right neck and a single positive lymph node in right parotid with extracapsular extension. No perineural invasion was identified on any pathology specimen.

that EGFR inhibition may be of value with concurrent RT in the adjuvant setting for high-risk cSCC. In locally advanced unresectable cSCC, cetuximab has been investigated as a single agent, demonstrating 69% disease control rate at 6 weeks by RECIST criteria.[16] Seventy-eight percent of patients developed grade 2 acneiform rash, which was associated with prolonged disease-free survival. To date, cetuximab has not been prospectively investigated in the adjuvant setting with concurrent RT for cSCC.

Currently, there is much interest in the role of immunotherapy in aggressive cSCC and current trials of anti-PDL1 in metastatic cSCC are ongoing. Genomic studies have shown high mutational burden in cSCC caused by cumulative UV exposure, which may be associated with high response rates to immunotherapy regimens.[17]

MELANOMA

The incidence of cutaneous melanoma is increasing at an alarming rate and cutaneous melanoma is responsible for most skin cancer–related deaths.[18,19] Primary head and neck melanoma represents almost 30% of all cutaneous melanoma, although the head and neck represent only 9% of the total body surface area, possibly attributable to higher melanocyte concentration and increased sun exposure in the head and neck. The role of RT in melanoma is largely adjuvant therapy for advanced nodal or primary disease after definitive resection and lymph node dissection. Other roles of RT include palliation in distant metastases and rarely definitive treatment of primary lesions.

Although melanoma has historically been considered a radioresistant tumor, high rates of locoregional control have been achieved with surgery and postoperative RT. In the primary site, definitive management is wide excision with up to 2-cm margins and appropriate sentinel lymph node biopsy (SLNB) or nodal dissection.[20] Adjuvant RT is typically not recommended to the primary site after adequate resection because of low rates of local recurrence. However, definitive or adjuvant RT to the primary may be considered for medically inoperable patients, cases where surgical morbidity may be extremely high, or for positive margins where further resection is not possible, or tumors with extensive neurotropism. Desmoplastic melanoma is associated with high local recurrence rates and superior local control rates have been seen with resection and postoperative RT.[21,22] Additionally, lentigo maligna has been selectively treated with RT most commonly with Grenz rays or superficial RT demonstrating high local control rates of greater than 90%.[23]

In regional nodal disease, risk factors for regional recurrence after appropriate surgical management include two or more cervical nodes, one or more parotid lymph node, greater than or equal to 3 cm cervical lymph node, or extranodal extension based on the TROG 02.01 study of adjuvant nodal RT (48 Gy in 20 fractions). This study demonstrated adjuvant RT to be associated with reduced regional recurrence in the previously mentioned high-risk patients, but without overall survival or disease-free survival benefit.[24] MD Anderson published their experience with another popular fractionation scheme of 30 Gy in 5 fractions associated with loco-regional control (LRC) of 88% with only 3 of 174 patients experiencing late complications.[25]

In the era of immunotherapies and targeted agent use in melanoma, careful consideration should be given to the timing of RT and systemic therapy. National Comprehensive Cancer Network guidelines suggest that BRAF and/or MEK inhibitors should be held for 3 or more days before and after fractionated radiation and 1 or more day surrounding stereotactic radiosurgery (SRS).[26]

MERKEL CELL CARCINOMA

Merkel cell carcinoma represents a rare cutaneous neuroendocrine malignancy with increasing incidence in the United States since the 1990s. Merkel cell carcinoma is often rapid growing with up to 16% metastatic at diagnosis and up to 35% presenting with lymph node involvement. Over the course of their disease, larger series show that one-third of patients develop distant metastases.[27]

The initial treatment of Merkel cell carcinoma is typically surgical excision of the primary tumor with wide 2- to 3-cm margins and therapeutic dissection of clinically involved lymph nodes. SLNB is performed when there is no clear clinical lymphadenopathy. RT is indicated for unresectable disease to 60 to 66 Gy. RT may be given to the primary postoperative bed to 50 to 56 Gy in the setting of negative margins with a boost to 60 to 66 Gy for positive margins. However, improvement with RT in locoregional control or disease-specific survival is inconsistent in the literature. Observation may be recommended for tumors less than 1 cm without lymphovascular invasion or immunosuppression but is generally recommended for all other primary tumors.[28–30]

In the setting of negative SLNB, observation of the lymph node basin is appropriate. For positive SLNB, completion lymph node dissection is typically planned.[20] Adjuvant RT to the nodal basin is indicated after completion lymph node dissection for multiple positive nodes or extracapsular extension and is typically not performed for low nodal disease burden on completion lymph node dissection. In tumors of the head and neck, SLNB has an increased false-positive rate possibly because of multiple nodal basins or aberrant lymph node drainage. RT is often considered to nodal basins of the head and neck at risk for subclinical disease. For regional nodal areas, RT is prescribed to 60 to 66 Gy for clinical evident lymphadenopathy without dissection, and 46 to 50 Gy for nodal basins at risk for microscopic disease according to National Comprehensive Cancer Network guidelines 2018. These dose ranges reflect institutional series because there are no prospective randomized trials of RT adjuvantly for Merkel cell carcinoma. Delays in adjuvant RT have been associated with worse outcomes, and thus RT is recommended to start 4 to 6 weeks postoperatively.

TECHNICAL ASPECTS OF RADIOTHERAPY

The method by which skin cancers are treated with RT depends on the target area. For primary superficial tumors, orthovoltage, superficial radiation or electron beam are frequently used. Orthovoltage or superficial radiation have long been used to treat skin cancers and the advantage of these techniques for lesions less than 1 cm deep are (1) less lateral margin of normal tissue is exposed, (2) maximum dose at skin surface, and (3) the beam may be collimated or shaped at skin surface. Orthovoltage has a 10% to 20% higher relative biologic effectiveness compared with electron and photon energies. For lesions up to 4 cm in depth, electrons have been more frequently used in recent years. Electrons are produced in linear accelerators along with photon energies commonly used to treat other areas of the body. The physical properties of electron beam therapy including high superficial dose and steep dose fall-off with distance into tissue make electron beam therapy attractive to target primary skin tumors. D_{max} for 6 to 15 MeV electrons is 1.4 to 3.0 cm deep in tissue. Electrons are best used on a uniform surface with the treatment gantry perpendicular to the treated surface. Generally, electron energy is chosen such that the 90% isodose line encompasses the tumor and deep margin.

When nodal regions are targeted or the depth of treatment needs is greater than 5 cm, photon beams are used in addition to electrons or photon intensity modulated radiation therapy (IMRT) plans are used to encompass all areas of disease. Patients undergo simulation where the area to be treated is defined: for superficial primary tumors only, this frequently encompasses the tumor plus 1- to 2-m margin lateral and deep. Generous margins should be used for high-grade histologies, recurrent tumors, sclerosing BCC histology, and tumors with indistinct margins. With electron treatments, the target may be drawn on the skin and this image is then transferred to create a custom beam block of Cerrobend for use during treatment. An Aquaplst mask may be created to immobilize patients for head and neck treatment when multiple fractions are planned. Depth dose calculations are then performed to plan the electron energy that will be used for treatment (higher energy electrons deliver dose deeper into tissue). For more complex treatments and those involving photons, CT simulation is performed. A CT-compatible wire may be placed around the skin lesion to help define the target area, and CT is used to delineate tumor clinical target margin laterally and deep.

In the planning phase, the radiation oncologist defines the target area and dose to be delivered. Dosimetry aids in the creation of a plan to encompass the desired volumetric target with the desired dose while limiting normal tissue dose.

RT may be delivered in nonmelanoma skin cancers over diverse fraction schemes and the optimal dosing has not been determined. Because acute and late toxicities of RT are related to the volume of tissue irradiated, smaller superficial volumes

Table 2
Common radiation fractionation schemes for nonmelanoma skin cancers treated definitively or adjuvantly

Tumor Size	Dose Per Fraction (Gy)	Total Dose (Gy)
<2 cm	3–5	40–51
2 cm without cartilage involvement	2.5	50–55
2 cm with cartilage involvement	2	60–66

may be treated in three to five fractions, whereas postoperative courses are typically treated over 30 to 33 fractions. Palliative cases of large tumors may be treated in 10 to 20 fractions. Common fractionation schemes are shown in **Table 2**.

Specific Anatomic Site Considerations

Ear
RT can offer cosmetic advantages compared with surgery in tumors of the pinna and deeper tumors may be treated adjuvantly. Tissue or water-equivalent material may be placed in the ear to minimize dose inhomogeneity and irregular contours when electrons are used to treat superficial tumors. For more infiltrative tumors with bone or cartilage involvement, millivolt photons are often used with IMRT or volumetric modulated arc therapy (VMAT) technique.

Lip
Electrons may be used to treat more common lower lip lesions. Dental rolls may be placed between the treated lip and underlying oral cavity mucosa to minimize dose to these structures. Upper lip lesions may involve to columella or nasal ala and interstitial brachytherapy implant may be used.

Nose
The sloping surface of the nose may require tissue-equivalent compensation to ensure adequate uniform dose distribution to tumor at depth. Tissue equivalent "bolus" material may be placed directly on the skin surface for two purposes: to deliver maximum RT dose to skin surface by drawing isodose lines up to skin surface; or for nonhomogeneous surfaces, to deliver a uniform dose to a nonuniform surface (**Fig. 3**). Nasal vestibule cancers are more often of squamous cell histology and may have elevated risk of lymph node involvement up to 15% in the submandibular and or facial lymph nodes.

Radiation Toxicity and Treatment

Acute toxicities of skin RT, which typically begin in Weeks 3 to 4 of RT, include erythema and desquamation, edema, and hair loss in the treatment field. Patients should avoid shaving, sun exposure, and scratching during and shortly after RT. Applications of creams, perfumes, cosmetics, or harsh cleansers should be avoided and a mild steroid cream may improve symptoms. Silver sulfadiazine 1% cream is used to treat moist desquamation. When cervical lymph nodes are targeted during RT, acute toxicities also include dysphagia, odynophagia, pharyngeal or laryngeal mucositis, temporary taste changes, and increased thick mucus. These acute toxicities are attributable to radiation damage in the rapidly dividing epithelial cells of

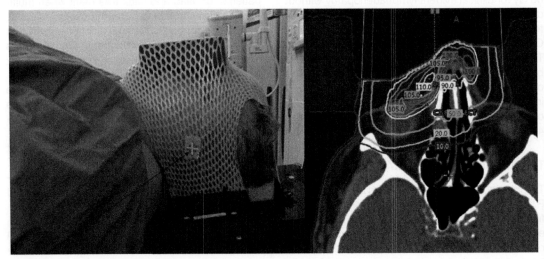

Fig. 3. Custom-fit tissue compensator is constructed to treat cSCC of the cheek and nose, whereby the bolus material is molded over the patient's nose and uniform dose to tumor at skin surface.

the skin and mucosa, and typically begin to recover 14 to 21 days after completion of RT as surviving stem cells in the basal layer move to the surface. Late toxicities of skin irradiation include telangiectasias, skin atrophy, hair loss and loss of sweat glands in the treatment field, and hypopigmentation with lower risk of skin necrosis (3%) or osteoradionecrosis/chondronecrosis (1%–2%). Late toxicities of neck RT may also include iatrogenic hypothyroidism, long-term dysphagia, xerostomia, soft tissue fibrosis, and osteoradionecrosis.

Relative contraindications to radiotherapy include a history of connective tissue disorder including active lupus or scleroderma, Gorlin syndrome, postradiation tumor recurrences, young age less than 40 because of the risk of second malignancy and declining cosmesis over time, and anatomic areas prone to repeated trauma or poor circulation including below the elbow or knee.

REFERENCES

1. Rowe D, Carroll R, Day C, et al. Prognostic factors for local recurrence, metastases and survival rates in squamous cell carcinoma of the skin,ear and lip. J Am Acad Dermatol 1992;26(6):976–90.

2. Garcia-Serra A, Hinerman R, Mendenhall W, et al. Carcinoma of the skin with perineural invasion. Head Neck 2003;25:1027–33.

3. O'Brien CJ, McNeil EB, McMahon JD, et al. Significance of clinical stage, extent of surgery and pathology findings in metastatic cutaneous squamous cell carcinoma of the parotid gland. Head Neck 2002;24: 417–22.

4. Audet N, Palme CE, Gullane P. Cutaneous metastatic squamous cell carcinoma of the parotid: analysis and outcome. Head Neck 2004;26:727–32.

5. Marcen R, Pascual J, Tato AM, et al. Influence of immunosuppression on the prevalence of cancer after kidney transplantation. Transplant Proc 2003;35: 1714–6.

6. Smith KJ, Hamza S, Skelton H. Histologic features in primary cutaneous squamous cell carcinoma in immunocompromised patients focusing on organ transplantation. Dermatol Surg 2004;30:634–41.

7. Manyam BV, Garsa AA, Chin RI, et al. A multi-institutional comparison of outcomes of immunosuppressed and immunocompetent patients treated with surgery and radiation therapy for cutaneous squamous cell carcinoma of the head and neck. Cancer 2017;123(11):2054–60.

8. Goepfert H, Dichtel W, Medina J, et al. Perineural invasion in squamous cell skin carcinoma of the head and neck. Am J Surg 1984;148:542.

9. Sapir E, Tolpadi A, McHugh J, et al. Skin cancer of the head and neck with gross or microscopic

10. Lee W, Mendenhall W, Parsons J, et al. Radical radiotherapy for T4 carcinoma of the skin of the head and neck: a multivariant analysis. Head Neck 1993;15(4):320–4.

11. Hinerman RW, Indelicato DJ, Amdur RJ, et al. Cutaneous squamous cell carcinoma metastatic to parotid-area lymph nodes. Laryngoscope 2008; 118:1989–96.

12. Givi B, Andersen PE, Diggs BS, et al. Outcome of patients treated surgically for lymph node metastases from cutaneous squamous cell carcinoma of the head and neck. Head Neck 2011;10: 999–1004.

13. Wang JT, Palme CE, Morgan GJ, et al. Predictors of outcome in patients with metastatic cutaneous head and neck squamous cell carcinoma involving cervical lymph nodes: improved survival with the addition of adjuvant radiotherapy. Head Neck 2012;34(11): 1524–8.

14. Gluck I, Ibrahim M, Popovtzer A, et al. Skin cancer of the head and neck with perineural invasion: defining the clinical target volumes based on the pattern of failure. Int J Radiat Oncol Biol Phys 2009;74(1):38–46.

15. Porceddu S, Bressel M, Poulsen M, et al. Postoperative concurrent chemoradiotherapy versus postoperative radiotherapy in high-risk cutaneous squamous cell carcinoma of the head and neck: the randomized phase III TROG 05.01 trial. J Clin Oncol 2018;36: 1275–83.

16. Maubec E, Petrow P, Scheer-Senyarich I. Phase II study of cetuximab as first line single drug therapy in patients with unresectable squamous cell carcinoma of the skin. J Clin Oncol 2011;29(25):3419–26.

17. Pickering C, Zhou J, Lee J, et al. Mutational landscape of aggressive cutaneous squamous cell carcinoma. Clin Cancer Res 2014;20(24):6582–92.

18. Simard EP, Ward EM, Seigel R, et al. Cancers with increasing incidence trends in the United States: 1999 through 2008. CA Cancer J Clin 2012;62(2): 118–28.

19. Jemal A, Saraiya M, Patel P, et al. Recent trends in cutaneous melanoma incidence and death rates in the United States, 1992-2006. J Am Acad Dermatol 2011;65:S17–25.

20. 2018 NCCN guidelines. Available at: nccn.org.

21. Guadagnolo B, Prieto V, Weber R, et al. The role of adjuvant radiotherapy in the local management of desmoplastic melanoma. Cancer 2014;120:1361–8.

22. Strom T, Caudell J, Han D, et al. Radiotherapy influences local control in patients with desmoplastic melanoma. Cancer 2014;120:1369–78.

23. Fogarty G, Hong A, Scolyer R, et al. Radiotherapy for lentigo maligna: a literature review and recommendations for treatment. Br J Dermatol 2014;170: 52–8.

24. Henderson M, Burmeister B, Ainslie J, et al. Adjuvant lymph node field radiotherapy versus observation only in patients at high risk for further lymph-node field relapse after lymphadenectomy (ANZMTG 01.02/TROG 02.01). Lancet Oncol 2015; 16:1049–60.

25. Ang K, Peters L, Weber R. Postoperative radiotherapy for cutaneous melanoma of the head and neck region. Int J Radiat Oncol Biol Phys 1994;30: 795–8.

26. Anker C, Grossmann K, Atkins M, et al. Avoiding severe toxicity from combined BRAF inhibitor and radiation treatment: consensus guidelines from the Eastern Cooperative Group. Int J Radiat Oncol Biol Phys 2016;95:632–46.

27. Medina-Franco H, Urist MM, Fiveach J, et al. Multimodality treatment of Merkel cell carcinoma: case series and literature review of 1024 cases. Ann Surg Oncol 2001;8:204–8.

28. Tarantola T, VAllow L, Halyard M, et al. Prognostic factors in Merkel cell carcinoma: analysis of 240 cases. J Am Acad Dermatol 2013;68:425–32.

29. Smith F, Yue B, Marzban S, et al. Both tumor depth and diameter are predictive of sentinel lymph node status and survival in Merkel cell carcinoma. Cancer 2015;121:3252–60.

30. Johnson M, Zhu F, Li T, et al. Absolute lymphocyte count: a potential prognostic factor for Merkel cell carcinoma. J Am Acad Dermatol 2014;70: 1028–35.

31. Chan S, Dhadda AL, Snidell R. Single fraction radiotherapy for small superficial carcinoma of the skin. Clin Oncol 2007;19(4):256–9.

32. Schulte K, Lippold A, Auras C, et al. Soft x-ray therapy for cutaneous basal cell and squamous cell carcinoma. J Am Acad Dermatol 2005;53(6): 993–1001.

33. Locke J, Karimpour S, Young G, et al. Radiotherapy for epithelial skin cancer. Int J Radiat Oncol Biol Phys 2001;51(3):748–55.

34. Cognetta A, Howard B, Heaton H, et al. Superficial x-ray in the treatment of basal and squamous cell carcinoma: a viable option in selected patients. J Am Acad Dermatol 2012;67:1235–41.

Adjuvant and Neoadjuvant Treatment of Skin Cancer

Assuntina G. Sacco, MD*, Gregory A. Daniels, MD, PhD

KEYWORDS

- Basal cell carcinoma • Cutaneous squamous cell carcinoma • Melanoma • Adjuvant • Neoadjuvant
- Systemic therapy • Checkpoint inhibitors • Hedgehog inhibitor

KEY POINTS

- Basal cell carcinoma is caused by dysregulated signaling of the sonic hedgehog pathway, with inhibitors such as vismodegib and sonidegib displaying promising activity.
- Cutaneous squamous cell carcinoma has overexpression of the epidermal growth factor receptor pathway and a similar mutational profile to mucosal head and neck squamous cell carcinoma.
- Immune checkpoint inhibition and targeted therapies (inhibitors of BRAF and MEK) have led to new adjuvant standards in melanoma.

INTRODUCTION

Skin cancer represents a broad classification of malignancies, which can be further refined by histology, including basal cell carcinoma, squamous cell carcinoma, and melanoma. Because these three cancers are distinct entities, this article reviews each one separately, with a focus on their epidemiology; cause, including relevant genomic data (**Table 1**); and the current evidence-based recommendations for adjuvant and neoadjuvant therapy. Future directions and opportunities for continued therapeutic advances are also discussed.

BASAL CELL CARCINOMA

Basal cell carcinoma (BCC) is the most common cancer worldwide, with a rapidly increasing incidence, increased treatment-related health care expenditures, and a cumulatively significant burden on patient-related quality of life.[1] Despite the low rate of metastatic potential (<0.1% of cases), BCCs can cause significant disfigurement and local destruction, involving extensive areas of soft tissue, bone, and cartilage.[2–4] The current mainstay of treatment involves localized therapies, such as surgery and radiation. Systemic therapy is often reserved for the management of metastatic or locally advanced BCC for which localized therapies have failed or are not an option. Given the rarity of advanced disease, there is a paucity of literature regarding the role of cytotoxic chemotherapy, which is often platinum-based, and now being used less frequently since the advent of targeted therapies.

Inappropriate activation of the sonic hedgehog (SHH) signaling pathway plays a pivotal role in the pathogenesis of sporadic BCC and BCC secondary to the heritable condition known as basal cell nevus syndrome (Gorlin syndrome).[5,6] Patched 1 (PTCH1) is a tumor suppressor gene that forms a receptor complex with a second protein, smoothened (SMO). This receptor complex is activated by SHH, resulting in activation of the SHH pathway. Germline or acquired mutations in PTCH1 or SMO results in dysregulation

Disclosure: Dr A.G. Sacco has the following relevant disclosures: Merck, Pfizer. Dr G.A. Daniels has the following relevant disclosures: Regeneron, Sanofi Aventis, Array.
Division of Hematology-Oncology, University of California San Diego, Moores Cancer Center, 3855 Health Sciences Drive, La Jolla, CA 92093-0658, USA
* Corresponding author.
E-mail address: agsacco@ucsd.edu

Table 1
Common mutations and available drug therapies by skin cancer type

Skin Cancer Type	Common Mutations	FDA-Approved Therapies
BCC	Patched 1 (PTCH1)	—
	Smoothened (SMO)	Vismodegib
		Sonidegib
Squamous cell carcinoma	p53	—
	EGFR overexpression	Cetuximab[a]
	CDKN2a	—
	NOTCH 1	—
	NOTCH 2	—
	HRAS	—
Melanoma		Approved irrespective of mutational status:
		Ipilimumab
		Pembrolizumab
		Nivolumab
	BRAF	Vemurafenib
		Dabrafenib
		Trametinib (MEKi)
		Cobimetinib (MEKi approved in combination with vemurafenib for unresectable/metastatic disease)
	NRAS	MEKi
	NF1	—
	c-kit	—

Abbreviation: MEKi, MEK inhibitor.
 [a] Off-label use.

of hedgehog signaling, leading to constitutive activation and subsequent tumorigenesis (see **Table 1**).[5,6]

Vismodegib is a first-in-class SMO antagonist and SHH pathway inhibitor that was approved by the US Food and Drug Administration (FDA) in 2012 for the following indications: metastatic BCC, locally advanced BCC that has failed surgery, or BCC that is not amenable to surgery or radiation. Sonidegib, a second SMO antagonist, has also been approved for similar indications and carries a comparable toxicity profile to vismodegib. Objective response rates noted in clinical trials for these two agents have ranged from 38% to 67% and 15% to 38% for locally advanced and metastatic BCC, respectively.[7–11] Key limitations of SHH inhibitors include poor tolerance secondary to on-target toxicities, which often require treatment disruptions or ultimately discontinuation, and the development of acquired resistance, which affects duration of response.

Adjuvant Treatment

The role of adjuvant therapy for BCC is primarily governed by risk for recurrence, dictated by clinical and pathologic risk features. These risks include location, size, borders, de novo versus recurrent disease, underlying immunosuppression, prior radiation, and pathologic subtype.[12–14] Pathologic risk features include positive surgical margins and neural involvement (perineural or large-nerve invasion).[15,16] Low-risk BCC with surgical margin involvement should preferentially undergo reresection, or receive radiation (for nonsurgical candidates). Adjuvant therapy for high-risk BCC also includes reresection for positive margins, or radiation for positive margins or presence of extensive perineural and/or large-nerve involvement. Because of the reduced efficacy of superficial therapies such as topical 5-fluorouracil, imiquimod, photodynamic therapy, and cryotherapy, these modalities should be reserved for patients in whom surgery or radiation is contraindicated, impractical, or declined by the patient.[1,17]

The role of systemic therapy in the adjuvant setting is less well-defined and primarily restricted to settings in which there is residual disease following surgery and/or radiation. Decisions surrounding systemic therapy should involve multidisciplinary consultation. Clinical trial participation (when feasible) should be recommended. The adjuvant use of SHH inhibitors may be considered, however, there is a lack of clinical trial evidence to support early application.

Neoadjuvant Treatment

Utilization of a neoadjuvant approach for locally advanced disease in a functionally sensitive anatomic location represents an attractive treatment strategy. In theory, such an approach may result in preoperative tumor cytoreduction, reduced surgical morbidity, and improved oncologic efficacy. A phase II trial evaluated vismodegib for reduction of existing tumor burden and as chemoprevention for patients with BCC secondary to basal cell nevus syndrome.[18] In this randomized, double-blind, placebo-controlled trial, 41 patients were treated with vismodegib or placebo for a mean of 8 months (range, 1–15 months). Pertinent findings included significantly reduced per-patient rates of new surgically eligible BCCs after 1 month of vismodegib. There was also significantly reduced size of existing clinically significant BCCs compared with placebo. Biopsy samples were obtained from sites of clinically regressed BCCs; 83% of these samples had no residual BCC. Although no tumors progressed during treatment with vismodegib, BCCs did recur following its discontinuation. In addition, slightly more than half (54%) of patients had to discontinue treatment secondary to toxicity. These findings were promising because they showed that vismodegib is effective not only in decreasing the number of new lesions but also in reducing the size of existing surgically eligible BCC in patients with basal cell nevus syndrome.

In a trial of 15 patients with sporadic, locally advanced, or recurrent BCC amenable to surgical resection, reduction in surgical defect area was evaluated after 3 to 6 months of neoadjuvant vismodegib.[19,20] Of 13 patients who underwent target tumor excision after a mean of 4 months (range 2–6 months) of vismodegib, the surgical defect area was reduced by 34%, primarily in de novo tumors. Vismodegib was not effective in patients receiving less than 3 months of treatment and had to be discontinued after 3 months in 29% of patients because of toxicity. With a mean follow-up of 22 months (range 12–28 months), only 1 patient developed recurrence 17 months postoperatively. Of note, this patient was only able to complete 2 months of vismodegib secondary to hepatotoxicity for a recurrent, infiltrative BCC.

In a phase II, nonrandomized, 3-cohort, open-label trial of patients with de novo nodular BCC amenable to surgical resection, 3 different schedules of neoadjuvant vismodegib were studied (cohort 1, 3 months of vismodegib; cohort 2, 3 months of vismodegib followed by 6 months of observation before surgery; cohort 3, vismodegib given 2 months on, 1 month off, then 2 additional months).[21] Twenty-four patients were enrolled in cohort 1 and 25 in cohorts 2 and 3. The primary end point (complete histologic clearance rate of >50% in cohorts 1 and 3, and >30% in cohort 2) was not met, because clearances rates were 42% in cohort 1, 16% in cohort 2, and 44% in cohort 3. Safety and tolerability were comparable irrespective of dosing schedule (continuous vs intermittent dosing).

These trials highlight the potential utility of a neoadjuvant approach for patients with locally advanced, high-risk BCC. The greatest benefit may be for those patients whose disease affects a functionally sensitive location. Clinical trials are currently underway to further validate these findings in a larger population with longer follow-up to ensure low rates of recurrence. It remains possible that lesions regress in a discontinuous fashion, thus the routine use of SHH inhibitors in the neoadjuvant setting is not recommended and should be performed in the context of a clinical trial or after careful evaluation by a multidisciplinary team.

Future Directions

Identification of the SHH pathway's role in BCC development, and the understanding of the multiple signaling cascades involved in this pathway, marks a watershed of opportunity for future research. The SMO inhibitors are certainly the furthest along in development, but they have limitations related to overall response rate, duration of response, potential resistance, and toxicity. Development of hedgehog pathway inhibitors with downstream targets (such as itraconazole, inhibitor of Gli transcription factor activated following SMO agonism) or combinatory strategies with drugs affecting other signaling cascades may afford an opportunity to generate higher response rates, more durable responses, use in less advanced BCC, or as second-line therapies following SHH inhibitor resistance.[1,22]

Immunotherapy represents an attractive target in the management of BCC for a variety of factors. The immune system already plays a critical role in the prevention and elimination of BCCs, as shown by the development of BCCs in immunosuppressed patients, likely because of loss of immune surveillance and elimination of early transformed cells.[23] The high immunogenicity (high mutational burden, high rate of cancer-testis antigen expression, and tumor infiltrating CD8+ T cells), potential for immune escape (low levels of MHC-1 expression and high levels of regulatory T cells in the microenvironment), and high levels of PD-L1 expression also suggest that immune checkpoint inhibition may be efficacious.[23,24] In addition, SHH pathway signaling reduces T-cell activation, whereby SHH inhibition upregulates major histocompatibility complex expression to attract T cells, suggesting that SHH inhibitors may downregulate tumor-mediated immune suppression.[23] At present, trials are underway to assess the efficacy of immunotherapy in the management of locally advanced, unresectable, or metastatic disease. Synergism of SHH inhibitors combined with anti–programmed death 1 (anti-PD1) therapy is also being evaluated.

In addition, the use of targeted therapies in a neoadjuvant treatment paradigm represents an attractive strategy (as outlined earlier), for which clinical trials are also underway.

CUTANEOUS SQUAMOUS CELL CARCINOMA

Cutaneous squamous cell carcinoma (cSCC) is the second most common skin cancer, representing approximately 20% of nonmelanoma skin cancers.[25,26] Some studies have suggested that the incidence rates of cSCC are increasing much more rapidly than BCC, with the most frequent implicated site of disease involving the head and neck.[27,28] Although cSCC metastasizes more frequently than BCC, overall metastatic potential still remains low, with an estimated 3.7% risk of regional metastasis and 2.1% risk of disease-specific death.[29] However, cSCC can cause significant disfigurement and local destruction, and, in cases of regional or distant involvement, can result in severe morbidity and poor survival outcomes. The current mainstay of treatment involves localized therapies such as surgery or radiation. Systemic therapy is typically administered concurrently with definitive radiation for locally advanced disease, in certain adjuvant settings, and for the management of metastatic disease. Given the limited data available, systemic agents are often extrapolated from management of mucosal head and neck squamous cell carcinoma (HNSCC).

The epidermal growth factor receptor (EGFR) pathway, which is overexpressed in about half of all cSCC, is involved in signaling pathways responsible for cell proliferation, survival, invasion, angiogenesis, and metastasis.[30] EGFR inhibition with monoclonal antibodies (such as cetuximab) and small tyrosine kinase inhibitors (such as erlotinib or gefitinib) have shown modest antitumor activity in advanced cSCC.[31–33] Interestingly, response to EGFR inhibition does not appear to correlate with EGFR mutation status nor immunohistochemical expression of the receptor. Except for the ultraviolet signature, the mutational landscape of aggressive cSCC is similar to that of mucosal HNSCC, with a predominance of tumor suppressor genes, such as TP53 (most common), CDKN2A, NOTCH1 and 2, and HRAS (see **Table 1**).[34]

Adjuvant Treatment

The role of adjuvant therapy for cSCC is primarily governed by the presence of high-risk features. Risk features are categorized by clinical factors (location, size, borders, de novo vs recurrent disease, underlying immunosuppression, prior radiation, and neurologic symptoms) and pathologic features (surgical margin involvement, degree of differentiation, pathologic subtype, and perineural involvement).[35,36] Low-risk cSCC with surgical margin involvement should preferentially undergo reresection or receive radiation (for nonsurgical candidates). High-risk lesions typically require multimodality treatment to optimize cure rates. Although definitive recommendations for adjuvant radiation are lacking, it is generally recommended that patients with locally advanced disease, surgical margin involvement (not amenable to reresection), extensive perineural or large-nerve involvement, multiply recurrent disease, nodal involvement, or multiple high-risk factors would benefit from adjuvant radiation.[37–39]

Data for the use of adjuvant chemotherapy concurrent with radiation in cSCC are even further limited, with case reports and small studies showing activity with platinum and cetuximab.[40,41] A recent phase III randomized trial of 310 immunocompetent patients with high-risk cSCC receiving adjuvant radiation with or without carboplatin (area under the curve, 2) showed no benefit from the addition of carboplatin with respect to locoregional control, disease-specific survival, or overall survival.[42] At present, recommendations for the addition of chemotherapy concurrent with postoperative radiation in cSCC are still extrapolated from mucosal HNSCC, for which surgical margin involvement and/or extranodal extension are hard indications to support the addition of chemotherapy.[43]

Neoadjuvant Treatment

At present, a neoadjuvant approach for the management of locally advanced cSCC is not a recognized standard of care. In a trial of 34 consecutive patients with unresectable, locally advanced cSCC, patients initially received cetuximab as monotherapy or combined with platinum and 5-fluorouracil to determine whether an induction approach could facilitate surgical resectability.[44] In the combination arm (median age, 70 years), 23 of 25 patients (92%) were able to proceed to surgery, with 15 of these patients experiencing a complete pathologic response. In the cetuximab monotherapy arm (median age, 86 years), 5 of 9 patients were able to proceed to surgery, with 3 having a complete pathologic response. These findings suggest that cetuximab-based induction may represent a reasonable option for patients with unresectable locally advanced disease, particularly given the good tolerability in a primarily elderly population; however, prospective evaluation is warranted.

In a phase II, prospective trial of patients with primary or recurrent cSCC amenable to curative intent therapy with surgery and/or radiation, neoadjuvant gefitinib was administered to determine disease control rate and toxicity.[45] Of 22 patients evaluable for response before definitive local treatment, 18.2% of patients had a complete response (CR) and 27.3% of patients had a partial response. Toxicity (grade 2–3) was noted in 59.1% of patients, with on-target effects. The investigators concluded that neoadjuvant gefitinib was active, well tolerated, did not interfere with receipt of definitive treatment, and showed the potential for CR, warranting further investigation of EGFR inhibitors for aggressive cSCC. However, the recent introduction of immunotherapy may quickly change the area of adjuvant and neoadjuvant options (discussed later).

Future Directions

Similar to BCC, immunotherapy also represents an attractive treatment strategy for cSCC, because these tumors possess prerequisites, such as tumor-associated antigens (high somatic mutation burden) and tumor-specific immune response, that are needed for immune intervention.[46] The development of cSCC in immunosuppressed patients also shows the critical role of the immune system in its prevention and elimination. cSCC has shown loss of human leukocyte antigen-A, B-monomorphic determinants, downregulation of total surface class I expression, and differential heavy chain and beta-2 microglobulin expression.[46] In addition, there are data to suggest that cSCC can abrogate immune recognition through the production of various immunosuppressive Th2-type cytokines, thus resulting in inhibition of the cell-mediated immune response, depletion of antigen-presenting cells (APCs), and downregulation of costimulatory molecules (CD80 and CD86) on APCs.[46] A phase I expansion and a phase II cohort of cemiplimab, a programmed cell death protein 1 (PD-1) inhibitor, induced durable responses in nearly half of patients with unresectable, locally advanced or metastatic cSCC.[47] These initial results are promising, providing justification for further exploration of immunotherapy in immunocompetent patients with aggressive or locally advanced cSCC.

The promising early results of immune checkpoint inhibitors and EGFR inhibitors (either alone or in combination) could also lead to more effective neoadjuvant or adjuvant treatment paradigms in this disease, with active trials currently underway.

CUTANEOUS MELANOMA

Melanoma is the most aggressive form of skin cancer and is the sixth most common cancer in both genders.[48,49] The dramatically increasing incidence of melanoma is such that it is now increasing in men more rapidly than any other cancer and is only second to lung cancer in women.[49] Most patients present with localized disease, for which curative intent surgery remains the mainstay of treatment. High-risk pathologic features such as increasing Breslow thickness, high mitotic rate, presence of ulceration, and nodal involvement are prognostic factors used to define patient subsets at increased risk for disease recurrence.[50–54] Until recently, systemic therapy played a limited role, largely because of marginal benefits. Innovations in both targeted therapies (based on mutational status) and immunotherapies have ushered in a new era of systemic therapies for melanoma that has drastically changed treatment paradigms and significantly improved outcomes.

Dysregulation of the mitogen-activated protein kinase (MAPK) pathway is implicated in nearly all cases of melanoma. BRAF (downstream mediator of activated RAS) and NRAS (G-protein member of RAS family) mutations are the most commonly observed in cutaneous melanoma.[55,56] Mutation of NF1 (tumor suppressor gene that suppresses NRAS signaling) is considered the third most common genomic subset behind BRAF and NRAS.[56,57] Mutations in c-kit have also been noted, occurring most often in patients with chronic skin damage.[57] With rare exceptions, activating mutations in BRAF, NRAS, and c-kit are mutually exclusive.[58] Mutations of the BRAF gene can be further subdivided into V600E and V600K, with the former accounting for 90% of cases.[59] Understanding the critical role of how MAPK dysregulation drives oncogenesis, targeted therapies (BRAF and MEK inhibitors) have subsequently been developed, resulting in significantly improved outcomes for advanced disease (see **Table 1**). Additional therapies targeting other components of the pathway are also in development.

The high somatic mutation burden of cutaneous melanomas results in numerous cancer-specific antigens being subjected to immune surveillance, possibly making melanoma an especially attractive target for cancer immunotherapy. Tumor cells are known to co-opt certain immune checkpoint pathways (particularly against T cells specific for tumor antigens) as a major mechanism of immune resistance.[60] Thus, the development of immune checkpoint inhibitors has been a key breakthrough in the management of cancer, with successes in melanoma at the forefront. Targeting the immunologic synapses of the cytotoxic T-lymphocyte-associated antigen 4 (CTLA-4; ipilimumab) and the PD1 molecule (pembrolizumab and nivolumab) either alone or in combination has significant activity in advanced melanoma, dramatically changing the treatment landscape and significantly improving survival outcomes. These major advances have marked a seminal moment in drug development to further enhance antitumor immunity.

Adjuvant Treatment

High-dose interferon
Given that most melanoma-related deaths are secondary to distant failure after initial surgical resection, the use of adjuvant systemic therapies to reduce recurrence risk has been a focus of extensive research over the past few decades.[61] ECOG (Eastern Cooperative Oncology Group) 1684, the landmark trial showing that adjuvant high-dose interferon improved both relapse-free and overall survival in patients with surgically resected stage IIb/III disease, led to its FDA-approved adjuvant indication in 1995.[62] Since then, a large body of evidence has amassed evaluating the benefits of adjuvant interferon, with contrasting survival outcomes. Varying doses of interferon (low or intermediate), pegylated formulation, and combinations with various cytotoxic agents have also been widely evaluated and shown to lack superiority to high-dose interferon.[63–67] Thus, high-dose interferon remained the best option for nearly 20 years, until it was toppled by the emergence of checkpoint inhibitors. Interferon no longer has a well-defined role in the adjuvant setting, except perhaps as a treatment consideration for high-risk, node-negative disease if clinical trial participation is not an option.

Checkpoint inhibitors
The overwhelming success of checkpoint blockade in metastatic melanoma naturally drove the evaluation of these agents in the adjuvant setting for patients with high-risk disease. In recent years, there have been multiple, pivotal phase III randomized trials that have established the role of both checkpoint blockade and targeted therapy as the new adjuvant landscape (**Table 2**).

Ipilimumab (CTLA-4 inhibitor) received its FDA-approved adjuvant indication in 2015 based on the results of the European Organisation for Research and Treatment of Cancer (EORTC) 18071 trial, in which ipilimumab at 10 mg/kg reduced the risk of recurrence by 25% and showed an 11% overall survival benefit compared with placebo in patients with resected, stage III melanoma.[68] Given that the dosing of ipilimumab was higher than the approved dosing in the metastatic setting (3 mg/kg), a second phase III trial is underway to evaluate adjuvant ipilimumab at each dose level (3 mg/kg and 10 mg/kg) compared with high-dose interferon. An unplanned exploratory analysis was presented at the 2017 annual American Society of Clinical Oncology (ASCO) meeting, in which ipilimumab-related toxicity was considerably reduced in the patients receiving 3 mg/kg, and relapse-free survival was comparable at 3 years for both dosing levels.[69] Given these are preliminary findings, when adjuvant ipilimumab is used, the dosing should still remain at 10 mg/kg at this time. However, it is important to highlight that toxicity of 10 mg/kg dosing is high (53.3% of patients in EORTC 18071 discontinued treatment because of toxicity) and benefit of therapy varies across different subgroups (patients with stage IIIA disease seemed to derive less benefit than those with stage IIIB–IIIC disease). Taken together, these findings emphasize the need to have a careful discussion with the patient regarding risks and benefits of therapy. In addition, these data should guide treatment selection by providers, particularly in light of the improved efficacy and toxicity profiles of PD-1 inhibitors, specifically nivolumab and pembrolizumab.

The CheckMate 238 trial showed the superiority of nivolumab compared with ipilimumab in patients with resected stage III to IV disease.[70] Recurrence-free survival (RFS) at 2 years, the primary end point, was significantly higher (63% vs 50%) in patients who received nivolumab versus ipilimumab, respectively. This improvement was also sustained when they evaluated prespecified major groups (stage III vs IV, presence/absence of ulceration, microscopic vs macroscopic node involvement), PD-L1 expression (< vs ≥5%), and BRAF mutation status. Nivolumab also had a more favorable toxicity profile, with 14% of patients having grade 3 to 4 treatment-related adverse events compared with 46% of patients who received ipilimumab. In addition, treatment discontinuation because of toxicity was reduced in patients receiving nivolumab (4%) compared with ipilimumab (30%). Nivolumab subsequently received its FDA-approved adjuvant indication in 2017 and is considered the preferred regimen rather than ipilimumab.

Table 2
Adjuvant phase III randomized trials for cutaneous melanoma

Trial	Stage Inclusion	Patients (n)	Drug Therapy	Primary End Point	Results
EORTC 18071	Resected, IIIA–IIIC	951	Ipilimumab 10 mg/kg vs placebo	RFS	5-y rate of RFS: 40.8% ipilimumab vs 30.3% placebo (HR, 0.76; 95% CI, 0.64–0.89; P<.001) 5-y rate of OS: 65.4% ipilimumab vs 54.4% placebo (HR, 0.72; 95% CI, 0.58–0.88; P = .001) 5-y rate of DMFS: 48.3% ipilimumab vs 38.9% placebo (HR, 0.76; 95% CI, 0.64–0.92; P = .002)
Checkmate 238	Resected, IIIB–IV	130	Nivolumab 3 mg/kg vs ipilimumab 10 mg/kg	RFS	1-y rate of RFS: 70.5% nivolumab vs 60.8% ipilimumab (HR, 0.65; 95% CI, 0.51–0.83; P<.001)
EORTC 1345 (KEYNOTE 054)	Resected, III	1019	Pembrolizumab 200 mg vs placebo	RFS	1-y rate of RFS: 75.4% pembrolizumab vs 61% placebo (HR, 0.57; 95% CI, 0.43–0.74; P<.001)
COMBI-AD	Resected, III, BRAF mutant	870	Dabrafenib + trametinib vs placebo	RFS	3-y rate of RFS: 58% BRAF/MEK combo vs 39% placebo (HR, 0.47; 95% CI, 0.39–0.58; P<.001)
BRIM8	Resected, IIC–III, BRAF mutant	498	Vemurafenib vs placebo	DFS	Median DFS for IIIC: 23.1 mo vemurafenib vs 15.4 mo placebo (HR, 0.8; 95% CI, 0.54–1.18; P = .026) Median DFS for IIC–IIIB NR for vemurafenib vs 36.9 mo placebo (HR, 0.54; 95% CI, 0.37–0.78; P = .001)

Abbreviations: DFS, disease-free survival; DMFS, distant metastasis-free survival; EORTC, European Organisation for Research and Treatment of Cancer; HR, hazard ratio; NR, not reached; OS, overall survival; RFS, recurrence-free survival.

Pembrolizumab also showed a statistically significant improvement in RFS compared with placebo in the phase III EORTC 1345/KEYNOTE-054 trial of patients with resected stage III disease.[71] At 18 months, there was an absolute benefit of 18% for patients who received pembrolizumab. PD-L1 expression was not a predictor of response, because RFS was improved in all patients irrespective of PD-L1 status. In a phase III cooperative group trial (S1404), pembrolizumab is being compared with high-dose interferon or high-dose ipilimumab for patients with resected stage III to IVA disease. The study has completed accrual and results are forthcoming.

Note that in the aforementioned trials of checkpoint blockade, patients with high-risk, stage IIC disease were excluded. In addition, all of the trials required mandatory completion lymph-node dissection (CLND) as an inclusion criterion. Recently, 2 pivotal phase III randomized controlled trials (Multicenter Selective Lymphadenectomy Trial II [MSLT-II] and German Dermatologic Cooperative Oncology Group Selective Lymphadenectomy Trial [DeCOG-SLT]) evaluating the utility of CLND in patients with sentinel node positivity have challenged this dogma.[72,73] DeCOG-SLT showed that CLND did not improve recurrence-free, distant metastasis-free, or melanoma-specific survival.[72] Similarly, in the MSLT-II trial, although CLND improved regional control, it did not improve melanoma-specific survival.[73] In light of these recent findings, CLND should no longer be compulsory for the decision to recommend adjuvant therapy.

Targeted therapies

Given that approximately one-half of cutaneous melanomas harbor an oncogenic BRAF mutation, and that BRAF and MEK inhibitors have shown improved survival outcomes in metastatic melanoma, the role of targeted therapy in the adjuvant setting has also been evaluated (see **Table 2**). COMBI-AD was the first clinical trial to combine targeted therapies as adjuvant treatment of patients with completely resected, BRAF-mutant (91% V600E, 9% V600K), stage III melanoma.[74] In this phase III, randomized controlled trial, patients received either 1 year of dabrafenib (BRAF inhibitor) plus trametinib (MEK inhibitor) or placebo. At a median follow-up of 2.8 years, the estimated 3-year rate of relapse-free survival (primary end point) was significantly longer in the combination group (58%) versus placebo (39%; P<.001). Although the 3-year overall survival rate was also significantly higher in the combination group (86%) versus placebo (77%), it did not meet a prespecified interim analysis boundary. The combination therapy also led to improved rates of distant metastasis-free survival and freedom from relapse. Very few patients experienced early relapses during treatment with the drug combination, suggestive of an immediate benefit, akin to the rapid responses seen in advanced disease. Approximately 41% of patients receiving the combination therapy experienced grade 3 to 4 adverse events, and 26% of patients stopped treatment because of toxicity. Based on the positive results of this trial, dabrafenib plus trametinib has been approved as an adjuvant treatment in patients with resected, stage III, BRAF-mutant melanoma.

Vemurafenib, a BRAF inhibitor, was evaluated as a single agent versus placebo (1 year of therapy) in a phase III trial of patients with completely resected stage IIC to III melanoma.[75] The primary

end point, disease-free survival, was not reached. A secondary end point, disease-free survival in stage IIC to IIIB disease, was prolonged with vemurafenib; however, these findings should be considered exploratory.

For patients with BRAF-mutant stage III melanoma, adjuvant options include checkpoint blockade as well as combination BRAF/MEK inhibition with dabrafenib/trametinib. Given the recent approvals of both options, a direct comparison has not been completed yet. Provider decisions surrounding which adjuvant option to select may be based on toxicity profiles and patient comorbidities, although the authors would generally recommend consideration of immunotherapy unless otherwise contraindicated.

Radiation

Adjuvant radiation is generally not recommended to the primary site, given the low risk of local recurrence, except for perhaps in suboptimally resected desmoplastic neurotropic melanomas because of the high propensity for local failure.[76] The utility of adjuvant radiation to the nodal basins remains controversial. In the only phase III randomized trial of adjuvant nodal basin radiotherapy (RT) versus observation, although in-field nodal recurrence was significantly reduced in the adjuvant radiation group (primary end point), there was no difference in relapse-free survival or overall survival between the groups (secondary end points).[77] There was also an increased incidence of toxicity caused by pain and swelling in the radiation group. With systemic therapies as the new adjuvant standards, the role of adjuvant RT will likely further diminish, and it should not be routinely recommended.

Neoadjuvant Treatment

Early neoadjuvant trials evaluating the use of high-dose interferon, biochemotherapy, or ipilimumab showed the ability to induce tumor responses and augment the tumor's immune microenvironment. With the development of more active therapies, such as checkpoint inhibitors and BRAF/MEK inhibitors, neoadjuvant approaches have garnered a resurgence of interest. The first phase II randomized control trial involved neoadjuvant and adjuvant use of dabrafenib and trametinib versus standard of care in patients with high-risk, surgically resectable melanoma.[78] Twenty-one patients with surgically resectable stage III to IV disease were randomized (1:2) to receive standard of care (upfront surgery followed by consideration of adjuvant therapy) or 8 weeks of neoadjuvant dabrafenib and trametinib followed by surgery and then up to 1 year of adjuvant therapy. With only one-quarter of patients accrued, the study was stopped early when the prespecified interim safety analysis determined that the neoadjuvant approach led to significantly improved event-free survival. The randomization was dropped and the study continued with the single neoadjuvant arm. This trial shows proof of concept for further investigations of neoadjuvant approaches in melanoma. Multiple studies evaluating neoadjuvant checkpoint blockade are currently underway.

Future Directions

Immunotherapy and molecularly targeted therapies have revolutionized the management of melanoma; thus, the future remains promising. Clinical advances will include determination of the appropriate multimodality treatment paradigm for patients with resectable, high-risk disease. These future directions include neoadjuvant approaches as well as further refinement of adjuvant therapies.

REFERENCES

1. Lanoue J, Goldenberg G. Basal cell carcinoma: a comprehensive review of existing and emerging nonsurgical therapies. J Clin Aesthet Dermatol 2016;9(5):26–36.
2. Nguyen-Nielsen M, Wang L, Pederson L, et al. The incidence of metastatic basal cell carcinoma (mBCC) in Denmark, 1997-2010. Eur J Dermatol 2015;25(5):463–8.
3. Von Domarus H, Stevens PJ. Metastatic basal cell carcinoma. Report of five cases and review of 170 cases in the literature. J Am Acad Dermatol 1984; 10(6):1043–60.
4. Lo JS, Snow SN, Reizner GT, et al. Metastatic basal cell carcinoma: report of twelve cases with a review of the literature. J Am Acad Dermatol 1991;24(5): 715–9.
5. Aszterbaum M, Rothman A, Johnson RL, et al. Identifications of mutations in the human PATCHED gene in sporadic basal cell carcinomas and in patients with the basal cell nevus syndrome. J Invest Dermatol 1998;110(6):885–8.
6. Bale AE, Yu KP. The hedgehog pathway and basal cell carcinomas. Hum Mol Genet 2001;10(7): 757–62.
7. Sekulic A, Migden MR, Oro AE, et al. Efficacy and safety of vismodegib in advanced basal-cell carcinoma. N Engl J Med 2012;366:2171–9.
8. Sekulic A, Migden MR, Lewis K, et al. Pivotal ERIVANCE basal cell carcinoma (BCC) study: 12-month update of efficacy and safety of vismodegib in advanced BCC. J Am Acad Dermatol 2015;72:1021–6.
9. Chang AL, Solomon JA, Hainsworth JD, et al. Expanded access study of patients with advanced basal cell carcinoma treated with the Hedgehog pathway inhibitor, vismodegib. J Am Acad Dermatol 2014;70:60–9.
10. Basset-Seguin N, Hauschild A, Grob JJ, et al. Vismodegib in patients with advanced basal cell carcinoma (STEVIE): a pre-planned interim analysis of an international, open-label trial. Lancet Oncol 2015;16: 729–36.
11. Migden MR, Guminski A, Gutzmer R, et al. Treatment with two different doses of sonidegib in patients with locally advanced or metastatic basal cell carcinoma (BOLT): a multicentre, randomised, double-blind phase 2 trial. Lancet Oncol 2015;16:716–28.
12. Dubin N, Kopf AW. Multivariate risk score for recurrence of cutaneous basal cell carcinomas. Arch Dermatol 1983;119:373–7.
13. Rigel DS, Robins P, Friedman RJ. Predicting recurrence of basal-cell carcinomas treated by microscopically controlled excision: a recurrence index score. J Dermatol Surg Oncol 1981;7:807–10.
14. Connolly AH, Baker DR, Coldiron BM, et al. AAD/ACMS/ASDSA/ASMS 2012 appropriate use criteria for Mohs micrographic surgery: a report of the American Academy of Dermatology, American College of Mohs Surgery, American Society for Dermatologic Surgery Association, and the American Society for Mohs Surgery. Dermatol Surg 2012;38:1582–603.
15. Bartos V, Pokorny D, Zacharova O, et al. Recurrent basal cell carcinoma: a clinicopathological study and evaluation of histomorphological findings in primary and recurrent lesions. Acta Dermatovenerol Alp Pannonica Adriat 2011;20:67–75.
16. Ratner D, Lowe L, Johnson TM, et al. Perineural spread of basal cell carcinomas treated with Mohs micrographic surgery. Cancer 2000;88:1605–13.
17. Braathen LR, Szeimies RM, Basset-Seguin N, et al. Guidelines on the use of photodynamic therapy for nonmelanoma skin cancer: an international consensus. International Society for Photodynamic Therapy in Dermatology, 2005. J Am Acad Dermatol 2007;56(1):125–43.
18. Tang JY, Mackay-Wiggan JM, Aszterbaum M, et al. Inhibiting the hedgehog pathway in patients with the basal-cell nevus syndrome. N Engl J Med 2012;366(23):2180–8.
19. Ally MS, Aasi S, Wysong A, et al. An investigator-initiated open-label clinical trial of vismodegib as a neoadjuvant to surgery for high-risk basal cell carcinoma. J Am Acad Dermatol 2014;71(5):904–11.
20. Kwon GP, Ally MS, Bailey-Healy I, et al. Update to an open-label clinical trial of vismodegib as neoadjuvant before surgery for high-risk basal cell carcinoma (BCC). J Am Acad Dermatol 2016;75(1):213–5.
21. Sofen H, Gross KG, Goldberg LH, et al. A phase II, multicenter, open-label, 3-cohort trial evaluating the efficacy and safety of vismodegib in operable basal cell carcinoma. J Am Acad Dermatol 2015;73(1): 99–105.

22. Dreier J, Dummer R, Felderer L, et al. Emerging drugs and combination strategies for basal cell carcinoma. Expert Opin Emerg Drugs 2014;19(3): 353–65.

23. Fenton SE, Sosman JA, Chandra S. Current therapy for basal cell carcinoma and the potential role for immunotherapy with checkpoint inhibitors. Clin Skin Cancer 2017;2(1):59–65.

24. Lipson EJ, Lilo MT, Ogurtsova A, et al. Basal cell carcinoma: PD-L1/PD-1 checkpoint expression and tumor regression after PD-1 blockade. J Immunother Cancer 2017;5(1):23–7.

25. Rogers HW, Weinstock MA, Harris AR, et al. Incidence estimates of nonmelanoma skin cancer in the United States, 2006. Arch Dermatol 2010; 146(3):283–7.

26. Alam M, Ratner D. Cutaneous squamous-cell carcinoma. N Engl J Med 2001;344:975–83.

27. Sella T, Goren I, Shalev V, et al. Incidence trends of keratinocytic skin cancers and melanoma in Israel 2006-11. Br J Dermatol 2015;172(1):202–7.

28. Athas WF, Hunt WC, Key CR. Changes in nonmelanoma skin cancer incidence between 1977-1978 and 1998-1999 in northcentral New Mexico. Cancer Epidemiol Biomarkers Prev 2003;12:1105–8.

29. Schmults CD, Karia PS, Carter JB, et al. Factors predictive of recurrence and death from cutaneous squamous cell carcinoma: a 10-year, single-institution cohort study. JAMA Dermatol 2013; 149(5):541–7.

30. Sweeny L, Dean NR, Magnuson JS, et al. EGFR expression in advanced head and neck cutaneous squamous cell carcinoma. Head Neck 2012;34(5): 681–6.

31. Maubec E, Petrow P, Scheer-Senyarich I, et al. Phase II study of cetuximab as first-line single-drug therapy in patients with unresectable squamous cell carcinoma of the skin. J Clin Oncol 2011;29(25):3419–26.

32. William WN, Feng L, Ferrarotto R, et al. Gefinitib for patients with incurable cutaneous squamous cell carcinoma: a single-arm phase II clinical trial. J Am Acad Dermatol 2017;77(6):1110–3.

33. Gold KA, Kies MS, William WN, et al. Erlotinib in the treatment of recurrent or metastatic cutaneous squamous cell carcinoma: a single-arm phase 2 clinical trial. Cancer 2018;124(10):2169–73.

34. Pickering CR, Zhou JH, Lee JJ, et al. Mutational landscape of aggressive cutaneous squamous cell carcinoma. Clin Cancer Res 2014;20(24): 6582–92.

35. Skulsky SL, O'Sullivan B, McArdle O, et al. Review of high-risk features of cutaneous squamous cell carcinoma and discrepancies between the American Joint Committee on Cancer and NCCN Clinical Practice Guidelines in Oncology. Head Neck 2017;39(3): 578–94.

36. Baum CL, Wright AC, Martinez JC, et al. A new evidence-based risk stratification system for cutaneous squamous cell carcinoma into low, intermediate, and high risk groups with implications for management. J Am Acad Dermatol 2018;78(1): 141–7.

37. Koyfman SA, Cooper JS, Beitler JJ, et al. ACR appropriateness criteria aggressive nonmelanomatous skin cancer of the head and neck. Head Neck 2016;38(2):175–82.

38. Jambusaria-Pahlajani A, Miller CJ, Quon H, et al. Surgical monotherapy versus surgery plus adjuvant radiotherapy in high-risk cutaneous squamous cell carcinoma: a systematic review of outcomes. Dermatol Surg 2009;35(4):574–85.

39. Waxweiler W, Sigmon JR, Sheehan DJ. Adjunctive radiotherapy in the treatment of cutaneous squamous cell carcinoma with perineural invasion. J Surg Oncol 2011;104(1):104–5.

40. Tanvetyanon T, Padhya T, McCaffrey J, et al. Postoperative concurrent chemotherapy and radiotherapy for high-risk cutaneous squamous cell carcinoma of the head and neck. Head Neck 2015;37(6):840–5.

41. Nottage MK, Lin C, Hughes BG, et al. Prospective study of definitive chemoradiation in locally or regionally advanced squamous cell carcinoma of the skin. Head Neck 2017;39(4):679–83.

42. Porceddu SV, Bressel M, Poulsen MG, et al. Postoperative concurrent chemoradiotherapy versus postoperative radiotherapy in high-risk cutaneous squamous cell carcinoma of the head and neck: the randomized phase III TROG 05.01 trial. J Clin Oncol 2018;36(13):1275–83.

43. Bernier J, Cooper JS, Pajak TF, et al. Defining risk levels in locally advanced head and neck cancers: a comparative analysis of concurrent postoperative radiation plus chemotherapy trials of the EORTC (#22931) and RTOG (#9501). Head Neck 2005; 27(10):843–50.

44. Reigneau M, Robert C, Routier E, et al. Efficacy of neoadjuvant cetuximab alone or with platinum salt for the treatment of unresectable advanced nonmetastatic cutaneous squamous cell carcinomas. Br J Dermatol 2015;173(2):527–34.

45. Lewis CM, Glisson BS, Feng L, et al. A phase II study of gefitinib for aggressive cutaneous squamous cell carcinoma of the head and neck. Clin Cancer Res 2012;18(5):1435–46.

46. Urosevic M, Dummer R. Immunotherapy for nonmelanoma skin cancer: does it have a future? Cancer 2002;94(2):477–85.

47. Migden MR, Rischin D, Schmults CD, et al. PD-1 blockade with cemiplimab in advanced cutaneous squamous-cell carcinoma. N Engl J Med 2018; 379(4):341–51.

48. Siegel RL, Miller KD, Jemal A. Cancer statistics, 2018. CA Cancer J Clin 2018;68(1):7–30.

49. National Cancer Institute. Surveillance epidemiology and end results. 2008. Available at: http://seer.cancer.gov/statfacts/html/melan.html#ref11. Accessed August 13, 2018.

50. Balch CM, Gershenwald JE, Soong SJ, et al. Final version of 2009 AJCC melanoma staging and classification. J Clin Oncol 2009;27:6199–206.

51. Lyth J, Hansson J, Ingvar C, et al. Prognostic subclassifications of T1 cutaneous melanomas based on ulceration, tumour thickness and Clark's level of invasion: results of a population-based study from the Swedish Melanoma Register. Br J Dermatol 2013;168:779–86.

52. In 't Hout FE, Haydu LE, Murali R, et al. Prognostic importance of the extent of ulceration in patients with clinically localized cutaneous melanoma. Ann Surg 2012;255:1165–70.

53. Thompson JF, Soong SJ, Balch CM, et al. Prognostic significance of mitotic rate in localized primary cutaneous melanoma: an analysis of patients in the multi-institutional American Joint Committee on Cancer melanoma staging database. J Clin Oncol 2011;29:2199–205.

54. Maurichi A, Miceli R, Camerini T, et al. Prediction of survival in patients with thin melanoma: results from a multi-institution study. J Clin Oncol 2014;32:2479–85.

55. Omholt K, Platz A, Kanter L, et al. NRAS and BRAF mutations arise early during melanoma pathogenesis and are preserved throughout tumor progression. Clin Cancer Res 2003;9(17):6483–8.

56. Krauthammer M, Kong Y, Bacchiocchi A, et al. Exome sequencing identifies recurrent mutations in NF1 and RASopathy genes in sun-exposed melanomas. Nat Genet 2015;47(9):996–1002.

57. Cancer Genome Atlas Network. Genomic classification of cutaneous melanoma. Cell 2015;161(7):1681–96.

58. Hodis E, Watson IR, Kryukov GV, et al. A landscape of driver mutations in melanoma. Cell 2012;150(2):251–63.

59. Wellbrock C, Hurlstone A. BRAF as therapeutic target in melanoma. Biochem Pharmacol 2010;80(5):561–7.

60. Pardoll DM. The blockade of immune checkpoints in cancer immunotherapy. Nat Rev Cancer 2012;12(4):252–64.

61. Agha A, Tarhini A. Adjuvant therapy for melanoma. Curr Oncol Rep 2017;19(5):36.

62. Kirkwood JM, Strawderman MH, Ernstoff MS, et al. Interferon alfa- 2b adjuvant therapy of high-risk resected cutaneous melanoma: the Eastern Cooperative Oncology Group Trial EST 1684. J Clin Oncol 1996;14:7–17.

63. Kirkwood JM, Ibrahim JG, Sosman JA, et al. High-dose interferon alfa-2b significantly prolongs relapse-free and overall survival compared with the GM2-KLH-QS-21 vaccine in patients with resected stage IIB-III melanoma: results of intergroup trial E1694/S9512/C509801. J Clin Oncol 2001;19(9):2370–80.

64. Mocellin S, Pasquali S, Rossi CR, et al. Interferon alpha adjuvant therapy in patients with high-risk melanoma: a systematic review and meta-analysis. J Natl Cancer Inst 2010;102(7):493–501.

65. Eggermont AM, Suciu S, MacKie R, et al. Post-surgery adjuvant therapy with intermediate doses of interferon alfa 2b versus observation in patients with stage IIb/III melanoma (EORTC 18952): randomised controlled trial. Lancet 2005;266(9492):1189–96.

66. Eggermont AM, Suciu S, Santinami M, et al. Adjuvant therapy with pegylated interferon alfa-2b versus observation alone in resected stage III melanoma: final results of EORTC 18991, a randomised phase III trial. Lancet 2008;372(9633):117–26.

67. Eigentler TK, Gutzmer R, Hauschild A, et al. Adjuvant treatment with pegylated interferon α-2a versus low-dose interferon α-2a in patients with high-risk melanoma: a randomized phase III DeCOG trial. Ann Oncol 2016;27(8):1625–32.

68. Eggermont AM, Chiarion-Sileni V, Grob JJ, et al. Adjuvant ipilimumab versus placebo after complete resection of high-risk stage III melanoma (EORTC 18071): a randomised, double-blind, phase 3 trial. Lancet 2015;16(5):522–30.

69. Tarhini AA, Lee SJ, Hodi FS, et al. A phase III randomized study of adjuvant ipilimumab (3 or 10 mg/kg) versus high-dose interferon alfa-2b for resected high-risk melanoma (U.S. Intergroup E1609): preliminary safety and efficacy of the ipilimumab arms. [abstract: 9500]. Paper presented at: American Society of Clinical Oncology annual meeting. Chicago, June, 2017. Available at: http://ascopubs.org/doi/abs/10.1200/JCO.2017.35.15_suppl.9500. Accessed August 13, 2018.

70. Weber J, Mandala M, Del Vecchio M, et al. Adjuvant nivolumab versus ipilimumab in resected stage III or IV melanoma. N Engl J Med 2017;377:1824–35.

71. Eggermont AM, Blank CU, Mandal M, et al. Adjuvant pembrolizumab versus placebo in resected stage III melanoma. N Engl J Med 2018;378:1789–801.

72. Leiter U, Stadler R, Mauch C, et al. Complete lymph node dissection versus no dissection in patients with sentinel lymph node biopsy positive melanoma (DeCOG-SLT): a multicentre, randomised, phase 3 trial. Lancet Oncol 2016;17(6):757–67.

73. Faries MB, Thompson JF, Cochran AJ, et al. Completion dissection or observation for sentinel-node metastasis in melanoma. N Engl J Med 2017;376:2211–22.

74. Long GV, Hauschild A, Santinami M, et al. Adjuvant dabrafenib plus trametinib in stage III

BRAF-mutated melanoma. N Engl J Med 2017;377: 1813–23.

75. Maio M, Lewis K, Demidov L, et al. Adjuvant vemurafenib in resected, BRAF^{V600} mutation-positive melanoma (BRIM8): a randomised, double-blind, placebo-controlled, multicentre, phase 3 trial. Lancet Oncol 2018;19(4):510–20.

76. Strom T, Caudell JJ, Han D, et al. Radiotherapy influences local control in patients with desmoplastic melanoma. Cancer 2014;120:1369–78.

77. Henderson MA, Burmeister BH, Ainslie J, et al. Adjuvant lymph- node field radiotherapy versus observation only in patients with melanoma at high risk of further lymph-node field relapse after lymphadenectomy (ANZMTG 01.02/TROG 02.01): 6-year follow-up of a phase 3, randomised controlled trial. Lancet Oncol 2015;16(9): 1049–60.

78. Amaria RN, Prieto PA, Tetzlaff MT, et al. Neoadjuvant plus adjuvant dabrafenib and trametinib versus standard of care in patients with high-risk, surgically resectable melanoma: a single-centre, open-label, randomized, phase 2 trial. Lancet Oncol 2018; 19(2):181–93.

Tissue Engineering and 3-Dimensional Modeling for Facial Reconstruction

Kyle K. VanKoevering, MD[a],*, David A. Zopf, MD[b],
Scott J. Hollister, PhD[c]

KEYWORDS

• Facial reconstruction • 3D printing • Tissue engineering • Scaffolds • Prosthetics • Bioprinting

KEY POINTS

• Three-dimensional (3D) printing has dramatically impacted advancements in personalized medicine, with craniofacial reconstruction pioneering many of the key developments in the last decade.
• Facial reconstruction is an ideal field for 3D technologies, owing to the intricate and highly personalized anatomic constraints, along with the concepts of mirroring symmetry and restoring cosmetic contours.
• Digital anaplastology has rapidly advanced over the last 5 years thanks to improved access to high-quality desktop 3D printing technology and 3D modeling/design software, making complex prosthetics potentially more affordable and with faster turnaround in production.
• Three-dimensional printing allows for the development of highly complex, microporous 3D scaffolds that have allowed tissue engineering to rapidly expand from traditional 2-dimensional planar concepts into organic 3D constructs.
• The Food and Drug Administration continues to provide guidelines and recommendations that have fostered innovation while maximizing safety for patients in this rapidly evolving field and will continue to assist in guiding the implementation of clinical applications.

INTRODUCTION

The recent push toward personalized medicine has driven several important advancements across facial plastic surgery. The facial shape and features provide an integral part of patients' fundamental identify, necessitating meticulous high-fidelity reconstructive options for craniofacial defects. This need for personalized reconstruction has been significantly impacted by the rapid growth of 3D modeling and printing technologies, which are allowing for more anatomically accurate reconstructive outcomes for complex craniofacial defects. More recently, the power of 3D printing has merged with tissue engineering as medicine works toward more biological, precise solutions to facial reconstruction via regenerative medicine. This article aims to highlight the current state of 3D printing and tissue engineering as it applies to

Disclosure Statement: Dr S.J. Hollister has a patent for airway reconstruction that has been licensed for manufacturing. Dr D.A. Zopf and Dr S.J. Hollister have a preliminary patent filed for the 3D printed auricular scaffold described in the article.
[a] Department of Otolaryngology–Head and Neck Surgery, University of Michigan Medical Center, 1500 East Medical Center Drive, 1904 Taubman Center, Ann Arbor, MI 48109, USA; [b] Department of Otolaryngology–Head and Neck Surgery, Division of Pediatric Otolaryngology, University of Michigan Medical Center, 1500 East Medical Center Drive, Ann Arbor, MI 48109, USA; [c] Wallace H. Coulter Department of Biomedical Engineering, Georgia Institute of Technology, 313 Ferst Drive Northwest, Atlanta, GA 30332, USA
* Corresponding author.
E-mail address: kylevk@med.umich.edu

Facial Plast Surg Clin N Am 27 (2019) 151–161
https://doi.org/10.1016/j.fsc.2018.08.012
1064-7406/19/© 2018 Elsevier Inc. All rights reserved.

facial reconstruction and review current trends for the future of the technology.

BACKGROUND

Three-dimensional printing was first described in the mid-1980s by Charles Hull[1] and was pioneered for use in the aerospace and automotive industries. At the time, 3D printing, synonymously referred to as additive manufacturing or rapid prototyping, used an early computer-aided design (CAD) modeling software to develop a 3D model of an object to be manufactured. The model is then digitally sliced into thin 2-dimensional (2D) planar layers. The printer then builds the 3D object by printing each of these 2D slices stacked atop each other. The initial technology used a UV laser light to solidify, or cure, a liquid photopolymer resin as it traced out the design of each layer in 2D space.[1]

Although the technology has expanded greatly since the initial conception in the 1980s, the principles of 3D printing remain constant: virtual 3D design, digital slicing, and layered manufacturing.[2] Three-dimensional printing technologies have expanded since this time to include nozzle-based deposition, laser-based sintering of powdered materials, laser-based polymerization, and extrusion-based methods. Although the detailed technological principles of 3D printing are beyond the scope of this review, the recent decade has seen an impressive expansion in a variety of new technologies and materials available for 3D printing.[3–7] New desktop printers have simplified the design and modeling process, making the technology affordably accessible to a wide range of medical providers.[8] New materials have been adapted into printing technology, promoting biologically compatible constructs with a wide variety of structural properties.[9,10] Printing technology is now capable of directly depositing biological materials, including protein hydrogels and cellular suspensions, through a variety of bioprinting techiques[11,12] as regenerative medicine has fused with 3D printing.

Compared with traditional machining technologies, 3D printing allows for the creation of highly complex internal design configurations that can be manufactured with very few limitations, depending on the particular 3D printing machine used. Yet, the real power in the technology ultimately stems from the capacity to turn traditional medical imaging technologies (such as computed tomography [CT] ad MRI) into high-resolution, *patient-specific*, 3D models of complex anatomy. This capacity, in turn, allows for craniofacial anatomy to be digitally refined using principles of mirroring symmetry, smoothing functions, and virtual molding tools, whereas devices can be designed to perfectly compliment patients' anatomy.

As the technology for 3D printing and digital design becomes more readily accessible to medical providers, the authors are seeing substantial changes in customized solutions to complex craniofacial defects. From evolving techniques with digital anaplastology to virtually planned and executed surgical resection and reconstruction, cutaneous oncologic surgeons have impactful new tools in their armamentarium; the evolution of tissue engineering solutions, as it merges with the power of 3D printing, is a promising new horizon that is rapidly evolving.

BONY CRANIOFACIAL RECONSTRUCTION

Although reconstruction of significant bony defects is not frequently encountered by the cutaneous oncologic surgeon, when such malignancies require large bony resection, precise rigid reconstruction is critical to both functional and cosmetic outcomes for these patients. This demand for precision and symmetry, particularly in the facial skeleton, has helped drive several technologies over the last 2 decades combining digital modeling, 3D printing, and tissue engineering to provide unique, customized reconstruction for patients undergoing large craniofacial resection and reconstruction. These bony reconstructive challenges have served as the foundation merging 3D printing and facial plastic surgery in the recent past; highlighting this recent evolution, the currently available options and future horizons in bony reconstruction are important for surgeons who may tackle large cutaneous malignancies.

3-Dimentional Printed Bone Models

Perhaps one of the first strongholds of 3D printing technology in craniofacial reconstruction evolved from preoperative planning techniques for bony reconstruction. Initial operative planning techniques were first reported in the early 1990s whereby 3D models of skull defects were used to plan grafting procedures.[13,14] The technology has advanced substantially since this initial inception, whereby the bony anatomy of the craniofacial skeleton is modeled and printed, sterilized, and used as reference in the operating room (OR). Operative models are now commonplace in microvascular reconstruction and can be used to plan reconstructive geometry, prebend reconstructive plates, and practice alignment of bone grafts to oncologic resections.[15–19] While prospective studies with definitive outcomes are still lacking, reports have demonstrated faster reconstruction with good subjective cosmetic results. Today, as the technology becomes more readily accessible, several options exist for these models to be made in-house with potentially reduced cost (**Fig. 1**).

Virtual Surgical Planning and Cutting Guides

To further assist with the complex geometric osteotomies and reconstruction, surgical guides and prebent customized reconstructive plates are now offered through a concept called virtual surgical planning (VSP).[20] Commercial services are now offered through several companies, including 3D Systems (VSP, 3D Systems, Rock Hill, SC) and Materialise (ProPlan and Patient-Specific Guides, Materialise, Leuven, Belgium). Through these systems, surgeons planning a craniofacial reconstruction after proposed onco-logic resection first participate in a virtual recon-struction via teleconference with oncologic margins and the bone graft of choice. Surgical guides are then designed to fit onto the native bone to guide the osteotomies (aligning the saw blade at the planned location and angle) for the oncologic resection as well as the osteotomies required for the grafted bone to precisely align with the reconstruction. This process can also include a custom-bent plate to assist with the reconstruction. The cutting guides are 3D printed and sterilized for temporary implantation in the OR.

Customized Implants for Bony Defects

In addition to expediting bony reconstruction, oc-casionally a synthetic implant is a more feasible option for reconstruction of a large bony defect. This concept was initially developed from neuro-surgical patients who underwent large craniecto-mies for trauma or tumor resection. Traditionally the bony void was covered with a semirigid, crudely fitted titanium mesh.

More recently, cranioplasty is being performed via more precise customized synthetic grafts. A CT scan of the patients' skull is performed after the initial craniectomy. A 3D reconstruction of the bony anatomy is then performed. Using the con-cepts of 3D modeling, a customized graft is then designed to smoothly reconstruct the skull. The graft is designed to perfectly fit into the bony defect, with ledges overhanging the outer cortex to secure the graft in place.[16]

Using this concept, a wide variety of cranioplasty implants have been described.[21] Custom implants fabricated from hydroxyapatite were described early with good results,[22] as well as 3D print molds, which were sterilized and filled with poly (methyl methacrylate) intraoperatively.[23] Polyetheretherke-tone (PEEK) has become a standard choice for custom cranioplasty owing to its strong, light-weight properties. Using the same 3D design con-cepts, a custom implant is then manufactured with traditional machining technology from the polymer, sterilized, and implanted with reliable results[24,25] and offered as a commercial service. Custom tita-nium implants have also been reported for cranial reconstruction using similar concepts but using the biomaterial properties of titanium blended with 3D printing technology or traditional molding techniques with promising results.[26–28]

With the success of cranioplasty reconstruction, several groups have further expanded custom implant design into the facial skeleton, particularly with PEEK.[29–31] Materialise (Leuven, Belgium) of-fers customized titanium plates and implants to augment bone graft reconstruction related to oncologic and orthognathic reconstruction. More recently, Oxford Performance Materials (Windsor,

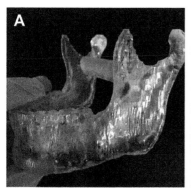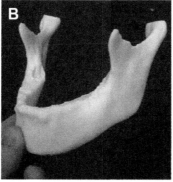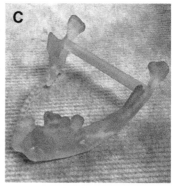

Fig. 1. Three-dimensional printed models of mandible anatomy, which were all created in-house for planning and plate bending of mandibular defects. (*A*) Normal mandibular anatomy printed on stereolithography printer. (*B*) Fused Deposition Modeling (FDM) (FDM 3000, Stratasys, Minnesota) printed digitally reconstructed mandible after comminuted mandibular fracture. (*C*) Complex revision mandibulectomy planned after prior composite resection and plate reconstruction.

CT) received Food and Drug Administration (FDA) clearance for customized 3D printed polyetherketoneketone (PEKK) implants manufactured with selective laser sintering printing technology. These implants are approved to replace large bony defects of the non–load-bearing craniofacial skeleton, including naso-orbital, zygomatic, and cranial defects.[32] Polycaprolactone (PCL) is a bioresorbable implant material that has also been 3D printed for patient-specific cranial and midface implants.[33,34]

The trend of customized solutions to facial bony defects, such as those incurred after oncologic resection of large cutaneous malignancies, continues to advance with new, innovative, and clinically relevant options for patients whereby the complex geometry or anatomic constraints limit traditional reconstructive techniques. Implants such as those noted earlier have shown excellent bio-integration with low rates of infection; however, care must be taken when these are to be used in a radiated field or adjacent to mucosal surfaces where seeding and infection could occur.

SOFT TISSUE (NASAL AND AURICULAR) RECONSTRUCTION

The cutaneous oncologic reconstructive surgeon is frequently presented with the challenge of resecting and replacing underlying support structures. Highest rates of recurrence in facial cutaneous malignancies are those of the ear and nose.[35] As a result, the recommendation is for tumor-free margins erring on larger resection. The geometry of support structures needing reconstruction, associated with partial or total auricular or nasal excision, can be extremely complex. Auricular and nasal reconstruction demand significant experience, training, and the utmost artistic and detail-oriented precision and skill.

The current gold standard for auricular and nasal reconstruction uses autologous cartilage as foundational support for overlying soft tissue, which is classically harvested from the nasal septum, auricle, or rib depending on the support required. Subsequently sculpting the undulating apices and ascents of this intricate anatomy demands in-depth experience and innate artistic ability. Even in the most experienced of hands, outcomes are short of exact. Inconsistent results have led to low patient and family satisfaction in many surgeons' hands. Alternatively, implantable high-density porous polyethylene, approved under the trade name MedPor (Stryker, Kalamazoo, MI, USA) or SuPor (Poriferous LLC, Newnan, GA, USA), has been used for ear reconstruction, though predominantly for reconstruction in congenital microtia. MedPor was approved for use by the FDA as a class

II device through the 510k pathway. However, only a single size implant is available for a wide range of pediatric and adult patients needing reconstruction. Importantly, this alloplastic approach depends highly on the vascularity and quality of adjacent soft tissue and the availability and viability of the temporoparietal fascial flap, all of which may be in jeopardy in cutaneous malignancy.

Although outcomes with these traditional approaches can be quite good, the inherent challenges in achieving satisfactory results for these complex anatomic defects has opened the door for 3D printing, digital 3D design, and tissue engineering alternatives to rapidly and precisely reconstruct structures with ease.

Digital Prosthodontics and Anaplastology

Traditional facial prosthodontics use an artistic, though rudimentary, facial impression, molding and sculpting approach to ultimately develop a silicone prosthesis that can provide excellent cosmetic outcomes.[36] However, prosthodontics can, at times, be costly, require frequent replacement, and require multiple revisions to improve fit and limit skin irritation and gapping.[37–39] Prosthetics are most widely used for complex nasal and auricular reconstruction. Over the last 10 years, there has been a notable increase in the marriage of 3D printing and virtual design concepts to expedite the molding and prosthesis design process, while expanding to more and more complex prosthetic options. Using 3D modeling techniques with cross-sectional imaging, mirroring and digital sculpting can be used to design a new prosthesis that perfectly integrates with the patients' underlying anatomy. The prosthesis or molds can be 3D printed for subsequent silicone molding.[40–42] Palousek and colleagues[43] used this similar approach to rapidly design and manufacture a nasal prosthesis after a complex subtotal rhinectomy. The entire manufacturing process required only 19 hours, a substantial improvement over traditional approaches with excellent cosmesis. Grant and colleagues[44] reported a large naso-facial prosthesis digitally designed for a pediatric patient who sustained an explosive trauma to the face. They used an optical scan from a virtual facial donor, which was then modified and digitally integrated into the facial defect. A mold was designed and 3D printed for the prosthesis and, after detailed silicone pouring and coloring, was applied with adhesive and had good cosmetic results. Perhaps most publicized was a very large mandibulofacial prosthesis for a patient with a remote near-total mandibulectomy defect who had never been able to fit a prosthesis. Dubbed the Shirley technique (as described earlier), a prosthesis was digitally sculpted onto his 3D facial model, then molds were printed to fabricate the prosthesis.[45] Taking a slightly different approach, Sultan and Byrne[46] describe the use of 3D printing technology to create intraoperative masks for patients undergoing large nasal reconstruction. First, a wax model of the patient's ideal reconstructed nose was made by an anaplastologist. This model was then scanned into a virtual design, where a mask was modeled based on the ideal nasal structural anatomy. This mask was then 3D printed and used intraoperatively to guide the geometric orientation of the structural nasal framework. All 3 patients were pleased with the reconstructive outcomes. New and innovative concepts continue to evolve as 3D printing has become more readily accessible to anaplastologists for complex prosthetic design.

TISSUE ENGINEERING

Tissue engineering is a rapidly evolving field that aims to combine cellular biology, organogenesis, and biomaterials into regenerative medicine. Although tissue engineering is a concept garnering high-profile and somewhat futuristic attention in the media, many of the key concepts are becoming well defined as efforts to streamline and safely define standards for clinical implementation continue to evolve. The remainder of this article highlights some of the key concepts in tissue engineering as coupled with 3D printing and focus on the current state of the technology as it pertains to complex craniofacial reconstruction.

Key Concepts in Tissue Engineering, Scaffold Design, and Fabrication for Craniofacial Reconstruction

Tissue engineering traditionally used 2D culture wells and a variety of growth factors to control the fate of cellular differentiation. In more recent decades, it became apparent that 3D spatial orientation was critical not only in organizing cellular growth into an organic construct but also providing a structural framework for vascular and intercellular communication. These 3D constructs, or scaffolds, serve as a lattice of structural material along which cells can theoretically grow and divide as they develop into functional organ subunits.[47] Ever since the first pictures of a human auricle on the back of a mouse was published in the 1990s,[48] the auricle has served as a poster child for many of the tissue engineering efforts in cartilaginous scaffold development.

There are 3 significant challenges for craniofacial soft tissue engineering based on reconstruction scaffolds: matching the complex geometry of facial structures, fabricating a scaffold from a biocompatible material with appropriate mechanical properties that provide structure, resist contracture, and avoid dehiscence, and delivering appropriate types and doses of biologics to regenerate craniofacial soft tissues. The first challenge requires software to design porous structures directly from patient image data creating a surface that can be 3D printed from a biomaterial. The second challenge requires computational models the can predict the mechanical response and biomaterials that can be 3D printed into the final designed form. The last challenge requires choosing appropriate biologics (cells, proteins, and/or genes) that can be efficiently delivered to the manufactured scaffold.

Matching Patient Anatomy

Several groups have developed approaches to design scaffolds to match complex craniofacial anatomy, primarily for bone reconstruction.[49–55] Designing such complex scaffolds necessitates volume image data (CT or MRI) be converted to a surface stereolithography (STL) file. There are several commercially available software (MimicsTM, www.materialise.com; SimplewareTM, www.synopsis.com) and shareware (3Dslicer, www.slicer.org) that can perform this conversion. Initial patient image data, such as voxels, are segmented into a set or mask. This voxel set/mask defines the patient anatomy. A separate voxel database representing the intended scaffold pore structure is then imported followed by a Boolean intersection of the patient anatomy and the pore architecture database to create a scaffold that matches the desired patient anatomy, with the final result as a STL model of a porous, scaffold anatomic construct.[50,56]

Providing Appropriate Mechanical Properties

Matching patient anatomy is only the first step in creating patient specific scaffolds for tissue reconstruction. Ideally, the scaffolds should possess effective mechanical properties stiff enough to provide structure and avoid contracture, while also compliant enough to avoid dehiscence. Contracture is a significant problem and can result in a final construct having 20% to 30% of the original construct volume. Preventing contracture requires a scaffold with sufficient stiffness to resist cellular contraction forces.[57,58] On the other hand, structures that are too stiff may engender significant strain on the overlying skin during surgical reconstruction, inhibiting vascularity and causing dehiscence. Thus, the effective scaffold mechanical properties must strike a balance to avoid complications of contracture and dehiscence. Designing mechanical properties to track native craniofacial cartilage and skin properties may be an appropriate design target.[59,60] Finally, these scaffolds designed with appropriate mechanical properties must be fabricated with a porous architecture in the correct anatomic shape from a biocompatible material. A wide range of potential biocompatible materials for craniofacial tissue engineering have been investigated, and include titanium alloy, PEEK, PEKK, synthetic polymers including polyesters (poly (L-Lactic Acid), PCL, poly (Glycerol Sebacate), poly(Glycerol-Dodecanoate)), and hydrogels.[61] Titanium alloy, PEEK, and PEKK are likely too stiff for soft tissue applications, increasing the risk for dehiscence unless sufficient architectural porosity is introduced to reduce construct stiffness. Hydrogels are advantageous for cell delivery but are too soft and will likely allow contracture. In all likelihood, a composite synthetic polymer/hydrogel scaffold will have to be used to optimize craniofacial soft tissue reconstruction. Finally, such scaffolds will have to be reproducibly manufactured according to FDA design controls to achieve clinical use in the United States. Because of the microscale and macroscale complexity, this will certainly require 3D printing techniques.

Achieving Robust Biological Delivery

The third requirement for tissue engineering of craniofacial structures is achieving robust biological delivery. These biologics may include chondrocytes and adult stem cells, harvested from patients, likely from within the OR because of regulatory hurdles.[62] There will be a need to encapsulate such cells in a natural or synthetic hydrogel to contain them within the stiffer structural scaffold. As demonstrated previously,[56] the structural scaffold will require interconnected pore structures to facilitate cell seeding and enhance tissue regeneration. Later incarnations of craniofacial scaffolds may include surface modifications for tethering growth factors.

Auricular Reconstruction with Tissue Engineering

Vacanti and colleagues[48] first reported implantation of a human-shaped ear cartilage framework on the dorsum of rodents. Although a visually impressive image penetrated media, what was not highlighted were the challenges for tissue engineering in ear reconstruction that has limited translation to date. Vacanti's group found contraction of the scaffold to be a significant issue resulting in framework distortion. This group's scaffold manufacturing methods involved clay negative molds with polyglycolic acid (PGA) fill coated with poly lactic acid (PLA) and poly lactic-co-glycolic acid (PLGA).

Additive manufacturing emerged as holding great potential for ear tissue engineering, as it allows an intricate and complex scaffold geometry to be manufactured within a complex 3D dimensional shape. Cai and colleagues[63] were the first to describe an early investigative use for scaffold-based engineering in ear tissue reconstruction. Acrylonitrile/butadiene/styrene (ABS) scaffolds (not biocompatible) were manufactured through Fused Deposition Modeling (FDM) (FDM 3000, Stratasys, Minnesota). Scaffolds were then coated with fibronectin to promote cell adhesion and then incubated with fibroblasts with and without keratinocytes.

The use of CAD/computer-aided manufacturing to generate negative molds for scaffold production has also been described.[64,65] The manufacturing method was achieved by compressing PLA/PGA in negative ear-shaped molds and in a separate report using collagen as the infill material. Multipod photography was used to generate 3D models and imported into SolidWorks (Dassault Systems Corp, Waltham, MA). The components were printed out of ABS plastic using a Stratasys FDM 2000 3D printer (Eden Prairie, MN). Cartilage growth was demonstrated by each group, though distortion over time was again a concern.

Zopf and colleagues[56] proposed a workflow for patient-specific, 3D-printed, positive porous scaffold-based designs for partial and total ear and nose reconstruction. The proposed pathway is aimed at feasible clinical translation, using a hierarchical image design for the patient-specific ear or nasal scaffold using the technique highlighted earlier.

They describe a variety of micropore structures can be designed into the scaffold, such as spherical or random porosities, using specially written MATLAB codes (The Mathworks, Natick, MA). These codes map the pore structure over a region that encompasses the final size of the anatomic region (**Fig. 2**A). Once a final design is achieved, the scaffold is 3D printed using laser sintering of PCL in a similar fashion to the manufacturing of airway splints previously described[66] (PCL, Polysciences, Warrington, PA; PCL Preparation, Jet Pulverizer, Moorsetown, NJ). The laser sintering process can fabricate feature sizes on the order of 700 μm (0.7 mm) (**Fig. 2**C). Using this approach and seeding with hydrogel and chondrocytes, the authors' team has demonstrated consistent and robust chondrogenesis with small and large preclinical in vivo animal models (**Fig. 2**B, D).

A potential landmark in auricular tissue engineering has been the first-in-human description by Zhou and colleagues[67] as a part of 5 case series. Tissue-engineered cartilage was implanted with excellent

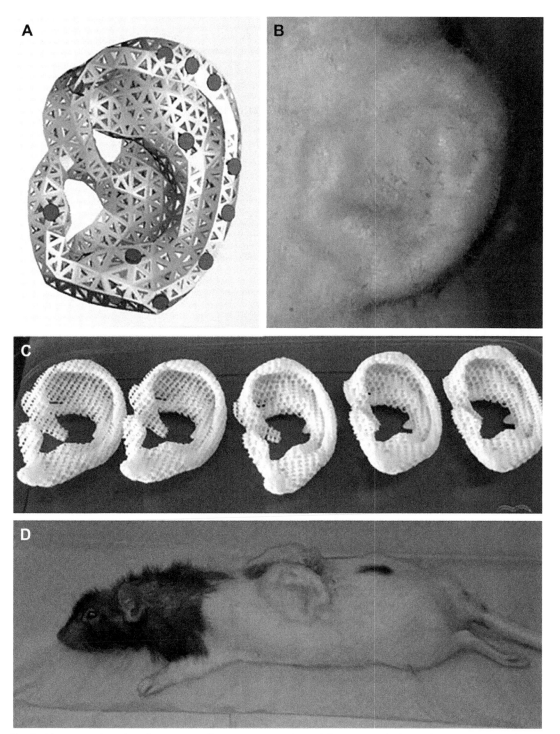

Fig. 2. Tissue engineering for ear cartilage reconstruction. (*A*) CAD rendering of a patient-specific ear including designed porous architecture. (*B*) Preclinical in vivo implant at 2 months after implantation showing preservation of scaffold dimensions and well-vascularized overlying soft tissue. (*C*) 3D printed, biocompatible, good manufacturing practices grade, laser sintered, PCL ear scaffolds. (*D*) Preclinical in vivo implant at 2 months after implantation demonstrating excellent anterior and posterior definition. Scaffolds consistently facilitate robust cartilage growth. (*Courtesy of* David A. Zopf, MD, Ann Arbor, MI; and Scott J. Hollister, PhD, Atlanta, GA.)

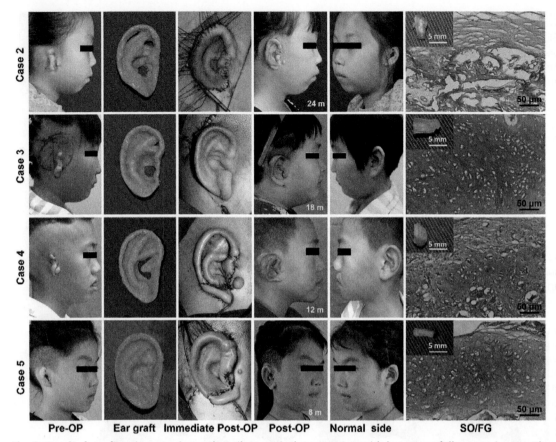

Fig. 3. Results from first tissue engineered cartilage auricular constructs with long-term follow-up pictures. The image demonstrates the engineered auricular construct, immediate postoperative result, and long-term result with good cosmetic results with good cartilage ingrowth on the constructs (*far right*). FG, fast green stains for cartilage matrix; OP, operative (ie, post-operative and pre-operative); SO, safranin-O. (*From* Zhou G, Jiang H, Yin Z, et al. In vitro regeneration of patient-specific ear-shaped cartilage and its first clinical application for auricular reconstruction. EBioMedicine 2018;28:298; with permission.)

outcomes at 2.5 years (**Fig. 3**). Caveats exist with the report. Some evidence of contraction is noted in some of these patients; although the follow-up is an impressive duration with adequate structural preservation, additional follow-up will be critical to assess maintenance beyond the anticipated period of scaffold resorption. Furthermore, although the methods used were performed under the Chinese Clinical Trial Registry, these methods may not meet the regulatory demands of other bodies, such as the FDA. Nonetheless, the significance of this report undoubtedly signals that progress is occurring and that tissue engineering, with the aid of 3D printing, will be a likely component of craniofacial soft tissue reconstruction.

Nasal reconstruction, either partial or total, poses a significant challenge to the most experienced reconstructive surgeon. Total nasal reconstruction, in particular, requires significant effort and technical skill. In the best of hands, unpredictable and undesirable outcomes are characteristic.

Nasal reconstruction is frequently necessary as a result of cutaneous oncologic resections. The authors' group was the first to propose a patient-specific, 3D-printed, porous scaffold-based design for nasal reconstruction. Design and manufacturing methods are analogous to the production of ear scaffolds; however, the microporous architecture is fitted into a patient-specific nasal framework.

Using this approach, nasal scaffolds have been tested in rodent and porcine animal models with robust demonstration of cartilage growth and short-term maintenance of scaffold dimensions.[56] The authors have seeded their craniofacial scaffolds with primary auricular chondrocytes as well as in a coculture environment with adipose-derived stem cells, both exhibiting robust cartilage growth. Long-term data are necessary before human use; however, the authors' proposed manufacturing methods are designed for near-future translation.

Bio-printing

Bio-printing involves direct deposition of cellular suspensions and organic hydrogels into 3D constructs. Although the details are beyond the scope of this article, there are several technologies used in bio-printing, including extrusion, ink jetting, laser-induced forward transfer, and integrated tissue-organ printing (ITOP).[68] Cell printing typically involves a hydrogel carrier, providing a viable, biocompatible environment and more predictable transfer methods. Each existing method has had limitations secondary to difficulty with manufacturing stable significant anatomic structures, limitations of structural stability, and flow rate limitations.

Of the methods listed, only the ITOP method has reported production of larger-scale facial soft tissue constructs. Although ear geometries were successfully bio-printed, these constructs were approximately one-half the size of an average adult ear. Kang and colleagues[69] described a multi-nozzle extrusion system producing composite scaffolds composed of internal PCL, gelatin/fibrinogen/hyaluronic acid/auricular chondrocyte hydrogel, and an external sacrificial Pluronic F-127 hydrogel. PCL is chosen for its previously stated property of stable structural support, prolonged degradation time of approximately 2 years, as well as its low melting temperature of 60°C, conducive to coprinting with cell containing hydrogels. The group used Pluronic F-127, despite poor biocompatibility, for added structural support. Gelatin was selected for its thermosensitive properties, solidifying at less than 25°C and liquefying at greater than 37°C. Fibrinogen was chosen to encourage cell adhesion and proliferation. Hyaluronic acid and glycerol were used to facilitate flow and homogeneity. The materials are delivered via a 3-axis stage, whereby the PCL nozzle included a heating unit allowing polymerization. CT imaging was used as the basis for CAD models, though presumably scaled down, as scaffolds measured only 3.2 × 1.6 × 0.9 cm.

Standard outcomes were reported, including glycosaminoglycan content, histologic comparison with native auricular cartilage (hematoxylin-eosin, safranin O, alcian blue, and collagen II), and biomechanical characteristics. Although gross appearance of the explanted ear scaffold at 1 month is provided, in vivo subcutaneous appearance in situ was not displayed. Nonetheless, this impressive report further details the ITOP method for manufacturing mandibular bone segments, calvarial bone, and skeletal muscle.

Although still short of direct clinical applications, tissue engineered scaffolds for facial reconstruction hold promise to give individuals their sense of wholeness or restore individuals to their original form in a manner that may avert poor surgical outcome, mitigate surgical risk, and limit operative and anesthetic time.

SUMMARY

Reconstruction of the craniofacial anatomy, particularly after an oncologic resection, demands precision, creativity, and attention to detail to obtain adequate symmetry, cosmetic outcomes, and functional results. Apart from the critical role of the facial anatomy in patients' identity, the cutaneous oncologic surgeon faces unique challenges particularly in reconstruction of nasal and auricular defects related to compromised vascularity and radiation, limited grafting options, and the intricate details that can be difficult to recreate. Three-dimensional printing and tissue engineering strategies have already demonstrated significant, clinically translatable impacts in these complex reconstructions. Digital prosthetic design and manufacture, along with 3D-printed surgical guides are becoming commonplace techniques for improved outcomes. Several groups have demonstrated impressive preliminary results with various tissue engineering approaches, particularly for auricular reconstruction fueled by 3D printed scaffolds. Although encouraging, additional work will be needed to transition these experimental approaches into feasible translatable clinical applications.

REFERENCES

1. Hull CW. Apparatus for production of three-dimensional objects by stereolithography. US Patent 4,575,330. March 11, 1986.
2. VanKoevering KK, Hollister SJ, Green GE. Advances in 3-dimensional printing in otolaryngology: a review. JAMA Otolaryngol Head Neck Surg 2017;143(2):178–83.
3. Melchels FP, Feijen J, Grijpma DW. A review on stereolithography and its applications in biomedical engineering. Biomaterials 2010;31(24):6121–30.
4. Pham DT, Gault RS. A comparison of rapid prototyping technologies. Int J Mach Tool Manu 1998;38(10–11):1257–87.
5. Kuang M, Wang L, Song Y. Controllable printing droplets for high-resolution patterns. Adv Mater 2014;26(40):6950–8.
6. Boland T, Xu T, Damon B, et al. Application of inkjet printing to tissue engineering. Biotechnol J 2006;1(9):910–7.
7. Campbell PG, Weiss LE. Tissue engineering with the aid of inkjet printers. Expert Opin Biol Ther 2007;7(8):1123–7.

8. AlAli AB, Griffin MF, Butler PE. Three-dimensional printing surgical applications. Eplasty 2015;15:e37.

9. Youssef A, Hollister SJ, Dalton PD. Additive manufacturing of polymer melts for implantable medical devices and scaffolds. Biofabrication 2017;9(1):012002.

10. Kelly CN, Miller AT, Hollister SJ, et al. Design and structure-function characterization of 3D printed synthetic porous biomaterials for tissue engineering. Adv Healthc Mater 2018;7(7):e1701095.

11. Jammalamadaka U, Tappa K. Recent advances in biomaterials for 3D printing and tissue engineering. J Funct Biomater 2018;9(1) [pii:E22].

12. Gungor-Ozkerim PS, Inci I, Zhang YS, et al. Bioinks for 3D bioprinting: an overview. Biomater Sci 2018; 6(5):915–46.

13. Mankovich NJ, Samson D, Pratt W, et al. Surgical planning using three-dimensional imaging and computer modeling. Otolaryngol Clin North Am 1994; 27(5):875–89.

14. Stoker NG, Mankovich NJ, Valentino D. Stereolithographic models for surgical planning: preliminary report. J Oral Maxillofac Surg 1992;50(5): 466–71.

15. D'Urso PS, Barker TM, Earwaker WJ, et al. Stereolithographic biomodelling in cranio-maxillofacial surgery: a prospective trial. J Craniomaxillofac Surg 1999;27(1):30–7.

16. Parthasarathy J. 3D modeling, custom implants and its future perspectives in craniofacial surgery. Ann Maxill Surg 2014;4(1):9–18.

17. Valentini V, Agrillo A, Battisti A, et al. Surgical planning in reconstruction of mandibular defect with fibula free flap: 15 patients. J Craniofac Surg 2005; 16(4):601–7.

18. Hannen EJ. Recreating the original contour in tumor deformed mandibles for plate adapting. Int J Oral Maxillofac Surg 2006;35(2):183–5.

19. Hallermann W, Olsen S, Bardyn T, et al. A new method for computer-aided operation planning for extensive mandibular reconstruction. Plast Reconstr Surg 2006;117(7):2431–7.

20. Chim H, Wetjen N, Mardini S. Virtual surgical planning in craniofacial surgery. Semin Plast Surg 2014;28(3):150–8.

21. Bonda DJ, Manjila S, Selman WR, et al. The recent revolution in the design and manufacture of cranial implants: modern advancements and future directions. Neurosurgery 2015;77(5):814–24 [discussion: 824].

22. Staffa G, Barbanera A, Faiola A, et al. Custom made bioceramic implants in complex and large cranial reconstruction: a two-year follow-up. J Craniomaxillofac Surg 2012;40(3):e65–70.

23. Gerber N, Stieglitz L, Peterhans M, et al. Using rapid prototyping molds to create patient specific polymethylmethacrylate implants in cranioplasty. Conf Proc IEEE Eng Med Biol Soc 2010;2010:3357–60.

24. Chacon-Moya E, Gallegos-Hernandez JF, Pina-Cabrales S, et al. Cranial vault reconstruction using computer-designed polyetheretherketone (PEEK) implant: case report. Cir Cir 2009;77(6):437–40.

25. Brandicourt P, Delanoe F, Roux FE, et al. Reconstruction of cranial vault defect with polyetheretherketone implants. World Neurosurg 2017;105:783–9.

26. Lopez-Heredia MA, Goyenvalle E, Aguado E, et al. Bone growth in rapid prototyped porous titanium implants. J Biomed Mater Res A 2008;85(3):664–73.

27. Park EK, Lim JY, Yun IS, et al. Cranioplasty enhanced by three-dimensional printing: custom-made three-dimensional-printed titanium implants for skull defects. J Craniofac Surg 2016;27(4):943–9.

28. Honeybul S, Morrison DA, Ho KM, et al. A randomized controlled trial comparing autologous cranioplasty with custom-made titanium cranioplasty. J Neurosurg 2017;126(1):81–90.

29. Alonso-Rodriguez E, Cebrian JL, Nieto MJ, et al. Polyetheretherketone custom-made implants for craniofacial defects: report of 14 cases and review of the literature. J Craniomaxillofac Surg 2015;43(7): 1232–8.

30. Gerbino G, Zavattero E, Zenga F, et al. Primary and secondary reconstruction of complex craniofacial defects using polyetheretherketone custom-made implants. J Craniomaxillofac Surg 2015;43(8): 1356–63.

31. Rammos CK, Cayci C, Castro-Garcia JA, et al. Patient-specific polyetheretherketone implants for repair of craniofacial defects. J Craniofac Surg 2015;26(3):631–3.

32. FDA. US Food and Drug Administration 510(k) Premarket Notification. K121818 osteofab patient specific cranial device. 2013. Available at: http://www.accessdata.fda.gov/scripts/cdrh/cfdocs/cfpmn/pmn.cfm?ID=K121818. Accessed September 25, 2015.

33. Teo L, Teoh SH, Liu Y, et al. A novel bioresorbable implant for repair of orbital floor fractures. Orbit 2015;34(4):192–200.

34. Schantz JT, Lim TC, Ning C, et al. Cranioplasty after trephination using a novel biodegradable burr hole cover: technical case report. Neurosurgery 2006; 58(1 Suppl):ONS-E176 [discussion: ONS-E176].

35. Yoon M, Chougule P, Dufresne R, et al. Localized carcinoma of the external ear is an unrecognized aggressive disease with a high propensity for local regional recurrence. Am J Surg 1992;164(6): 574–7.

36. Becker C, Becker AM, Dahlem KKK, et al. Aesthetic and functional outcomes in patients with a nasal prosthesis. Int J Oral Maxillofac Surg 2017;46(11): 1446–50.

37. Kiat-Amnuay S, Gettleman L, Goldsmith LJ. Effect of multi-adhesive layering on retention of extraoral maxillofacial silicone prostheses in vivo. J Prosthet Dent 2004;92(3):294–8.

38. Eleni PN, Krokida MK, Frangou MJ, et al. Structural damages of maxillofacial biopolymers under solar aging. J Mater Sci Mater Med 2007;18(9):1675–81.

39. Sanchez-Garcia JA, Ortega A, Barcelo-Santana FH, et al. Preparation of an adhesive in emulsion for maxillofacial prosthetic. Int J Mol Sci 2010;11(10):3906–21.

40. Watson J, Hatamleh MM. Complete integration of technology for improved reproduction of auricular prostheses. J Prosthet Dent 2014;111(5):430–6.

41. Qiu J, Gu XY, Xiong YY, et al. Nasal prosthesis rehabilitation using CAD-CAM technology after total rhinectomy: a pilot study. Support Care Cancer 2011;19(7):1055–9.

42. Goiato MC, Santos MR, Pesqueira AA, et al. Prototyping for surgical and prosthetic treatment. J Craniofac Surg 2011;22(3):914–7.

43. Palousek D, Rosicky J, Koutny D. Use of digital technologies for nasal prosthesis manufacturing. Prosthet Orthot Int 2014;38(2):171–5.

44. Grant GT, Aita-Holmes C, Liacouras P, et al. Digital capture, design, and manufacturing of a facial prosthesis: clinical report on a pediatric patient. J Prosthet Dent 2015;114(1):138–41.

45. FormLabs I. Shirley technique: cancer survivor receives new jaw. 2016. Available at: https://formlabs.com/blog/shirley-technique-facial-prosthesis/. Accessed April 8, 2018.

46. Sultan B, Byrne PJ. Custom-made, 3D, intraoperative surgical guides for nasal reconstruction. Facial Plast Surg Clin North Am 2011;19(4):647–53. viii-ix.

47. Jessop ZM, Javed M, Otto IA, et al. Combining regenerative medicine strategies to provide durable reconstructive options: auricular cartilage tissue engineering. Stem Cell Res Ther 2016;7:19.

48. Cao Y, Vacanti JP, Paige KT, et al. Transplantation of chondrocytes utilizing a polymer-cell construct to produce tissue-engineered cartilage in the shape of a human ear. Plast Reconstr Surg 1997;100(2):297–302 [discussion: 303–4].

49. Giannitelli SM, Accoto D, Trombetta M, et al. Current trends in the design of scaffolds for computer-aided tissue engineering. Acta Biomater 2014;10(2):580–94.

50. Hollister SJ, Levy RA, Chu TM, et al. An image-based approach for designing and manufacturing craniofacial scaffolds. Int J Oral Maxillofac Surg 2000;29(1):67–71.

51. Hollister SJ. Porous scaffold design for tissue engineering. Nat Mater 2005;4(7):518–24.

52. Rajagopalan S, Robb RA. Schwarz meets Schwann: design and fabrication of biomorphic and durataxic tissue engineering scaffolds. Med Image Anal 2006;10(5):693–712.

53. Smith MH, Flanagan CL, Kemppainen JM, et al. Computed tomography-based tissue-engineered scaffolds in craniomaxillofacial surgery. Int J Med Robot 2007;3(3):207–16.

54. Sun W, Starly B, Darling A, et al. Computer-aided tissue engineering: application to biomimetic modelling and design of tissue scaffolds. Biotechnol Appl Biochem 2004;39(Pt 1):49–58.

55. Yoo D. New paradigms in hierarchical porous scaffold design for tissue engineering. Mater Sci Eng C Mater Biol Appl 2013;33(3):1759–72.

56. Zopf DA, Mitsak AG, Flanagan CL, et al. Computer aided-designed, 3-dimensionally printed porous tissue bioscaffolds for craniofacial soft tissue reconstruction. Otolaryngol Head Neck Surg 2015;152(1):57–62.

57. Visscher DO, Bos EJ, Peeters M, et al. Cartilage tissue engineering: preventing tissue scaffold contraction using a 3D-printed polymeric cage. Tissue Eng Part C Methods 2016;22(6):573–84.

58. Otto IA, Melchels FP, Zhao X, et al. Auricular reconstruction using biofabrication-based tissue engineering strategies. Biofabrication 2015;7(3):032001.

59. Joodaki H, Panzer MB. Skin mechanical properties and modeling: a review. Proc Inst Mech Eng H 2018;232(4):323–43.

60. Zopf DA, Flanagan CL, Nasser HB, et al. Biomechanical evaluation of human and porcine auricular cartilage. Laryngoscope 2015;125(8):E262–8.

61. Tevlin R, McArdle A, Atashroo D, et al. Biomaterials for craniofacial bone engineering. J Dent Res 2014;93(12):1187–95.

62. Morrison RJ, Kashlan KN, Flanangan CL, et al. Regulatory considerations in the design and manufacturing of implantable 3D-printed medical devices. Clin Transl Sci 2015;8(5):594–600.

63. Cai H, Azangwe G, Shepherd DE. Skin cell culture on an ear-shaped scaffold created by fused deposition modelling. Biomed Mater Eng 2005;15(5):375–80.

64. Liu Y, Zhang L, Zhou G, et al. In vitro engineering of human ear-shaped cartilage assisted with CAD/CAM technology. Biomaterials 2010;31(8):2176–83.

65. Reiffel AJ, Kafka C, Hernandez KA, et al. High-fidelity tissue engineering of patient-specific auricles for reconstruction of pediatric microtia and other auricular deformities. PLoS One 2013;8(2):e56506.

66. Zopf DA, Hollister SJ, Nelson ME, et al. Bioresorbable airway splint created with a three-dimensional printer. N Engl J Med 2013;368(21):2043–5.

67. Zhou G, Jiang H, Yin Z, et al. In vitro regeneration of patient-specific ear-shaped cartilage and its first clinical application for auricular reconstruction. EBioMedicine 2018;28:287–302.

68. Shafiee A, Atala A. Printing technologies for medical applications. Trends Mol Med 2016;22(3):254–65.

69. Kang HW, Yoo JJ, Atala A. Bioprinted scaffolds for cartilage tissue engineering. Methods Mol Biol 2015;1340:161–9.

Health Outcome Studies in Skin Cancer Surgery

Cristen E. Olds, MD*, Jon-Paul Pepper, MD[1]

KEYWORDS

- Nonmelanoma skin cancer • Melanoma • Quality of life • Health care utilization • Health outcomes

KEY POINTS

- Cutaneous malignancy is a significant public health issue that continues to increase in magnitude, underscoring the importance of utilization, accurate outcomes assessment, and targeted cost research to guide therapeutic decision-making.
- Despite the wide variety of techniques available to manage nonmelanoma skin cancer, there is a paucity of data characterizing the utilization patterns and long-term outcomes.
- Social determinants of health are intimately linked to patient outcomes after management of cutaneous malignancy, and they represent a potential target for public education and focused screening.
- Patient-reported outcome measures are a crucial component of outcomes research, particularly in patients with facial lesions, as these may be disfiguring or compromise functional status.

INTRODUCTION

Cutaneous cancers are the most common malignancy in the United States, with more than 3 million nonmelanoma skin cancers (NMSCs) and more than 70,000 melanomas diagnosed every year.[1,2] The incidence of cutaneous malignancy is rapidly increasing in the United States, with an estimated increase of approximately twofold between 1974 and 2010.[3] This is partially explained by increased sun-seeking behaviors in combination with the increasing mean age of the American population.[3] Given the large number of patients seeking care for cutaneous malignancy yearly, this presents a major public health issue and is responsible for significant health care costs, on the order of $8.1 billion per year.[4] Of head and neck skin cancers, basal cell carcinoma (BCC) is the predominant variety, with 70% to 80% of all BCCs found in the head and neck, and generally has a slowly progressive, locally aggressive course.[5] However, cutaneous squamous cell carcinoma (SCC) and melanoma of the scalp and neck are more likely to result in regional metastasis or mortality than lesions at other sites.[6–9] In addition, organ transplant recipients are a growing population (with more than 33,000 transplants in 2016), which is at particularly high risk of developing cutaneous malignancy, with up to a 10-fold to 65-fold risk of cutaneous NMSC and a tendency to develop multiple, more aggressive, tumors.[10–12]

In addition to a risk of mortality, given the functionally and cosmetically sensitive nature of the head and neck, cutaneous malignancies and their treatment can have significant detrimental impacts on appearance, function, patient satisfaction, and quality of life (QOL). Health outcomes research is a broad field involving study of the end results of disease interventions; outcomes studied are diverse and may include morbidity/mortality, safety, cost, QOL, and patient perception of disease and its treatment (**Fig. 1**). In turn, these outcomes are influenced by an array of factors, including patient access to care and variation in treatment received.

Department of Otolaryngology–Head and Neck Surgery, Stanford University, Palo Alto, CA, USA
[1] Present address: 801 Welch Road, Stanford, CA 94305.
* Corresponding author. 801 Welch Road, Stanford, CA 94305.
E-mail address: ceo@stanford.edu

Facial Plast Surg Clin N Am 27 (2019) 163–170
https://doi.org/10.1016/j.fsc.2018.08.013

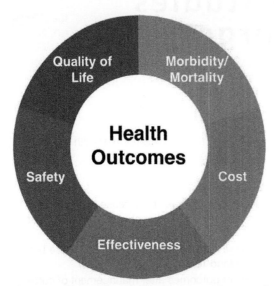

Fig. 1. Health outcomes research uses a wide array of measures to evaluate health interventions.

The management of cutaneous malignancy is a promising area of exploration for health care utilization and outcomes research given its high prevalence, wide variety of management options (with widely variable costs), and wide range of outcomes related to survival, cosmesis, and overall QOL. Here, we discuss disparities in access to health care and their impact on outcomes, describe utilization patterns and outcomes of various treatment modalities for head and neck NMSC and melanoma, and explore currently available patient-reported outcome measures (PROMs) as they relate to cutaneous malignancies of the head and neck.

SOCIAL DETERMINANTS OF HEALTH AND IMPACT ON HEALTH OUTCOMES OF CUTANEOUS MALIGNANCY

Social determinants of health span a broad range of interrelated topics, including socioeconomic context, sociodemographic factors, individual behaviors/predisposition for disease, and patients' interactions with the health care system (**Fig. 2**). The vast majority of available data pertains to the relationship between social determinants of health and outcomes after intervention for melanoma. Overall, findings in the melanoma literature have remained consistent with trends established in many other oncologic fields, in that systematic health disparities with regard to race, sex, and socioeconomic status (SES) are correlated with more advanced disease at time of presentation, differences in management decisions, and increased morbidity and mortality. Given the paucity of available data regarding head and neck NMSC specifically, this discussion draws heavily from the general melanoma literature.

Although white patients account for most of melanoma diagnoses, a disproportionate number of deaths occur among minority groups. African American and Hispanic patients are more likely to present with advanced disease and have significantly increased mortality when compared with Caucasian patients.[13–15] African American patients less likely to be offered surgical treatment (including excision and sentinel lymph node biopsy [SLNB]) for melanoma, and those who undergo surgery experience increased mortality, with persistence in these differences despite statistical controls for disease stage at time of presentation.[16–18] In at least one study, this increased mortality among African American patients compared with Caucasian patients remains after adjustment for age, sex, histologic subtype, site, SES, and treatment type.[19] Some patients may present with more aggressive primary lesions with different pathologic behavior, which would only be further amplified in the presence of existing disparities in SES and barriers to health care.[19,20]

Although patients with low SES have a lower incidence of melanoma, low SES has been demonstrated as an independent risk factor for

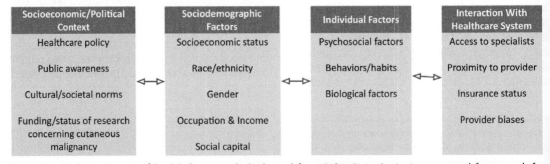

Fig. 2. Social determinants of health framework. (*Adapted from* Solar O, Irwin A. A conceptual framework for action on the social determinants of health. Social determinants of health discussion paper 2 [policy and practice]. Geneva (Switzerland): World Health Organization; 2010. p. 79; with permission.)

presentation with more advanced disease at time of diagnosis, as well as increased 5-year disease-specific mortality.[21-24] SES is intimately linked with many other social determinants of health that have been correlated with more advanced disease at time of presentation, including occupational exposures to ultraviolet radiation, high body mass index, single marital status, and increased distance to a medical provider who can provide a prompt diagnosis of melanoma.[23,25-27] Patients without a high school diploma are significantly less likely to undergo SLNB for melanoma than those with a high school diploma, with lack of this important staging and prognostic technique being linked to increased all-cause and disease-specific mortality.[18,28]

SURGICAL MANAGEMENT AND OUTCOMES FOR HEAD AND NECK MELANOMA
Mohs Microsurgery for Melanoma and Melanoma In Situ

Although the standard management of cutaneous melanoma is wide local excision of the primary lesion, use of Mohs microsurgery (MMS) for management of melanoma and melanoma in situ (MIS) is on the rise, particularly for regions of the head and neck where tissue preservation is important for function and tissue preservation. In a Surveillance, Epidemiology, and End Results Program (SEER) survey of patients treated for melanoma and MIS between 2003 and 2008, there was a 60% increase in the rate of MMS use, mainly in patients with lesions with a thickness of 1 mm or less.[29] One large retrospective study showed no significant difference in 5-year melanoma-specific or overall survival in patients with facial melanoma treated with MMS versus wide local excision.[30]

Sentinel Lymph Node Biopsy and Completion Lymphadenectomy

SLNB has emerged as the gold standard method for evaluation of nodal status in patients without clinical lymphadenopathy. The use of SLNB in the head and neck has been a matter of debate, given the complex lymphatic drainage of the region, resulting in up to 33% of lesions draining into more than one lymph node basin and a relatively high false-negative rate of SLNB in the head and neck compared with other sites.[31] A SEER database review of patients with head and neck melanoma did not show a significant correlation between SLNB and 5-year disease-free survival, regardless of melanoma thickness.[32] Data regarding the best course of action for patients with a positive SLNB has remained an area of

controversy.[33] In one randomized trial, 3-year melanoma-specific survival was not found to differ between patients who received completion lymphadenectomy (CLND) versus observation; of note, the number of included patients included in the head and neck subset was relatively small (241).[34,35] This is an important topic for future research, as the results of large randomized trials (with a focus on head and neck melanoma) are needed to guide therapeutic decision-making on this subject.

SURGICAL MANAGEMENT AND OUTCOMES FOR HEAD AND NECK NONMELANOMA SKIN CANCER

There are a multitude of options for management of NMSCs of the head and neck, including wide local excision, MMS, other procedural management (such as curettage, cryotherapy, electrosurgery and photodynamic therapy), and topical therapies (such as topical 5-flurouracil [5-FU] for BCC and SCC, and imiquimod for superficial BCC lesions), with radiation/systemic chemotherapy reserved for advanced cases or patients who are not surgical candidates (**Box 1**). There has been interest in the role of chemotherapy in management of high-risk head and neck SCC, with one recent randomized phase III trial demonstrating no added benefit in locoregional recurrence overall or disease-specific survival with the addition of carboplatin to postoperative radiation therapy.[36] Besides this study, there are very few quality prospective data to recommend treatment regimens and indications for systemic therapies, leading to calls for further randomized trials and development of a tumor registry.[37] In general, the literature regarding the multitude of management options for cutaneous NMSC predominantly consists of retrospective studies, or small prospective

---

Box 1
Treatment modalities for cutaneous nonmetastatic skin cancer

Wide/narrow local excision

Mohs microsurgery

Curettage and electrodessication

Cryosurgery

Brachytherapy

Photodynamic therapy

Topical medications

Radiation therapy

Systemic chemotherapy/targeted therapies

studies with relatively short follow-up periods, making for difficulty comparing the various methods and making inferences regarding recurrence rates.

The rate of MMS utilization for NMSC in the head and neck has increased with time, with current estimates describing a rate of Mohs surgery utilization of approximately 45% to 66% in the head and neck region. MMS is commonly used in this anatomic region, as it allows for sound oncologic control of tumors while decreasing the overall surface area of excised tissue.[38,39] The American Academy of Dermatology and American Academy of Mohs Surgery described appropriate use criteria for the use of MMS, which states that primary/recurrent BCC, SCC, MIS, and various other types of cutaneous malignancy arising in the mask areas of the face (as well as most lesions of the cheeks, scalp, neck, and forehead) are appropriate candidate lesions for MMS, as well as those with aggressive features histologically (Box 2, Fig. 3).[29,39,40] MMS is more likely to be used than excision in patients with BCC, younger patients, and with lesions of the lip or eyelid, as well as lesions with aggressive features.[41]

There are several studies comparing long-term outcomes of MMS with other management strategies. In a randomized trial of 612 high-risk facial BCC lesions (diameter >1 cm, location in the H-zone of the face, or an aggressive pathologic subtype), patients who underwent MMS had significantly lower 10-year recurrence rates than those who underwent narrow excision (with 3-mm margins), with a significant portion of recurrences occurring at least 5 years from initial treatment.[42] A prospective study comparing the use of MMS to narrow excision (with a mean margin of 3.8 mm) for facial cutaneous SCC yielded no significant difference in recurrence rates between the 2 groups.[43] In one prospective study (of 616 NMSC lesions), there was no statistically significant difference in more than 6-year NMSC recurrence rates among MMS, electrodessication with curettage, and excision.[43] There appears to be significantly increased rate of recurrence in patients who have undergone nonsurgical interventions (including cryotherapy, imiquimod, and 5-FU) for treatment of NMSC when compared with MMS, although recurrence rates for all methods were reported to be ≤5% and the aforementioned techniques are generally not favored over surgery.[39]

PSYCHOSOCIAL IMPACT OF FACIAL DEFECTS AND RECONSTRUCTION

There has been growing interest in quantitative measurement of psychosocial and QOL outcomes

Box 2
Histologic features of aggressive cutaneous nonmetastatic skin cancer lesions

Squamous Cell Carcinoma

Sclerosing

Basosquamous

Small cell

Poorly differentiated or undifferentiated

Spindle cell

Pagetoid

Infiltrating

Keratoacanthoma type (central facial)

Lymphoepithelial

Sarcomatoid

Perineural/perivascular invasion

Breslow depth ≥2 mm

Clark level IV or greater

Basal Cell Carcinoma

Morpheaform, fibrosing or sclerosing subtypes

Infiltrating

Perineural Invasion

Metatypical/keratotic

Micronodular

Adapted from Ad Hoc Task Force, Connolly SM, Baker DR, et al. AAD/ACMS/ASDSA/ASMS 2012 appropriate use criteria for Mohs micrographic surgery: A report of the American Academy of Dermatology, American College of Mohs Surgery, American Society for Dermatologic Surgery Association, and the American Society for Mohs Surgery. J Am Acad Dermatol. 2012;67(4):536; with permission.

related to reconstruction of facial defects, which is pertinent to management of cutaneous malignancy and the numerous options for management of resulting facial defects.[44] There is evidence that facial defects are correlated with negative social perception of facial attractiveness, particularly defects that are large and/or located on the central face; in addition, reconstruction of facial defects has been shown to significantly improve social perception of facial attractiveness, in some cases to near-normal values.[45] Furthermore, there is evidence that laypeople would theoretically be willing to pay significantly more for ideal reconstruction of larger and centrally located facial defects than smaller, peripheral ones, further emphasizing the perceived worsened QOL associated with presence of facial defects and the premium that patients place on adequate

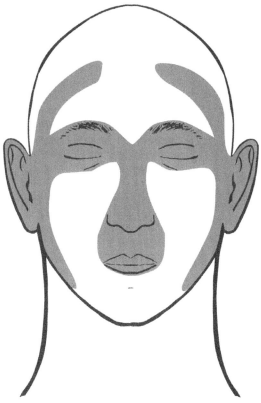

Fig. 3. Mask areas of face as defined in the American Academy of Dematology appropriate use criteria MMS guidelines.

reconstruction and resulting normalization of facial appearance.[46] Given the increasing emphasis on cost-effective clinical care and quality-based medicine, this is certainly an important topic for further study.[47] The findings demonstrate that patient psychosocial distress regarding their facial appearance normalizes with appropriate reconstruction.

PATIENT-REPORTED OUTCOME MEASURES

Although most investigations surrounding postoperative outcomes for cutaneous malignancy focus on the rate of lesion recurrence, spread, and morbidity/mortality, there is a growing interest in the use of PROMs, as they reflect the patient's satisfaction and perception of postintervention QOL.

Patient-Reported Outcome Measures and Nonmelanoma Skin Cancer

Several PROMs have been developed for use in patients with NMSC, whereas other, more generic PROMs have also been applied to this population. A common challenge that has been faced is validation of these tools across a diverse patient population with lesions of various head and neck sites,

and treatment options that present a wide variety of postoperative QOL concerns. The 2 PROMs that are most specific to head and neck NMSCs are the Facial Skin Cancer Index (FSCI) and the Skin Cancer Quality of Life Impact Tool (SCQOLIT). The FSCI is a 15-item questionnaire with emotional, appearance, and social subscales, and has been validated in a population of 211 patients who underwent MMS for cervicofacial NMSC.[48,49] It addresses fear of metastasis/recurrence, effects of the patient's skin cancer diagnosis on friends/family, and concerns about facial attractiveness and scarring, but does not address functional concerns or pain/discomfort. In a cohort of 183 patients with facial and neck NMSC, QOL in each subscale improved significantly 4 months after MMS compared with baseline, and poor QOL was significantly correlated with female sex and NMSCs of the lip. The SCQOLIT is a 10-item questionnaire that was developed for use in patients with nonmetastatic NMSC and melanoma and has been validated in 113 patients who underwent excision of an NMSC or melanoma.[50,51] In a cohort of patients with melanoma or NMSC, both groups of patients were equally concerned about scarring, disfigurement, and public perception; however, those with NMSC were significantly more likely to express concern over public awareness of skin cancer, whereas patients with melanoma were more likely to express feelings of anxiety, depression, and stress regarding their diagnosis.[50] Limitations to the SCQOLIT include a lack of items related to functional and appearance-related concerns specific to the head and neck.

PROMs that are less specific (and thus geared for use with a wide range of dermatologic conditions), such as Skindex-16, have also been applied to patients with NMSCs. Skindex-16 is a 16-question instrument that focuses on symptomatic, emotional, and functional domains.[52,53] However, it does not specifically address oncology-specific concerns or postoperative scarring/disfigurement, which is of particular concern in the head and neck. In a cohort of 633 patients undergoing electrodessication/curettage, excision, or MMS for all-site NMSC, there was a significantly higher emotional distress score among patients in the MMS group by Skindex-16, but otherwise no difference in appearance or functional outcomes.[52]

Patient-Reported Outcome Measures and Melanoma

Although there are several PROMs created specifically for evaluation of outcomes after management of melanoma, most studies focusing on health-related QOL in patients with melanoma have used generic cancer-related QOL questionnaires that do not account for cosmetic concerns, such as scarring, which is of particular importance for patients with facial lesions. There is a need for creation of validated PROMs designed for patients with head and neck melanoma and use of existing PROMs in studies focusing on head and neck melanoma; this is especially true given the morbidity associated with treatment of melanoma, particularly advanced disease.

The Functional Assessment of Chronic Illness Therapy–Melanoma (FACT-M) adds 24 melanoma-specific items to the functional, emotional, and social subscales described by the FACT-General.[54] Although melanoma-specific items include concerns related to swelling and sensation at the surgery site, functional and cosmetic concerns specific to the head and neck are not addressed, and there are not any known studies using this instrument specifically in patients with head and neck melanoma. One prospective study of 42 patients with head and neck melanoma who underwent wide local excision and reconstruction evaluated specific criteria of reconstructive outcomes (such as pain, stiffness, and scarring) and used a visual analog scale to assess satisfaction with postoperative appearance, perceived alteration in appearance, and emotional impairment.[55] Patients' emotional impairment was significantly correlated with the patient's perceived degree of appearance alteration, and patients who underwent skin grafts for reconstruction had significantly decreased satisfaction in their appearance and surgical outcome, and increased emotional impairment compared with local tissue transfer or free flap reconstruction; melanoma recurrence was found to have the largest negative impact on emotional impairment. Although promising, this instrument has not been validated or applied to studies with a larger patient cohort to our knowledge.

SUMMARY AND FUTURE DIRECTIONS

Diverse outcomes of head and neck cutaneous malignancy are worth consideration, from recurrence and mortality rates to patient perception of cutaneous malignancy and its treatment. Likewise, outcomes are influenced by social determinants that affect access to care and the type of care received from the multitude of available treatment options (particularly for NMSCs). There is significant need for additional research in the field, particularly large, randomized trials focused with long-term outcome data. Although there is an abundance of data related to the incidence of melanoma in socially vulnerable groups, the number

of large-scale outcome-related studies is scarce; this is even more true for similar research pertaining to NMSC-related outcomes in diverse patient populations. Last, there are a variety of PROMs pertaining to outcomes after management of melanoma and NMSCs, but there is significant opportunity for validation and use of head and neck–specific PROMs across a diverse patient population. Overall, there are a multitude of opportunities for impactful research in this field, given that cutaneous malignancy is a significant public health issue of ever-increasing magnitude.

REFERENCES

1. Rogers HW, Weinstock MA, Harris AR, et al. Incidence estimate of nonmelanoma skin cancer in the United States, 2006. Arch Dermatol 2010;146(3): 283–7.
2. U.S. Cancer Statistics Working Group. United States cancer statistics: 1999-2007 cancer incidence and mortality data. Atlanta (GA): GA Centers Dis Control Prev Natl Cancer Institute, US Dept Heal Hum Serv; 2017. Available at: http://apps.nccd.cdc.gov/uscs/.
3. Muzic JG, Schmitt AR, Wright AC, et al. Incidence and trends of basal cell carcinoma and cutaneous squamous cell carcinoma: a population-based study in Olmsted County, Minnesota, 2000 to 2010. Mayo Clin Proc 2017;92(6):890–8.
4. Guy GP, Machlin SR, Ekwueme DU, et al. Prevalence and costs of skin cancer treatment in the U.S., 2002-2006 and 2007-2011. Am J Prev Med 2015;48(2):183–7.
5. Chung S. Basal cell carcinoma. Arch Plast Surg 2012;39(2):166–70.
6. Jennings L, Schmults CD. Management of high-risk cutaneous squamous cell carcinoma. J Clin Aesthet Dermatol 2010;3(4):39–48. Available at: http://www.pubmedcentral.nih.gov/articlerender.fcgi?artid=2921745&tool=pmcentrez&rendertype=abstract.
7. Lachiewicz AM, Berwick M, Wiggins CL, et al. Survival differences between patients with scalp or neck melanoma and those with melanoma of other sites in the surveillance, epidemiology, and end results (SEER) program. Arch Dermatol 2008;144(4): 515–21.
8. Kang SY, Toland AE. High risk cutaneous squamous cell carcinoma of the head and neck. World J Otorhinolaryngol Head Neck Surg 2016;2(2):136–40.
9. Tseng WH, Martinez SR. Tumor location predicts survival in cutaneous head and neck melanoma. J Surg Res 2011;167(2):192–8.
10. 2016 annual report of the U.S. Organ Procurement and Transplantation Network and the Scientific Registry of Transplant Recipients: transplant data 2005-2016. Dep Heal Hum Serv Heal Resour Serv Adm Healthc Syst Bur Div Transplantation, Rockville,

MD; United Netw Organ Sharing, Richmond, VA; Univ Ren Res Educ Assoc. https://doi.org/10.1111/ajt.14563. Available at: https://optn.transplant.hrsa.gov/data/citing-data/.

11. O'Reilly Zwald F, Brown M. Skin cancer in solid organ transplant recipients: advances in therapy and management: part II. Management of skin cancer in solid organ transplant recipients. J Am Acad Dermatol 2011;65(2):253–61.

12. Mittal A, Colegio OR. Skin cancers in organ transplant recipients. Am J Transplant 2017;17(10):2509–30.

13. Harvey VM, Patel H, Sandhu S. Social determinants of racial and ethnic disparities in cutaneous melanoma outcomes. Cancer Control 2014;21(4):343–9.

14. Cormier J. Ethnic differences among patients with cutaneous melanoma. Arch Intern Med 2006;166(17):1907.

15. Wu XC, Eide MJ, King J, et al. Racial and ethnic variations in incidence and survival of cutaneous melanoma in the United States, 1999-2006. J Am Acad Dermatol 2011;65(5 SUPPL. 1):S26.e1-e13.

16. Collins KK, Fields RC, Baptiste D, et al. Racial differences in survival after surgical treatment for melanoma. Ann Surg Oncol 2011;18(10):2925–36.

17. Ward-Peterson M, Acuña JM, Alkhalifah MK, et al. Association between race/ethnicity and survival of melanoma patients in the United States over 3 decades: a secondary analysis of SEER data. Medicine (Baltimore) 2016;95(17):e3315.

18. Murtha TD, Han G, Han D. Predictors for use of sentinel node biopsy and the survival impact of performing nodal staging in melanoma patients. Ann Surg Oncol 2017;24(1):S16.

19. Zell JA, Cinar P, Mobasher M, et al. Survival for patients with invasive cutaneous melanoma among ethnic groups: the effects of socioeconomic status and treatment. J Clin Oncol 2008;26(1):66–75.

20. Agbai ON, Buster K, Sanchez M, et al. Skin cancer and photoprotection in people of color: a review and recommendations for physicians and the public. J Am Acad Dermatol 2014;70(4):748–62.

21. Reyes-Ortiz CA, Goodwin JS, Freeman JL, et al. Socioeconomic status and survival in older patients with melanoma. J Am Geriatr Soc 2006;54(11):1758–64.

22. Borghi A, Corazza M, Virgili A, et al. Impact of socioeconomic status and district of residence on cutaneous malignant melanoma prognosis: a survival study on incident cases between 1991 and 2011 in the province of Ferrara, Northern Italy. Melanoma Res 2017;27(6):619–24.

23. Jiang AJ, Rambhatla PV, Eide MJ. Socioeconomic and lifestyle factors and melanoma: a systematic review. Br J Dermatol 2015;172(4):885–915.

24. Clegg LX, Reichman ME, Miller BA, et al. Impact of socioeconomic status on cancer incidence and stage at diagnosis: selected findings from the surveillance, epidemiology, and end results: National Longitudinal Mortality Study. Cancer Causes Control 2009;20(4):417–35.

25. Stitzenberg KB, Thomas NE, Dalton K, et al. Distance to diagnosing provider as a measure of access for patients with melanoma. Arch Dermatol 2007;143(8):991–8.

26. Waggoner JK, Kullman GJ, Henneberger PK, et al. Mortality in the agricultural health study, 1993-2007. Am J Epidemiol 2011;173(1):71–83.

27. Samanic C, Gridley G, Chow W, et al. Obesity and cancer risk among white and black United States veterans. Cancer Causes Control 2016;15(1):35–43. Published by: Springer Stable URL. Available at: http://www.jstor.org/stable/3553913 cancer among.

28. Lange JR, Bilimoria KY, Balch CM, et al. Health care system and socioeconomic factors associated with variance in use of sentinel lymph node biopsy for melanoma in the United States. J Clin Oncol 2009;27(11):1857–63.

29. Viola KV, Rezzadeh KS, Gonsalves L, et al. National utilization patterns of Mohs micrographic surgery for invasive melanoma and melanoma in situ. J Am Acad Dermatol 2015;72(6):1060–5.

30. Trofymenko O, Bordeaux JS, Zeitouni NC. Melanoma of the face and Mohs micrographic surgery: nationwide mortality data analysis. Dermatol Surg 2018;44(4):481–92.

31. de Rosa N, Lyman GH, Silbermins D, et al. Sentinel node biopsy for head and neck melanoma: a systematic review. Otolaryngol Head Neck Surg 2011;145(3):375–82.

32. Sperry SM, Charlton ME, Pagedar NA. Sentinel lymph node biopsy for head and neck melanoma – survival analysis using SEER. JAMA Otolaryngol Head Neck Surg 2015;140(12):1101–9.

33. Schmalbach CE, Bradford CR. Completion lymphadenectomy for sentinel node positive cutaneous head & neck melanoma. Laryngoscope Investig Otolaryngol 2018;3(1):43–8.

34. Faries MB, Thompson JF, Cochran AJ, et al. Completion dissection or observation for sentinel-node metastasis in melanoma. Dermatol Ther 2017;376(23):2211–22.

35. Rosko AJ, Vankoevering KK, McLean SA, et al. Contemporary management of early-stage melanoma: a systematic review. JAMA Facial Plast Surg 2017;19(3):232–8.

36. Porceddu SV, Bressel M, Poulsen MG, et al. Postoperative concurrent chemoradiotherapy versus postoperative radiotherapy in high-risk cutaneous squamous cell carcinoma of the head and neck: the randomized phase III TROG 05.01 trial. J Clin Oncol 2018. https://doi.org/10.1200/JCO.2017.77.0941.

37. Trodello C, Pepper J-P, Wong M, et al. Cisplatin and cetuximab treatment for metastatic cutaneous

squamous cell carcinoma. Dermatol Surg 2017; 43(1):40–9.

38. Reeder VJ, Gustafson CJ, Mireku K, et al. Trends in Mohs surgery from 1995 to 2010: an analysis of nationally representative data. Dermatol Surg 2015; 41(3):397–403.

39. Drew BA, Karia PS, Mora AN, et al. Treatment patterns, outcomes, and patient satisfaction of primary epidermally limited nonmelanoma skin cancer. Dermatol Surg 2017;43(12):1423–30.

40. Connolly SM, Baker DR, Coldiron BM, et al. AAD/ ACMS/ASDSA/ASMS 2012 appropriate use criteria for Mohs micrographic surgery: A report of the American Academy of Dermatology, American College of Mohs Surgery, American Society for Dermatologic Surgery Association, and the American Society for Mohs Surgery. J Am Acad Dermatol 2012;67(4):531–50.

41. Jhaveri MB. Mohs micrographic surgery and surgical excision for nonmelanoma skin cancer treatment in the medicare population. Arch Dermatol 2012; 148(4):473.

42. Van Loo E, Mosterd K, Krekels GAM, et al. Surgical excision versus Mohs' micrographic surgery for basal cell carcinoma of the face: a randomised clinical trial with 10 year follow-up. Eur J Cancer 2014; 50(17):3011–20.

43. Chren M-M, Torres JS, Stuart SE, et al. Recurrence after treatment of nonmelanoma skin cancer: a prospective cohort study. Arch Dermatol 2011;147(5): 540–6.

44. Pepper JP, Baker SR. Local flaps: cheek and lip reconstruction. JAMA Facial Plast Surg 2013;15(5): 374–82.

45. Dey JK, Ishii M, Boahene KDO, et al. Impact of facial defect reconstruction on attractiveness and negative facial perception. Laryngoscope 2015;125(6): 1316–21.

46. Dey JK, Ishii LE, Joseph AW, et al. The cost of facial deformity: a health utility and valuation study. JAMA Facial Plast Surg 2016;18(4):241–9.

47. Pepper JP, Asaria J, Kim JC, et al. Patient assessment of psychosocial dysfunction following nasal reconstruction. Plast Reconstr Surg 2012;129(2):430–7.

48. Rhee JS, Matthews BA, Neuburg M, et al. Creation of a quality of life instrument for nonmelanoma skin cancer patients. Laryngoscope 2005;115(7): 1178–85.

49. Rhee JS, Matthews BA, Neuburg M, et al. Validation of a quality-of-life instrument for patients with nonmelanoma skin cancer. Arch Facial Plast Surg 2006;8(5):314–8.

50. Burdon-Jones D, Thomas P, Baker R. Quality of life issues in nonmetastatic skin cancer. Br J Dermatol 2010;162(1):147–51.

51. Burdon-Jones D, Gibbons K. The Skin Cancer Quality of Life Impact Tool (SCQOLIT): a validated health-related quality of life questionnaire for nonmetastatic skin cancers. J Eur Acad Dermatol Venereol 2013;27(9):1109–13.

52. Chren MM. The Skindex instruments to measure the effects of skin disease on quality of life. Dermatol Clin 2012;30(2):231–6.

53. Bates AS, Davis CR, Takwale A, et al. Patient-reported outcome measures in nonmelanoma skin cancer of the face: a systematic review. Br J Dermatol 2013;168(6):1187–94.

54. Cormier JN, Askew RL. Assessment of patient-reported outcomes in patients with melanoma. Surg Oncol Clin N Am 2011;20(1):201–13.

55. Buck D, Rawlani V, Wayne J, et al. Cosmetic outcomes following head and neck melanoma reconstruction: the patient's perspective. Can J Plast Surg 2012;20(1):e10–5. Available at: http://www. ncbi.nlm.nih.gov/pubmed/23598768%5Cnhttp:// www.pubmedcentral.nih.gov/articlerender.fcgi?artid= PMC3307686.

Printed and bound by CPI Group (UK) Ltd, Croydon, CR0 4YY

08/05/2025

01864738-0001